The International Library of Psychology

THE PSYCHOLOGY OF CHARACTER

Founded by C. K. Ogden

The International Library of Psychology

INDIVIDUAL DIFFERENCES
In 21 Volumes

THE PSYCHOLOGY OF CHARACTER

With a Survey of Personality in General

A A ROBACK

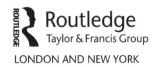
Routledge
Taylor & Francis Group

LONDON AND NEW YORK

First published in 1927 by
Routledge
2 Park Square, Milton Park, Abingdon, Oxfordshire OX14 4RN
711 Third Avenue, New York, NY 10017

First issued in paperback 2014

Routledge is an imprint of the Taylor and Francis Group, an informa business

British Library Cataloguing in Publication Data
A CIP catalogue record for this book
is available from the British Library

The Psychology of Character
ISBN 0415-21067-4
Individual Differences: 21 Volumes
ISBN 0415-21130-1
The International Library of Psychology: 204 Volumes
ISBN 0415-19132-7

ISBN 13: 978-1-138-87543-2 (pbk)
ISBN 13: 978-0-415-21067-6 (hbk)

PREFACE

THE appearance of a book on character should require no apology, although as may easily be seen from the bibliography, there is no dearth of such books. The subject of character or, in the wider sense, personality has within the last decade come to occupy the forefront of the psychological sciences and has been receiving the earnest attention of psychiatrists and social workers as well as of personnel experts.

The announcement of courses on personality, which at one time would have been greeted not without a perceptibly amused expression, is now rather welcomed by educators, at least in the United States ; and the students themselves often find that such courses broaden their outlook and reveal to them a sphere which the psychological textbook, even with its ready assimilation of psychoanalytic material, barely touches upon. The great handicap, however, has been the lack of a comprehensive volume which might be used as a suitable text showing what contributions have been made to the field of character in its widest sense, at the same time offering a tentative plan for handling the subject scientifically, so that the term " character " would be employed unambiguously and the concept analysed in such a way as to provide the reader with a workable criterion of character and a guide for its measurement.

Whether this work bears out the anticipation of the author is a matter to be judged later. I have at least spared myself no pains to follow religiously the project conceived. In order to illumine the numerous angles from which the subject has been approached, it was necessary to compress practically a whole library into the compass of a single volume, and, substituting the word " vocable " for that of " syllable " in the couplet of Cowper. " *Chase a panting vocable through time and space* " ; and even if this hunt involved making excursions into the psychological literature of half a dozen languages, besides the three principal mediums of scientific thought.

How much easier it would have been to follow the general practice of devoting less space to the views of other people and more to one's own presentation ! In an age especially when erudition is frowned upon, the survey of so many authors is apt to call forth the comment that I am crowding the canvas. But it should be borne in mind that the writer on a subject like character, unless he approaches his task from a purely literary avenue, must lay before the reader an assortment of representative doctrines and treatments so as to furnish a proper background which might serve also as a guide in gaining a perspective of the field as a whole.

Selection is by all means a wholesome method to adopt in dealing with a huge mass of material, but not selection of the kind which is determined by sheer chance, national bias, local propinquity, or the results of effective publicity. Unless we take the trouble to go out of our way in quest of data before making the actual choice, unless we realize that important papers and books may have appeared in other languages than our own, and that not only those writings which have been translated into English are worth referring to—unless, in other words, we make a thorough search of the literature, inasfar as circumstances permit, we are not justified in the claim to have carried out a selective policy.

Aside from that, there is the question of what to include and what to eliminate. The process may be considered from either the inclusive or the exclusive angle. I have rather stressed the positive phase of selection because of the wide diversity of views on the subject, which may be considered representative. This was in no way an easy undertaking ; and when a colleague, also interested in characterology, on glancing at one of the historical chapters on temperament remarked that " it is a good thing if one likes such work as this ", he was hardly appreciating the fact that the task of poring over old discussions on temperament in order to secure a basis of comparison was irksome beyond words. Nevertheless someone has to do it ; and although I do not flatter myself upon having covered all the ground exhaustively,

I feel at least reassured in the thought that I have made a sincere effort to omit nothing of value which was reasonably accessible.

A word of explanation is necessary with regard to the subject-matter incorporated in this volume. There is a seeming inconsistency about the book in that the historical part deals with character in the sense of personality minus the intellectual phase, while the constructive portion delimits the discussion in a way to comprehend character in the more restricted sense.

The reason for this apparent discrepancy is twofold. First, it is nigh impossible to dissever the strands in the various characterological writings so as to dwell exclusively on what should, strictly speaking, be termed character. In the second place, since the historical development of the subject took place in a somewhat protean fashion, sometimes in the guise of character, sometimes appearing in the shape of temperament, and at other times taking on the aspect of individuality and personality, it becomes clear that until the chameleon-like qualities of our subject are removed or at least reduced to a minimum, we have no right to prescind its history on the ground that our premise will be established later in the book. Above all, the outline of character must be visualized against a background which, though somewhat faint and blurred, lends it, if not enchantment, at least perspective.

Many libraries have placed me under obligation for the courtesy extended in forwarding or otherwise placing at my disposal books not available in the Harvard College Library. Among these are the Clark College Library, the John Crerar Library in Chicago, the Library of Congress in Washington, the Columbia University Library, the Boston Medical Library, and the library of the Boston Psychopathic Hospital, but the special accommodations offered by the Harvard College Library deserve particular mention.

My indebtedness to Dr. G. W. Allport, of Dartmouth College, who read a large part of the manuscript and whose numerous critical suggestions have been most helpful, cannot be adequately expressed in a general acknowledgment.

Mr. J. Kelson, who has read nearly all the book in proof,

has also been of considerable assistance in pointing out occasional obscurities in the language.

The bibliography, to which frequent reference has been made in this work, was intended for inclusion in the present volume, but as its compass grew so as to include about 3,500 titles besides other references, it was decided to publish this appendix as a companion volume, which is being brought out simultaneously with the *Psychology of Character* under the title of *A Bibliography of Personality and Character* (340 pp. Sci.-Art Publishers, Cambridge, Mass.).

A. A. Roback.

Cambridge, Mass.

PREFACE TO THE SECOND EDITION

THE demand for a second edition within eight months of the original publication of a work which certainly could not appeal to the proverbial running reader indicates that there are many thinking men and women who still look upon the subject of character as one worthy of investigation. Indeed, in some colleges, courses in personality have been initiated through the medium of the present volume.

Since the book was completed in manuscript, naturally many new articles and books have appeared on character and personality, but it would be out of the question to discuss them at present. A few of the more important publications, both recent and earlier writings which had escaped my notice, I commented upon in my *Bibliography of Character and Personality*, in several instances giving an epitome of the material.

There has been nothing specific said in the numerous reviews thus far which would call for revision on my part. Hence the changes in this edition are confined to the correction of a few misprints, the touching up of a phrase here and there (especially when cognizance is to be taken of altered circumstances in the course of the year), and finally the postscript which deals with the fundamental issues raised in the most extensive reviews of the book.

A. A. Roback.

Cambridge, Mass.
February, 1928.

PREFACE TO THE THIRD EDITION

THE MS. of *The Psychology of Character* was completed toward the end of 1926. Twenty-five years is a long period so far as scientific progress is concerned, but the last quarter of a century is incommensurable in terms of time. Perhaps more than the carnage and suffering on the part of the many millions, the dark outlook, the feeling of insecurity and the awareness that culture and civilization are no guarantee of justice and liberty, and that the very meaning of the word progress is no longer what it used to be—gnaw at our vitals, with telling consequences. Prior to the first World War there was a general belief in serious circles that we were going forward not only technologically but socially, ethically, and that gradually feuds on a large scale would be a matter of the past. In the year 1951 a bewildered world is anxiously wondering whether a World War III is not likely to envelop the globe in actual flames and reduce it to an arid desert. The discovery that our prospect was an illusion is perhaps one of the greatest drawbacks against attaining that sense of equilibrium which was the norm in the first decade of the century.

At present every reflective and productive individual cannot help consciously or unconsciously asking himself whether his effort is worth the pains, whether some cataclysm of global dimensions will not, in the near future, annul everything in a total devastation. We have been fortunate in wresting many great secrets from nature, but the secret of living peaceably with one another seems to be receding more and more beyond our reach in proportion to our conquest of nature.

This meditation is germane here because we have unfortu-

nately witnessed a most paradoxical phenomenon, viz., that
the simplest task, that of *laissez-faire*, is far more difficult
than analysing the nucleus of the atom and destroying a
whole city with its inhabitants in a single instant. It further
goes to prove that our own personality, or character, is less
manageable than any part of nature ; and whoever would
unravel the secret of unfailingly inducing coöperation and
reducing distrust to a negligible minimum will have accomplished much more than splitting the atom. But there is the
rub. Nature may be resistant, but cannot employ strategy,
will not devise a countermove each time you have made
another gain, while man will oppose at every step, and once
the opposition revolves around an idea, no matter how
egregiously absurd, or infernally wicked, this will gain mo-
mentum and turn into an *idée fixe*, which is no longer an idea
but a neurosis, if not a psychosis, spreading in every direction.
The *physical* substrate, whatever it is, the continuum of mass
and energy, is not working at cross purposes with science,
is not perverted by dogma but is governed by law. In the
physico-chemical world, *force obeys the laws* of nature ; in our
social world, *force often imposes the laws* upon mankind, and
therein lies the chief difference.

A preface, however, is not the place for even a restricted
discussion of this issue, which has been reserved for the chapter
headed " Character in an Atomic Age ". If the subject
has been broached at all, it is because of the need of emphasizing the concrete advance in the physical and natural
sciences as against the comparative standstill in the mental
and social sciences, *in their application to living*. Not that we
have lagged behind in pursuing research from all angles,
but we have not the facilities for clinching the results so that
they are incontrovertible, and, what is more unfortunate,
the results are beset with, if not steeped in, all sorts of emotion.

In the past twenty-five years psychological schools have

expanded, new ones have been established, while others, like the vaunted behavioristic movement, have subsided, but it is gratifying to know that the trend in general has been in the direction of the point of view developed in this volume a quarter of a century ago, despite the fact that at the time, the original portion of the book was regarded as out of keeping with the theories of the day. In 1927 the mechanistic conception had reached its peak. From all sides, there were cries to throw the instinct doctrine overboard. Psychoanalysis was still busy with number-juggling and exploring complexes. The core of character was not perceived because of the various fungi that had surrounded it, and the hormic nature of man was ignored (except by McDougall and Adler, the latter of whom, however, adulterated it with adventitious matter) ; and for a time it seemed as if I were taking refuge in an antiquated structure.

Things have changed since. The efficacy of the stimulus-response bond is now being questioned even in mechanistic circles. The holistic pattern is receiving more and more attention generally. Problems of motivation are again centred around the theory of instincts or drives, yes even in their hereditary connotation ; and psychoanalysis has veered from the study of neuroses to an analysis of character, as the more fundamental of the two. Freud himself has initiated the turn, but he had already been aware of the rumblings within his own camp, and the dissidents known as neo-Freudians (or, as I would call them, para-Freudians) have been occupying themselves less with the *id* and more with the *ego* and the *superego*. Thus the stone which once was rejected by the builders has become the cornice of the wall.

In the present edition the constructive portion, which represents the author's own conception, remains the same. If anything, the findings have been confirmed by recent work in the mental and social sciences, and perhaps some of those

B

who have, within the last decade, brought serious objections against accepted beliefs in psychology or psychoanalysis will be surprised to find that they had been anticipated in the first edition of *The Psychology of Character*, with which most of them are apparently unfamiliar, having lived then in German-speaking countries.

The historical part of the book remains naturally unchanged, as little has transpired to require revision in this connection. Many of the chapters, however, on contemporary activities have been amplified, and six new chapters have been added. Psycho-analysis and psychometrics, or the empirical approach to character and personality, have been especially exploited.

Since books published simultaneously on both sides of the Atlantic occasionally come out under different titles, some readers may well wonder whether *The Psychology of Personality*, by the same author, brought out last year (Cambridge, Mass., Sci-Art Publishers) covers the same material as the present volume. Let it be known, therefore, that the books are entirely different in presentation, scope, and even in subject-matter.

A. A. ROBACK.

CAMBRIDGE, MASS.
   1st June, 1951.

CONTENTS

PART IV

CONSTRUCTIVE

CHARTS

PART I

HISTORICAL

CHAPTER I

INTRODUCTION

" Von einem Menschen schlechthin sagen zukönnen: ' Er hat einen
Charakter' heisst sehr viel von ihm nicht allein *gesagt,* sondern auch
gerühmt : denn das ist eine Seltenheit, die Hochachtung gegen ihn
und Bewunderung erregt." [1]

Kant : *Anthropologie*, Part II, Sec. III.

THERE is one department in psychology in which no
progress seems to have been made for about two thousand
years, in spite of the fact that it was perhaps the first topic
to attract attention. It may be surmised that I am here
referring to the interlocked subjects of character and temperament which, though forming the core of any study of human
nature, have continued to remain in the speculative stage,
while other psychological material was being subjected to
experimental scrutiny. Only recently have these siblings been
examined anew under the more comprehensive head of
personality, and in this fresh survey the place assigned to
character has been so circumscribed as to portend the eventual
eviction of this concept from the study of psychology. It is
for this reason, at least in part, that its claim to consideration
should be championed.

Temperament has fared better, because of its falling
distinctly into the psychological field, but it would be a
difficult task to treat the one without introducing material
properly belonging to the other, inasmuch as the concepts
even to-day have not been sufficiently differentiated, as will
be evident in the course of this volume.

---

[1] "Simply to be able to say of a man: 'he has *character*' is not
only to *say* a great deal of him, but to *extol* him; for that is a rare
attribute which calls forth respect towards him and admiration."

3

Stern, drawing the distinction between differential psychology and characterology, remarks that of the latter's two
main problems only that of temperament is " about to be
made accessible to our exact methods ; as regards the difficult
and fundamental problem of character, however, there
has scarce been an attempt made to approach it according to
modern procedure." [1] For this reason, he explains, the topic
of character, in spite of its importance, is hardly touched on
in his book.

The ancients have given evidence of almost uncanny insight
in many of the scattered observations· on both character
and temperament to be found in the various books of wisdom.
Yet for centuries the psychology of character seems to have
made no advance—even after experimental psychology
was making prodigious strides in at least some of its departments ; and, what is more noteworthy, after the subject of
character had already become a central topic in ethics, religion,
and education.

But perhaps it is in the latter circumstance that the trouble
is to be sought.   Perhaps character, as some very recent
writers maintain or at any rate imply, is not closely bound up
with psychology, and is merely a concept to which are attached
the possibilities of moral predication, so that it can easily be
dispensed with in text-books on mind or behaviour.

Causes of Neglect.   Certainly this situation, at least in part,
explains the neglect of this important subject, but it does not
serve to excuse or justify it.   While we must concede that
character is not an introspective datum, nor even a subconscious fact, it nevertheless constitutes an integral part of
personality ; and the study of personality has been rather
in the ascendant than on the wane.   We can just as easily
dispose of intelligence from a psychological angle as character.
Even assuming that character possesses primarily an ethical
denotation, must we not realize that this unity of behaviour

[1] W. Stern : *Die differentielle Psychologie,* etc., p. 12 (1911 and 1921).

or uniform response which in most cases permits of prediction and in 'any case serves to illuminate past responses, especially in the legal sphere, is psychological subject matter *per se* and furthermore is grounded in psychological causes ? Whatever objections may be raised against the psychological treatment of character may also be brought against the discussion of intelligence in psychology.

Those who see in character nothing but a moral concept and a psychological fiction are oblivious to the fact that the unity and uniformity of certain behaviour forms, even in new situations (thus ruling out the mere operation of habit), cannot be considered in anything but a psychological light. Surely there is a definite integration, the result of innate dispositions and acquired tendencies, which corresponds to the concept under discussion.

Character—a Datum of Psychology. I should not find it difficult even to subscribe to the notion that we are introspectively, or rather analytically, aware of our character, both before and after action. It is not because he is regarded as a gentleman that the man of character can readily place himself on the scale of social agents, just as the man of intellect does not require a series of intelligence tests in order to become aware of his mental capacity.

On the practical side of life the study of character will always have its advocates. The plea of Fernald which begins with the words " It is herein attempted to indicate that personality studies should recognize character as an integral field of inquiry " and ends with the conclusion that " character study then is entitled to recognition as a categorical entity ; since it is an integral field of inquiry having its own locus, mechanisms and event . . ." [1] is encouraging especially in view of the negative attitude taken by the more behaviouristically-inclined psychologists.

[1] G. G. Fernald : " Character *vs.* Intelligence in Personality Studies," *Journal of Abnormal Psychology,* 1920. Vol. xv.

It is not to be overlooked, however, that in their general use of the word *character*, clinicians, social workers, administrators, and others who represent the practical sphere of life, have no clear-cut conception to work on, but understand by the term a conglomeration of numerous traits and qualities. Fernald, for instance, regards intelligence as the capacity or degree of personality, and character as the quality of personality, and on the strength of this division, he makes the rather suggestive remark that " character modifications continue to be reflected in behaviour after intelligence development ceases ".[1]

Spoilt by Ethical Atmosphere. The most general use of the word " character " in everyday life is invariably coloured with moral predicates. We may think of a man as having a poor memory, we may be aware that our friend cannot concentrate, that his perception is slow, without his incurring our displeasure, but no sooner do we discover some weakness about his character than we are led to take an altogether different attitude. Not only do we begin to rely less and less upon him, but we treat him as if he himself is to blame for the particular defect.

The popular mind has never distinguished more than two kinds of characters. They were either good or bad, strong or weak, noble or base, of a high or a low type ; and all these predicates are appraisals rather than statements of facts. To say that a man has no character is a euphemistic equivalent for the expression that he has a low type of character, and again, when Pope describes women as having no character at all, meaning that they are fickle and inconstant, the utterance again occurs in a slightly derogatory sense. All such references are calculated to evoke in the listener or reader a certain attitude or indicate that the speaker or writer has assumed such and such a position.

[1] G. G. Fernald : "Character as an Integral Mentality Function," *Mental Hygiene*, 1916. Vol. ii, p. 452.

It seems to be this very circumstance, however, that proved detrimental to the growth of the study of character. Just because it was born or bred in an ethical milieu, the psychologist would be apt to disown it as spurious, while the moralist, on the other hand, after fully adopting it, would be prone to spoil it through sheer over-indulgence. Thus we see that between the neglect of a prejudiced parent and the exaggerated attentions of a zealous foster-parent, an arrested development has been the lot of our subject. And the more strongly moralists emphasized the cardinal importance of character for ethics, and incidentally in so doing encroached on the territory of other people, the more were experimental psychologists inclined to dispose of the whole matter with a word or two, sometimes barely mentioning such terms as character, temperament, and even self and personality, although more recently the latter concept has come to swallow up the other three.

In the present work only the strictly psychological phase of character will be discussed. The ethical and pedagogical aspects that deal with character-building and for the most part contain hortatory appeals in behalf of the moral life do not enter here. Nor will the psychotechnical side of character be gone into at present. It is quite obvious that the theoretical examination of character must antedate both these inquiries, and more especially the latter.

CHAPTER II

Dawn of Characterology. The history of the study of character is probably as old as mankind. So soon as our remote ancestors began to associate with one another in various activities, it was inevitable that certain rough generalizations should be made and handed down from generation to generation. With the advent of Greek culture, the study became more articulate ; and the third century B.C. marks the beginning of a serious approach to the subject—but from two different avenues. This bifurcated course with occasional intertwining has continued to this very day.

Double Approach to Subject. The literary avenue which requires the penetration and intuitive synthesis of the worldly mind has been trodden on even by some of the biblical writers as may be attested by the wisdom of Ecclesiastes, Proverbs, and the utterances of Ben-Sirach in the Apocryphal books. These Hebrew authors in their quaint characterization of the fool, the scoffer, the wise man, the God-fearing person, the virtuous woman, etc., Plato in his dialogues, and more particularly Aristotle in his Nicomachean Ethics, present portraits of universal types. The fine delineation of the magnanimous man or the classification of angry people in his chapter on gentleness immediately tempts us to regard Aristotle as the founder of the dynasty which in reality began with his pupil and successor, the learned Theophrastus, who, in a series of thirty sketches of human types, took his place at once as the pioneer in characterology.

The semi-scientific path which, after considerable meandering, opened up into the highway of modern endocrinology was, as is well-known, cleared by Hippocrates, whose theory of the humors as the basis of our temperaments has, except for the modification of the Græco-Roman physician Galen, a few centuries later, withstood the onslaughts of time perhaps more successfully than any other ancient doctrine.

Theophrastus as Pioneer on Descriptive side. The tradition inaugurated by Theophrastus concerned itself with merely *describing* the various characters ; and its votaries certainly gave evidence of *understanding* the men and women they came in contact with. It is thanks to these writers of antiquity and their imitators that we can say with a high degree of confidence that human nature, though ages and oceans apart, is about the same wherever found, i.e., the same differences among individuals will be discovered whether they be ancient Greeks or twentieth century Americans—a fact which would have interested the ninety-nine year old Theophrastus (at the time he wrote his *Characters*) even more than that which, as he tells us in his proem, forever puzzled him, viz. " Why it is that while all Greece lies under the same sky and all the Greeks are educated alike, it has befallen us to have characters variously constituted ".

Take for instance the following portrayal of the flatterer, and ask yourself whether its remoteness in time and place from our present environment makes it a whit less realistic than any modern account could be.

Flattery may be considered as a mode of companionship degrading but profitable to him who flatters.

The Flatterer is a person who will say as he walks with another, " Do you observe how people are looking at you ? This happens to no man in Athens but you. A compliment was paid to you yesterday in the Porch. More than thirty persons were sitting there ; the question was started, Who is our foremost man ? Everyone mentioned you first, and ended by coming back to your name." With these and the like words, he will remove a morsel of wool from his patron's coat ; or if a speck of chaff has been laid on the other's hair by the wind, he will pick it off ; adding with a laugh, " Do you see ? Because I have not met you for two days, you have had your beard full of white hairs ; although no one has darker hair for his years than you." Then he will request the company to be silent while the great man is speaking, and will praise him, too, in his hearing, and mark his approbation at a pause with "True"; or he will laugh at a frigid joke, and stuff his cloak into his mouth as if he could not repress his amusement. He will request those whom he meets to stand still until "his Honour" has passed. He will buy apples and pears and bring them in and give to the children in the father's presence ; adding with kisses, "Chicks of a good father." Also when he assists at the purchase of slippers, he will declare that the foot is more shapely than the shoe. If his patron is approaching a friend, he will run forward and say, "He is coming to you," and then turning back, "I have announced you." He is just the person, too, who can run errands to the Women's Market without drawing breath. He is the first of the guests to praise the wine ; and to say, as he reclines next the host, "How delicate is your fare !" and (taking up something from the table) "Now this—how excellent it is !" He will ask his friend if he is cold, and if he would like to put on something more ; and before the words are spoken, will wrap him up. Moreover he will lean towards his ear and whisper with him ; or will glance at him as he talks to the rest of the company. He will take the cushions from the slave in the theatre, and spread them on the seat with his own hands. He will say that his patron's house is well built, that his land is well planted, and that his portrait is like.

In short the Flatterer may be observed saying and doing all things by which he conceives that he will gain favour.

Nature of Literary Method. What the literary characterologists have done, then, is to label a mode of behaviour according as it affects others and then proceed to describe the essentials of this mode of behaviour. The list of such modes of behaviour must naturally remain arbitrary, and as we shall presently see, this is the chief fault of that extensive school. The trend which the study of temperament has taken, on the other hand, is bound up with the more scientific purpose of *explaining* differences in types. Hence the classification, to begin with, must be condensed and attached to some correlational scheme. In this way, Galen was able to assign a definite cause for each of the four outstanding types of individuals in the preponderance of the so-called bodily humors. The sanguine person, always full of enthusiasm, was said to owe his temperament to the strength of the blood, the melancholic's sadness was supposed to be due to the over-functioning of the black bile, the choleric's irritability was attributed to the predominance of the yellow bile in the body, while the phlegmatic person's apparent slowness and apathy were traced to the influence of the phlegm.

But to revert to the fundamental differences between the two approaches to the study of individual types, the one leading to the *description* of a large number of characters, the other calling for the *explanation* of a limited number of qualities on a physical basis, we note that throughout its long history, the subject, or perhaps one should say the twin subjects, had its two lines of followers without it becoming apparent until comparatively recently that after all *temperament was bound up with the affective side of man, while character had its being in a universe of conduct.*

Limitations of Theophrastus' Method. The limitations of the literary and descriptive characterologists can be gathered from an analysis of the titles in Theophrastus' sketches and are even more obvious in the host of imitators who introduced many new characters. In the first place, no one could venture to claim that Theophrastus has included all, or the majority, or even the most important human characters in his book. Furthermore, in spite of his gift for definition which seems to have been peculiar to the Greek philosophers, the description which follows his definition does not always correspond with it. But worse still, a number of the statements made in the various sketches might fit any one of several characters. There is considerable overlapping in the relatively small number of sketches. Much of what the boastful man and the vulgarian are guilty of doing, the boor will do also ; and how can we draw the line, notwithstanding the topical definitions, between the unreasonable man and the offensive person, between the garrulous man and the loquacious man ?

In addition, Theophrastus' conception of character is a rather miscellaneous one. The offensive man who is charged with a " distressing neglect of the person " is treated in the same series as the flatterer and the patron of rascals. Yet a little reflection will make it clear that the flatterer is criticized, not because of his actions but for his motives, while the offensive man is blamed for his actions only, as he certainly does not intend to be offensive. Again, these qualities which are universal can hardly be compared with such a circum-scribed trait as the patronizing of rascals ; and the disciples of Theophrastus of whom there have been many, beginning with the Renaissance, are even more open to this objection.

It is extremely difficult to determine just where to begin in the history of modern characterology,[1] for there is much

---

[1] Aldington's *Book of Characters*, published quite recently, is the best source-book of that kind. In this painstaking compilation, the author has brought together some five hundred short character studies from the time of Theophrastus to the eighteenth century British and French writers. Had he chosen to expand the volume, he doubtless would have added to his material several sources which we now miss in his anthology, such as *The English Theophrastus (or the manners of the age being the modern characters of the court, the town and the city)*, published in 1702 and attributed to Abel Boyer ; *Characters—* transcript made by and for the Reverend Philip Bliss ; *Confused Characters of Conceited Coxcombs*, by " Verax Philobasileus " (1661) and some of the lively descriptions in *The Lover*, one of Steele's numerous periodicals.

George Eliot's *Impressions of Theophrastus Such*, Thackeray's *Book of Snobs*, and Gay's *Miniature Pictures* (1781) might be added to the list. Fawcett's *Social Silhouettes* portrays American characters of recent years, by throwing into relief some special foible of the heroes and heroines.

On the other hand, we must not suppose that every book labelled " Characters " or " Characteristics " properly falls into our discourse. Shaftesbury's *Characteristics*, and also his *Second Characters*, treat of subjects entirely different from that under discussion, as does Carlyle's depiction of traits to be found in nearly every genre of writing. It is possible to begin with Chaucer as at any rate the first English sketcher of characters. His portraits of the merchant, the lawyer, the nun, the haberdasher, the friar, etc., are vivid descriptions of those types, even though they are too highly saturated with local color and too deeply cast in a narrative mould to possess any psychological value for our purpose. *A fortiori* must the two pamphlets which appeared about the middle of the sixteenth century, Awdeley's *Fraternity of Vagabonds* and Harman's *Caveat or Warning for Cursetors*, be ruled out of this category. They possess the germ of this type of writing, but lack the synthesis of characterization.

First Attempts at Characterology in England. Ben Jonson, though not ostensibly engaged in character writing, is perhaps the first English man of letters to have tackled this type of literature, and both in his *Cynthia's Revels* and *Every Man Out of his Humor*, he has given some excellent sketches which are, however, on the whole bare outlines rather than finished portraits.

Hall's *Characterismes of Vertues and Vices*, published in 1608, while patterned after Theophrastus, not only lacks his directness but is influenced in its moralizing by some of the biblical books like Psalms, Proverbs, and Ecclesiastes—a fact which seems to have escaped the classical scholar Jebb in his introduction to the translation of Theophrastus ! Hence Hall's rhetoric and hankering after antithesis, which Jebb with all his fine critical sense is at a loss to explain.

Sir Thomas Overbury and his associates whose collection appeared in 1614 (*Characters or Witty Descriptions of the Properties of Sundry Persons*) have added a decided literary

Characteristics. Hazlitt's *Characteristics* offers some tangential contact at least with the main problems of motivation, while Madame De Puisieux' *Les Caractères*, spoken of again toward the end of this chapter, is apparently calculated to bring to mind the brilliancy of La Bruyère's famous work by that name, without, however, resembling the latter in any other respect.

flavor to the simple wisdom of their predecessors. In the eighty sketches which make up that collection, few are of universal characters. Many are odd and complex characterizations, such as "A Drunken Dutchman Resident in England ", " A Button Maker of Amsterdam ", " A Braggadochio Welshman ", " A French Cook ", " An Almanac Maker ". There has been a departure from the original plan of Theophrastus in that different callings and stations in life are introduced ; the tailor, the sailor, the soldier, the tinker, the footman, etc. Comparisons are instituted by Overbury in felicitous metaphor. " The virtuous widow," for instance, " is the palm tree that thrives not after the supplanting of her husband. For her children's sake she first marries, for she married that she might have children, and for their sakes she marries no more. She is like the purest gold, only employed for prince's medals, she never receives but one man's impression ". The ordinary widow, however, described in the next sketch, " is like the herald's hearse cloth ; she serves to many funerals, with very little altering the color. The end of her husband begins in tears, and the end of her tears begins in a husband . . . Her chiefest pride is in the multitude of her suitors ; and by them she gains ; for one serves to draw on another, and with one at last she shoots out another, as boys do pellets in eldern guns." (This last thought was borrowed by other character writers.)

For our purpose, perhaps the most important item in the collection going under the name of Overbury, is the explanation of the threefold sense of the word character : [1] (1) " a deep impression ", like a letter in the alphabet ; (2) " an impress or short emblem, in little comprehending much " ; (3) " a picture (real or personal) quaintly drawn, in various colors, all of them

---

[1] The Earl of Shaftesbury in *The Second Characters* (Rand's edition, p. 90) appears to have had these three senses in mind, hence the title of his book, but he fails to distinguish them clearly, and the third meaning as given by Overbury is entirely missing in Shaftesbury's definitions.

heightened by one shadowing " ; and the author synthesizes
all three senses with this harmonic turn, " It is a quaint and
soft touch of many strings, all shutting up in one musical
close ; it is wit's descant on any plain song."

The sermonizing note is again struck in Nicholas Breton's
collection, which though appearing the following year (1615),
is a relapse to a medieval conception.   What the author
thinks of a parasite, a drunkard, a coward, a fool, a beggar,
and an " atheist or most bad man " is much in the way of
plain invective, and his reflections are highly subjective.

Psychological Penetration of Earle's Sketches.   John
Earle, on the other hand, is a worthy descendant of
Theophrastus, but whereas the latter describes the behaviour
of his characters in particular instances, Earle tells us what
they do in general.   There is perhaps less wit in his *Micro-
cosmographie* (1628) than in the Overbury collection, . but
there is a great deal more poise and sound judgment. His titles
are less whimsically chosen and his pictures developed with
greater finish. If Overbury is more worldly, Earle is more of a
sage, displaying no cynicism. His paradoxes and epigrams
are of a scintillating kind and are yet not exaggerated.

> A self-conceited man is one that knows himself so
> well that he does not know himself. Too excellent well-
> dones have undone him . . . . He is now become his
> own book which he pores on continually, yet like a truant
> reader skips over the harsh places and surveys only that
> which is pleasant. In the speculation of his own good parts
> his eyes, like a drunkard, see all double, and his forces
> like an old man's spectacles, make a great letter in a small
> print . . . . His walk is still in the fashion of a march,
> and like his opinion unaccompanied, with his eyes most
> fixed upon his own person, or on others with reflection
> to himself.

" The world's wise man is an able and sufficient wicked
man. It is a proof of his sufficiency that he is not called wicked
but wise . . . His conclusion is commonly one of these two,
either a great man or hanged."

A flatterer is a dunce to him for he can tell him nothing but what he knew before : and yet he loves him too because he is like himself. . . .

" The pretender to learning is one that would make all others more fools than himself, for though he knows nothing, he would not have the world know so much. He conceits nothing in learning but the opinion, which he seeks to purchase without it, though he might with less labor cure his ignorance than hide it."

" The affected man is an extraordinary man in ordinary things, one that would go a strain beyond himself and is caught in it. A man that overdoes all things with great solemnity of circumstance and whereas with more negligence he might pass better, makes himself with a great deal of endeavor ridiculous."

Earle refers to the bowling alley as a place where there are three things thrown away besides bowls, viz., " time, money and curses " and the last ten for one. It is there that one can best discover friends " especially in the losers, where you have a fine variety of impatience, whilst some fret, some rail, some swear and others more ridiculously comfort themselves with philosophy ". In this sentence, Earle seems to allude to the four temperaments in this order : (a) the melancholic, (b) the sanguine, (c) the choleric and (d) the phlegmatic.

Typical Characterizations Display Analytic Sense. One is safe, I believe, in regarding Earle as the most psychological of all the British literary characterologists. First of all he is comprehensive in his characterizations, instead of selecting only two or three elements to enlarge on ; but more than that he is analytic. The pictures of his plausible man and meddling man which are reproduced here easily rank with any portrait drawn by Theophrastus.

A Plausible Man

Is one that would fain run an even path in the world, and jut against no man. His endeavor is not to offend, and his aim the general opinion. His conversation is a kind of continued compliment, and his life a practice of manners. The relation he bears to others, a kind of fashionable respect, not friendship but friendliness, which is equal to all and general, and his kindnesses seldom exceed courtesies. He loves not deeper mutualities, because he would not take sides, nor hazard himself on displeasures, which he principally avoids. At your first acquaintance with him he is exceeding kind and friendly, and at your twentieth meeting after but friendly still. He has an excellent command over his patience and tongue, especially the last, which he accommodates always to the times and persons, and speaks seldom what is sincere, but what is civil. He is one that uses all companies, drinks all healths, and is reasonable cool in all religions. (He considers who are friends to the company, and speaks well where he is sure to hear of it again.) He can listen to a foolish discourse with an applausive attention, and conceal his laughter at nonsense. Silly men much honour and esteem him, because by his fair reasoning with them as with men of understanding, he puts them into an erroneous opinion of themselves, and makes them forwarder hereafter to their own discovery. He is one rather well thought on than beloved, and that love he has is more of whole companies together than any one in particular. Men gratify him notwithstanding with a good report, and whatever vices he has besides, yet having no enemies, he is sure to be an honest fellow.

A Meddling Man

Is one that has nothing to do with his business, and yet no man busier than he, and his business is most in his face. He is one who thrusts himself violently into all employments, unsent for, unfeed, and many times unthankt ; and his part in it is only an eager bustling, that rather keeps ado than does anything. He will take you aside, and question you of your affair, and listen with both ears, and look earnestly, and then it is nothing so much yours as his. He snatches what you are doing out of your hands, and cries " Give it me ", and does it worse, and lays an engagement upon you too, and you must thank him for his pains. He lays you down an hundred wild plots, all impossible things, which you must be ruled by perforce, and he delivers them with a serious and counselling forehead ; and there is a great deal more wisdom in this forehead than his head.

D

He will woo for you, solicit for you, and woo you to suffer him ; and scarce anything done, wherein his letter, or his journey, or at least himself is not seen, if he have no task in it else, he will rail yet on some side, and is often beaten when he need not. Such men never thoroughly weigh any business but are forward only to show their zeal, when many times this forwardness spoils it, and then they cry they have done what they can, that is, as much hurt. Wise men still deprecate these men's kindnesses and are beholding to them rather to let them alone ; as being one trouble more in all business, and which a man shall be hardest rid of.

Similarly his characterization of the rash man, the affected man, the flatterer, the foolishly reserved man who is " a fool with discretion," the discontented man, the mere great man and the coward who himself " is most commonly fierce against the coward . . . for the opinion of valor is a good protection to those who dare not use it . . . " are all not without psychological interest.

Although Earle has been dwelt on at greater length than was intended, it will be in place perhaps to cite his description of the staid man who might, in our own day, be regarded as the man of character.

A Stayed Man

Is a man : one that has taken order with himself, and sets a rule to those lawlessnesses within him : whose life is distinct and in method, and his actions, as it were, cast up before : not loosed into the world's vanities, but gathered up and contracted in his station : not scattered into many pieces of businesses, but that one course he takes, goes through with. A man firm and standing in his purposes, not heaved off with each wind and passion : that squares his expence to his coffers, and makes the total first, and then the items. One that thinks what he does, and does what he says, and foresees what he may do before he purposes. One whose " if I can " is more than another's assurance ; and his doubtful tale before some men's protestations :—this is confident of nothing in futurity, yet his conjectures oft true prophecies :—that makes a

pause still betwixt his ear and belief, and is not too hasty
to say after others.   One whose tongue is strung up like
a clock till the time, and then strikes, and says much when
he talks little :—that can see the truth betwixt two
wrangles, and sees them agree even in that they fall
out upon : that speaks no rebellion in a bravery or talks
big from the spirit of sack.   A man cool and temperate in
his passions, not easily betrayed by his choler :—that vies
not oath with oath, nor heat with heat, but replies calmly
to an angry man, and is too hard for him too :—that can
come fairly off from captains' companies, and neither drink
nor quarrel.   One whom no ill hunting sends home discontented, and makes him swear at his dogs, and family.
One not hasty to pursue the new fashion, nor yet affectedly
true to his old round breeches ;   but gravely handsome,
and to his place, which suits him better than his taylor :
active in the world without disquiet, and careful without
misery ;   yet neither ungulphy in his pleasure, nor a seeker
of business, but has his hour for both.   A man that seldom
laughs violently, but his mirth is a cheerful look : of a
composed and settled countenance, not set, nor much
alterable with sadness or joy.   He affects nothing so wholly,
that he must be a miserable man when he loses it ;   but
fore-thinks what will come hereafter, and spares fortune
his thanks and curses.   One that loves his credit, not his
word reputation ;   yet can save both without a duel.   Whose
entertainments to greater men are respectful, not com-
plimentary ; . and to his friends plain, not rude.   A good
husband, father, master ;   that is, without doting, pampering
familiarity.   A man well poised in all humours, in whom
nature shewed most geometry, and he has not spoilt the
work.   A man of more wisdom than wittiness, and brain
than fancy ;   and abler to anything than to make verses.

The Logician of Characterologists.   The distinctive feature
of Thomas Fuller's few character studies is the classificatory
tendency.   The writers before him, and indeed even those
who followed him, spoke of whole classes with one sweep.
At most, they divided their characters into good or bad, or
excellent and ordinary, such as the virtuous widow and the
ordinary widow, the mere dull physician and the surgeon ;
but Fuller is the logician of the seventeenth century character
portrayers.   His definitions are cast in a philosophical mould.

" The liar is one that makes a trade to sell falsehoods with
intent to deceive." " The harlot is one that herself is both
merchant and merchandise which she selleth for profit and
hath pleasure given her into the bargain, and yet remains
a great loser." Thus he classifies and sub-classifies his liars
and favorites, and is always anxious to discriminate between
terms.

In Samuel Butler we have the most pretentious character
writer of the period. Some of his sketches are veritable essays.
The most psychological of these treat of the proud man, the
philosopher, the fantastic, the melancholy man, the curious
man, the fanatic, the prater, the medicine-taker (who in our
own day would be called the neurotic) and the over-doer.

Richard Flecknoe's *Enigmatical Characters* (1658) may be
cited here only because of one truly psychological drawing
which the book contains, viz., *Of One Who Troubles Herself
With Everything*.

Decline of Character Writing in Eighteenth Century. The
eighteenth century did not see such a luxuriant crop of
literary characterologists as its predecessor. *The English
Theophrastus or the Manners of the Age* (anonymous) published
in 1702, is far from bearing out its title. The book is rather
a collection of sparkling sayings and epigrams derived from
many sources, particularly from La Rochefoucauld ; and
even the author's own reflections are patterned after the
French so-called moralists, and adapted to the taste of the
English readers, with perhaps a pinch of stronger seasoning.
To quote only one or two remarks of this acute observer who
wrote more than two hundred years ago : " To give a true
reason of *constancy* and *inconstancy* is more the business of an
anatomist or *naturalist* than of a moral philosopher, for
they rather depend upon the frame of the *body* than the
constitution of the mind . . . If divorce was to be come by
without the trouble of suing for an Act of Parliament,
't would raise the pleasures of a married life and sink the delights

of intriguing." As a critic of society, the author can well take his place with the most uncompromising of to-day.

Character Drawing in the Periodical Essay. Steele and Addison, through the medium of the various periodicals which are associated with their names : the *Tatler*, the *Spectator*, the *Guardian*, and the *Lover*, have contributed a number of both character and portrait studies of which Addison's " Character of a Salamander " in the *Spectator* is a remarkable anticipation of modern sex pathology, as may be observed from the following quotation :

> There is a Species of Women, whom I shall distinguish by the name of Salamanders. Now a Salamander is a kind of Heroine in Chastity, that treads upon Fire and lives in the midst of Flames without being hurt. A Salamander knows no Distinction of Sex in those she converses with, grows familiar with a Stranger at first Sight, and is not so narrow-spirited as to observe whether the Person she talks to be in Breeches or in Petticoats. She admits a Male Visitant to her Bed-side, plays with him a whole Afternoon at Pickette, walks with him two or three Hours by Moon-light ; and is extremely Scandalized at the unreasonableness of an Husband, or the Severity of a Parent, that would debar the Sex from such innocent Liberties. Your Salamander is therefore a perpetual Declaimer against Jealousie, and Admirer of the French Good-breeding, and a great Stickler for Freedom in Conversation. In short, the Salamander lives in an invincible State of Simplicity and Innocence ; Her Constitution is preserv'd in a kind of natural Frost ; She wonders what People mean by Temptations ; and defies Mankind to do their worst. Her Chastity is engaged in a constant Ordeal, or fiery Trial ; (like good Queen Emma) the pretty Innocent walks blindfold among burning Plough-shares, without being scorched or singed by them.

Mandeville the Trenchant. If I make a slight digression here in the subject matter, while yet keeping to the chronological order of the authors, to consider the work of Bernard de Mandeville, it is because that fearless and ruthless dissector of society presents an unvarnished picture of human nature and offers, incidentally, some observations which may be

applied in the view on character set forth in this book.
Mandeville, whose fame is due to his *Fable of the Bees*, may
be regarded as the English counterpart of the French literary
moralists, La Rochefoucauld, La Bruyère and Rousseau,
to whom, as his name suggests, he is most probably related
racially. To the critical spirit which inspired the former
two writers, however, he brings a discursive method which
renders his quasi-nihilistic views even more efficacious. Like
his French fellow-believers, he indicts man *en masse*, claiming
that the " moral virtues are the political offspring which
flattery begot upon pride ".

" There is no man," he continues to say, " of what capacity
or penetration soever that is wholly proof against the
witchcraft of flattery, if artfully performed and suited to
his abilities

A Precursor of Nietzsche. In his thoroughgoing *Enquiry
into the Origin of Moral Virtue*, he as much as denies the
existence of this quality, except in an artificial sense. We
must keep this in mind as bearing on the central discussion
of character in Chapter IX. How does he achieve his end ?
By analyzing generally accepted virtues into their mental
components and in the light of the situation of which they
are a part.

> Pity, though it is the most gentle and the least
> mischievous of all our passions, is yet as much a frailty
> of our nature as anger, pride or fear. The weakest minds
> have generally the greatest share of it, for which reason
> none are more compassionate than women and children.
> . . . It is an impulse of nature that consults neither the
> public interest nor our own reason, it may produce evil
> as well as good. It has helped to destroy the honour of
> virgins, and corrupted the integrity of judges ; and whoever
> acts from it as a principle, what good soever he may bring
> to the society, has nothing to boast of but that he has
> indulged a passion that has happened to be beneficial
> to the public. There is no merit in saving an innocent
> babe ready to drop into the fire ; the action is neither
> good nor bad, and what benefit soever the infant

received we only obliged ourselves; for to have seen it fall, and not striven to hinder it, would have caused a pain, which self-preservation compelled us to prevent: nor has a rich prodigal, that happens to be of a commiserating temper, and loves to gratify his passions, greater virtue to boast of, when he relieves an object of compassion with what to himself is a trifle.

Asylum in Religion. Mandeville is ready to admit that the case of the man who, from his love of goodness, can part with what he values himself is different; yet even such a one derives pleasure out of the act by contemplating his own worth, which contemplation is a sign of pride. Thus has Spinoza's dictum that " virtue is its own reward " paled under the searchlight of Mandeville, who, however, fearing lest his negativism has led him too far, turns to " true religion " for his solution and salvation. To sum up Mandeville's position : Mankind has essentially one character, manifesting itself in various phases of weakness or frailty. Not reason but passions govern us, hence our only refuge is in guidance of the Deity. And if we doubt the sincerity of Mandeville's injunction, as there is reason to do, we must conclude that the author of the celebrated *Fable of the Bees* is a follower of Mephistopheles in his moral nihilism.

A SCEPTIC TO THE RESCUE OF HUMAN VALUES

It will be surprising to some that the great sceptic David Hume should come to the defence of human dignity in almost the same words as his French contemporary Vauvenargues, who was the sanest of the French literary moralists.[1] With his characteristic common sense, this philosopher, the chief opponent of the Common Sense School, recognizes that " it is that comparison " between one animal and another or others of the same species " which regulates our judgment concerning its greatness ". That there is a natural difference between merit and demerit, virtue and vice, wisdom and folly, he

---

[1] See further, section II of this chapter.

continues to say in one of his minor essays *Of the Dignity or Meanness of Human Nature*, "no reasonable man will deny: yet it is evident that in affixing the term, which denotes either our approbation or blame, we are commonly more influenced by comparison than by any fixed unalterable standard in the nature of things."

The incisive logic of Hume's argument to refute the cynicism of many literary philosophers is so rarely referred to in spite of its analytical masterliness that I cannot forbear to quote several passages from this essay. Perhaps no one has brought out the issue so clearly as did Hume, and no one has in my estimation been more successful in turning the tables on the doubting and therefore doubtful moralists than was this sceptic who was viewed with such concern by his racial fellow-philosophers, the members of the " Common Sense " School, which in principle could not but receive greater impetus and support from its adversary's endeavors than from the representations set forth by its own leaders. And it is largely this essay which shows many exponents of Hume's philosophy mistaken when they class him as a hedonist, or a utilitarian, and mention him in one breath with Bentham, the Mills, and Spencer. Indeed Hume's statement " I feel a pleasure in doing good to my friend, because I love him ; but do not love him for the sake of that ' pleasure ' " might well be mistaken for an utterance of Bishop Butler's.

A Relative Matter. " There is much of a dispute of words in this controversy," says Hume. " When a man denies the sincerity of all public spirit of affection to a country and community, I am at a loss what to think of him. Perhaps he never felt his passion in so clear and distinct a manner as to remove all his doubts concerning its force and reality. But when he proceeds afterwards to reject all private friendship, if no interest or self-love intermix itself ; I am then confident that he abuses terms, and confounds the ideas of things ; since it is impossible for any one to be so selfish or rather so stupid, as to make no difference between one man and another, and give no preference to qualities which engage his approbation and esteem. Is he also, say I, as insensible to anger as he pretends to be to friendship? And does injury and wrong no more affect him than kindness or benefits? Impossible: he does not know himself: he has forgotten the movements of his heart; or rather, he makes use of a different language from the rest of his countrymen, and calls not things by their proper names. What say you of natural affection? (I subjoin), Is that also a species of self-love? Yes; all is self-love. *Your* children are loved only because they are yours: *your* friend for a like reason; and *your* country engages you only so far as it has a connection with *yourself*. Were the idea of self removed, nothing would affect you: you would be altogether inactive and insensible: or, if you ever give yourself any movement, it would only be from vanity, and a desire of fame and reputation to this same self. I am willing, reply I, to receive your interpretation of human actions, provided you admit the facts. That species of self-love which displays itself in kindness to others, you must allow to have great influence over human actions, and even greater, on many occasions, than that which remains in its original shape and form. For how few are there, having a family, children, and relations, who do not spend more on the maintenance and education of these than on their own pleasures? This, indeed, you justly observe may proceed from their self-love, since the prosperity of their family and friends is one, or the chief, of their pleasures, as well as their chief honour. Be you also one of these selfish men, and you are sure of every one's good opinion and good-will; or, not to shock your ears with their expressions, the self-love of every one, and mine among the rest, will then incline us to serve you, and speak well of you.

Analysis of Fallacy. " In my opinion, there are two things which have led astray those philosophers that have insisted so much on the selfishness of man. In the *first* place, they found that every act of virtue or friendship was attended with a secret pleasure; whence they concluded, that friendship and virtue could not be disinterested. But the fallacy of this is obvious. The virtuous sentiment or passion produces the pleasure, and does not arise from it. I feel a pleasure in doing good to my friend, because I love him; but do not love him for the sake of that pleasure.

" In the *second* place, it has always been found, that the virtuous are far from being indifferent to praise; and therefore they have been represented as a set of vainglorious men, who had nothing in view but the applauses of others. But this also is a fallacy. It is very unjust in the world, when they find any tincture of vanity in a laudable action, to depreciate it upon that account, or ascribe it entirely to that motive. The case is not the same with vanity, as with other passions. Where avarice or revenge enters into any seemingly virtuous action, it is difficult for us to determine how far it enters, and it is natural to suppose it the sole actuating principle. But vanity is so closely allied to virtue, and to love the fame of laudable actions approaches so near the love of laudable actions for their own sake, that these passions are more capable of mixture, than any other kinds of affection; and it is almost impossible to have the latter without some degree of the former. Accordingly we find, that this passion for glory is always warped and varied according to the particular taste or disposition of the mind on which it falls. Nero had the same vanity in driving a chariot, that Trajan had in governing the empire with justice and ability. To love the glory of virtuous deeds is a sure proof of the love of virtue."

Importance of Outcome. Thus does Hume vindicate the values which were in danger of being relegated to the mythological limbo by a set of wits whose very brilliancy occluded their horizon. A fundamental issue is involved here, even if the term character should not be restricted in the narrower sense. Unless we recognize the significance of comparison and discrimination, especially as regards the strivings and intentions of different individuals, we might as well give up our quest ; for it will be quite easy by pursuing the same nihilistic method with respect to other qualities to show that they are essentially the same in all individuals, and differ but in circumstance. Clearly then there would be no room for a scheme of types on any basis, if we embrace this negativistic view-point. Hence our dwelling at length on the controversy between the deniers and the upholders of human values. That this question is in no way influenced by a religious *Weltanschauung* or decided by an ethic " from above " is amply proven by Hume's protagonism on the side of the values. Surely no one with so much as a smattering of his life and philosophy would venture to class him with the religious or moral dogmatists. It is just because Hume was the empiricist *par excellence* that he was able to pick out the flaws in the reasoning of the superficial empiricists who degraded the status of man only because they were thinking in terms of absolute standards.

Bucke Atomizes Behavior. Character writing, as an art, declined in the nineteenth century, but it did not disappear. In the *Book of Human Character* (1837), by Charles Bucke, which is a mine of wisdom, drawing for its ore on anecdotes and episodes from history and biography, we have a more useful type of sketch. No longer do we meet with the ribaldry and bias of the early British character writers. Bucke, who is a diminutive Montaigne, in his own way, has endeavored to be objective in his observations, and for that reason his work approaches a scientific inquiry.

In the four hundred and fifty odd thimble studies, almost the whole gamut of human foibles and fortunes is run. By means of apt illustrations, Bucke treats here of persons whom it is difficult to know, who see clearly and yet represent superficially, those who spin too finely, those who can do little things greatly, who waste great powers on subordinate

subjects, whose politeness is altered by the mention of money,
who think too much about the past, who are always concerning themselves about the future, who believe their own
lies, who break off in the middle, who have elegant manners
but vulgar minds, who are cruel in general yet clement in
particular, who suspend their natural characters, who being
innocent have no regard to appearances, etc. To be sure, the
subject-matter of these two volumes is not altogether so
distinctly psychological, but after due allowance is made for
such apparently, at least for our purpose, irrelevant reflections,
as those on " whose opinions we value only in part ", those
" who are valued at a distance ", " who can be judged only
in reference to their misfortune ", etc., there is still a valuable
residue left.

Approaches Psychoanalysis. Bucke still remains a psychological analyst of rare acuteness. Instead of treating
characters *en bloc*, and following especially the general notions
of the time, he has searched deeper into the recesses of man,
looking not for vices but for peculiarities, contradictions,
twists in the make-up of man, duality of character, in this
way really anticipating the Freudian movement, not forsooth
in its principles and methods, but in *noting bits of uniform
behavior in different people*, peculiarities which, though Bucke
did not go that far, call for explanation, and which in themselves are of great service in throwing important light on the
whole life of a given individual. It is, for instance, highly
significant that some men are great in minor things. The
fact that Gray could turn out perhaps the most perfect
poem in the English language, yet could not finish his poem on
Education because of its contemplated magnitude, is something to be reckoned with, not only theoretically, but practically in the guidance of talent.

Some of the section headings in Bucke's work seem strangely
familiar to followers of the new movement in psychology.
I mean such headings as " who give reasons for all they do " ;

" who give wise reasons for unwise actions " ; " wise men who give unwise counsel ", and the like.

Miscellaneous Addenda. Before concluding the portion on the British contribution to literary characterology, mention might be made of Hazlitt's *Characteristics*, inspired by La Rochefoucauld's maxims. We should also refer to Thackeray's *Book of Snobs*, which, though written in a light vein, is not without insight, and George Eliot's *Impressions of Theophrastus Such*, not in its entirety, but in her delineations of Mixtus and Scintilla in " A Half-Breed ", of Touchwood's behaviour in " A Bad Temper ", and in the essays, " A Man Surprised at His Originality ", " A Too Deferential Man ", and " The Watch-Dog of Knowledge ". Edgar Fawcett's *Social Silhouettes* is an excellent example of the narrative-sketch in American literature.

In addition, the various collections extant on both famous and notorious figures, such as biographies of eccentrics, of scoundrels (not necessarily convicted by law) and last, but not least, the short character studies and silhouettes of notables which the English literature of the seventeenth century abounds in.

ESTIMATE OF BRITISH CHARACTEROLOGISTS

The chief defect of the British character writers of the seventeenth century, with the possible exception of Earle and Overbury, is the want of a serious purpose in their approach, as is well illustrated by the fact that *The Whimsies*, published in 1631,[1] and attributed to Richard Brathwait, contains a series of twenty-four characters according to the alphabet, such as an " Almanack-maker ", " A Ballad-monger ", " A Corranto Coiner ", " A Decoy ", an " Exchange man ", a " Forester ", a " Gamester ", etc.

[1] Reprinted in twenty-six copies only, with a preface by J. O. Halliwell, 1859.

Essence of Character Sketch. The dedicatory epistle of this anonymous writer is from the present standpoint more significant than most of the characters depicted . " What else are characters," we read in this epistle, " but stamps or impressions, noting such an especial place, person or office ; and leaving such a mark or cognizance upon it, as the conceit may neither taste of too much lightness nor the close of so witty an observance leave too much bitterness, nor the whole passage or series incline to too much dullness ? . . . Strong lines have been in request ; but they grew disrelishing, because they smelled too much of the lamp and opinionate singularity. Clinchings likewise were held nimble flashes ; but affectation spoiled all, and discovered their levity."

Alas, this author, who knows so well what is desirable and yet adopts a puerile method in practice, may truly say of himself :

Video meliora proboque
Pejora sequor.

" He writes best " we are told by this sage, " that affects least and effects most. . . . This hath been ever my maxim, that singularity and affectations are antipodes to judgment and discretion.   Self-opinion makes a man's self his own minion. He is the true emblem of Narcissus, and dotes more on his own shadow than on others' substance."

As a matter of fact, "Clitus-Alexandrinus," the pseudonymous author, has put his finger on the weak spot of English character writing during that period, which for the most part consisted of squibs and lampoons often garnished with disgusting profanity and such devices as puns, assonance, alliteration, and other effects of a low order.

Chief Fault of British Character Writers. Such is true especially of books like *Confused Characters of Conceited Coxcombs* by " Verax Philobasileus ", published in 1661,[1]

[1] Reprinted in twenty-six copies only, with a preface by J. O. Halliwell, 1859.

and the motley transcript collection of Philip Bliss entitled *Characters*.[1] The former, addressing himself to the " facetious reader ", justifies his invective by pleading that since " characters are descriptions and when the persons described prove vicious and vain, excuse me gentle reader, if this treatise prove so likewise ".

It would be only right to state that most of the character writers discussed are possessed of a fine style, employing an excellent diction and happy metaphor. As pamphleteers they are in their element ; but as psychological draughtsmen they are failures because they express *their* own emotions instead of observing universal traits. At the bottom of this short-coming is *provinciality or perhaps insularity*. For the British, character writing is a game which may be started anywhere and left off anywhere. Their skill is incontestable, but what they lack is a sense of *direction*. The French writers manifest a far more serious purpose *seeking that which is common to men and women of all countries* even if they see them only through the medium of their own countrymen. The British, with the exception of Earle, are apt to make much of the *individual* idiosyncrasies ; the French perceive the peculiarities of the type, even where they depict an individual.

II

CHARACTER WRITING IN FRANCE

The nation which, next to the English, cultivated the portraiture of human traits is the French. It would take us too far afield to comment on the racial differences as revealed by the character writings of the two peoples, but one can hardly dispute the fact that there are such differences, one

[1] For good reasons this transcript though published was never printed.

of the most striking being the seriousness with which the French characterologists approach their task, as compared with the levity of the English, except in the case of the exhortative writers who border on tedious sermonizing.

La Rochefoucauld. The giant in French character portrayal is of course La Bruyère, but we must not forget that Molière's characters, for instance Alceste in *Le Misanthrope*, or Tartuffe, are life pictures whose behavior intrigues us as students of human character even more than their comical situations entertain us as spectators. Nor must we lose sight of that shrewd observer of society, La Rochefoucauld, whose shafts forever tend to hurt our self-regard. It is true he speaks of human nature in general and is apt to slur individual differences, yet in probing the mainsprings of action, he constantly brings before us certain principles of motivation which are germane to our subject. In this respect, curiously enough, he happens to come nearer our territory in his *Pensées* which he has either suppressed or materially altered in the later edition of his main work, than in the *Maximes* for which he is chiefly known.

How true, e.g., is this thought of La Rochefoucauld's even in our own day of alleged predictability of human behaviour. " Prudence is raised to the skies ; there is no end to the praises which are sung to it. It is the guide of our actions and conduct. It is the master of fortune. It shapes the destiny of empires. Without it, we are beset with all the evils. With it we have all the good in the world, and as a poet once said, if we but possess prudence we lack no divinity, as if to say that we find in prudence all the assistance which we ask of the gods. And yet the most consummate prudence cannot make any guarantees in regard to the slightest effect in the world, since operating on material so changing and so unknown as man is, it cannot execute with certainty a single one of his projects." (*Pensées*, 20.) In spite of this, the French wit seems to believe in a deterministic, or rather in this case, fatalistic philosophy, for, says he in another place, " notwithstanding a certain amount of uncertitude and variation which is apparent in the world, there may yet be observed a definite secret concatenation and order regulated for all times by Providence, which brings it about that everything marches along in proper place and follows the course of its destiny." (*Pensées*, 69.)

Needless to say, many of La Rochefoucauld's severe and most *parti pris* judgments in the interest of his doctrine that egoism is the sole root of all our actions may be taken with a grain of salt by modern psychology. When, for instance, he traces curiosity back to the selfish impulse of appearing superior to others, he fails to examine this universal tendency as manifested by infants, animals, and savages, who are not yet tainted with the vices of a civilization as La Rochefoucauld sees it. Nor does he appreciate that curiosity expresses itself in a variety of ways and is not confined to the object of scholarship.[1]

The nearest La Rochefoucauld comes to differentiating men is in the section " De la différence des esprits " of his *Réflexions Diverses*. The word " esprit " in French is practically untranslatable, and does not quite answer to our term " intelligence ". It partly includes what is sometimes spoken of as character in the recent literature. Thus the detailed classification of the various forms of *esprit*, such as *bel esprit, esprit adroit, bon esprit, esprit utile, esprit d'affaires, esprit fin, esprit de finesse, esprit de feu, esprit brilliant, esprit de détail*, etc., falls within our universe of discourse and may well be considered in the light of modern analysis.

La Rochefoucauld's observations give the impression that their author might have made a far more important psychological contribution, if he had only exerted himself. As it is,

[1] It is interesting to note that La Rochefoucauld's great contemporary, Pascal, remarks similarly in his *Pensées* that curiosity is but vanity. " Most commonly we desire knowledge only that we may talk of it. Otherwise people would not cross the sea if they could say nothing about it."

E

however, his thoughts should be given more prominence
in books dealing with motivation, especially as many of his
and La Bruyère's *aperçus* make their appearance in the more
recent psychological literature as newly-discovered facts.

La Bruyère's General Condemnation of the Species Man.
The richest material on the study of human nature is to
be found in La Bruyère's *Les Caractères*. While also judging
men collectively in the manner of La Rochefoucauld, he is
less of the doctrinaire and more inclined to recognize that there
is a variety of characters. Of the seventeen chapters constituting the book for which his name is justly famous, that
on Mankind is the most important. La Bruyère, if I may use
an *oxymoron* figure, is benevolently severe. " Let us not be
angry with men," he opens up this chapter, " when we see
them cruel, ungrateful, unjust, proud, egotists, and forgetful
of others ; they are made so, it is their nature, we might
just as well quarrel with a stone for falling to the ground
or with a fire when the flames ascend." It would be
possible, however, to take a less charitable view of our author.
He may be said to extenuate a minor fault of man in order
to heap a greater one on him, and what he says on that score
is highly significant, especially as it tends to corroborate
La Rochefoucauld's more direct conclusions. " In one sense
men are not fickle, or only in trifles ; they change their
habits, language, outward appearance, their rules of pro-
priety and sometimes their taste, but they always preserve
their bad morals and adhere tenaciously to what is ill and to
their indifference for virtue." To seek consistency in this
perspicacious Frenchman would be a futile task. After all,
a writer who does not aim to be discursive, is exempt from
the obligation to work out all the implications of his views.

Samples of La Bruyère's Outstanding Human Types.
But we must remember that La Bruyère is better known for
his character portrayals than for his general reflections, and
though his miniature sketches are rather portraits, often

composites of people he had known, they are, in spite of the fact that a number of them (especially that of Ménalque, the most elaborate of his characters) are sheer caricatures, valuable for the characterization which limns the portraits. There is for instance, Giton : " He speaks with confidence. He unfolds an ample handkerchief and blows his nose noisily. He spits to a great distance and sneezes very loudly. . . . At table and in walking he occupies more room than any one else. He takes the centre and walks with his equals . . . If he sits down you see him settle into an armchair, cross his legs, frown, pull his hat over his eyes and see on one or lift it up again and show his brow from pride and audacity. He is cheerful, a hearty laugher, impatient, presumptuous, quick to anger, irreligious, politic, mysterious about current affairs. He believes he has talent and wit. He is rich." Who can fail to see in this picture the representation of what Jung has called the extravert, of the lower variety, or perhaps as he would deport himself two and a half centuries ago ?

On the other hand, who will deny that Phédon is the true example of the introvert ?

Phédon has a bilious complexion. He is abstracted, dreamy, and with all his wit seems stupid. He forgets to say what he knows—and if he does so, he sometimes comes out badly. He thinks he is a nuisance to those he speaks to ; he relates things briefly but frigidly. He is not listened to ; he does not stir laughter. He is superstitious, scrupulous, timid. He walks gently and lightly ; he seems afraid to touch the ground ; he walks with lowered eyes and dares not raise them to the passers-by. He is never among those who form a circle for discussion ; he places himself behind the person who is speaking, furtively gathers what he says and goes away if he is looked at. He occupies no space, claims no place ; he walks with hunched shoulders, his hat pulled over his eyes so as not to be seen ; he shrinks and hides himself in his cloak ; there are no streets or galleries so overcrowded and filled with people but that he finds a means of traversing them easily, of slipping through them without being noticed. If he is asked to sit down, he places himself just on the edge of the chair ; he speaks in a low tone in conversation and articulates badly ; yet with his friends he is open about public affairs, bitter against the age, very little disposed in favor of the ministers of state and the government. He never opens his mouth except to reply ; he coughs and blows his nose behind his hat ; he spits almost on himself, and he waits until he is alone to sneeze, or if it happens to him, it is unperceived by the company present : he costs nobody a salute or a compliment. He is poor.

Where shall we find such succinct portrayals of the professional spectator, who is seen everywhere and can tell you everything trivial, of the humdrum Narcisse who will do to-morrow what he does to-day and what he did yesterday ; of Hermippe, with whom no one is to be compared for accomplishing quietly and easily a perfectly useless piece of work ?

This Hermippe had taken ten steps to go from his bed to his wardrobe and now by altering his room he only takes nine—how many steps saved in the course of his life ! Elsewhere you turn the door-knob, push it or pull and the door opens ; what a waste of labour ! Here is an unnecessary movement which he saves himself—and how ? That is a mystery he does not reveal. Indeed he is a great master in mechanics and machinery, at least in those everyone can get on without. Hermippe brings the daylight into his house otherwise than by the windows ; he has found a way of going up and down stairs otherwise than by the stairway, and he is looking for a better way of going in and out than by the door.

Of a more desultory kind is the depiction of character in Montesquieu's *Lettres Persanes*. Nevertheless the correspondence between Rica and Usbec, who are the heroes of the book, contain some allusions to various types of people, which at least deserve mention.

Passing over the feeble imitation of La Bruyère by Madame de Puisieux[1] (published in 1750) which, however, is not without

---

[1] Like most of her predecessors and contemporaries in France who discussed the broad subject of human nature, she magnifies on the trait of *amour-propre* which, to the writers, served as a sort of

merit as a mirror of the finer man and especially woman, we come to the most' philosophical of the French character writers, compared with whom La Rochefoucauld and La Bruyère are men of the world, penetrating and sparkling, but still without the feeling that there is something more to be sought than they were content in finding.

Vauvenargues—Philosopher of French Characterologists. Naturally we cannot expect of a man who died in his thirty-second year the same degree of maturity as of a middle-aged person.   His range of experience must necessarily be limited as compared with the other two masters, but that his insight and depth exceed theirs may be inferred from many passages. Decrying the sweeping condemnations of humanity by the illustrious epigrammatists just named, Vauvenargues in his essay, *Sur le caractère des différents siècles,* justly points out " I speak of this force and grandeur of the mind, which compared with the sentiments of weak spirits, deserve the names which I have given them. I speak of a relative grandeur, and not of anything else, for there is nothing great among men except by comparison ".   The twenty-eight characters which Vauvenargues drew are again nothing but miscellaneous portraits of unequal merit. As such they do not concern us here, but it is in his psychological work, *Introduction à la connaissance de l'esprit humain,* that we meet with some attempt at a more systematic differentiation of characters. Vauvenargues holds that character comprises everything which goes to make up " l'esprit et le coeur ", and it is marked by the most bizarre contrarieties. He warns us against confusing the qualities of the " mind " (*âme*) with that of the " spirit " (*l'esprit*) especially as the majority of people are apt to judge a thing by its covering. Take, for instance, such a general trait as seriousness. We often think of it as an absolute

explanation of all the virtues as well as of the vices ; in other words, character as such was to them only a higher phase of egoism, which they took it upon themselves to reduce to a common denominator.

category, but how many different ingredients might have composed it. You may be serious by temperament, because of too great or too little feeling, too many or too few ideas, because of timidity, habit or even money considerations. Vauvenargues then proceeds to distinguish the different serious types as they appear to an attentive observer. Tranquil-minded seriousness, e.g., carries with it a gentle and serene air. The seriousness of despondency reveals a languishing exterior, etc. To be sure, these correlations are common-place, but this French moralist, unlike those who had gone before him recognizes "*la nécessité indispensable de bien manier les principes les plus familiers, et de les mettre tous ensemble sous un point de vue qui en découvre la fécondité et la liaison*". In other words, Vauvenargues is probably the first Frenchman to look for a basis of classification which could be more or less rigidly applied.

RÉSUMÉ

In the rather comprehensive survey of literary characterology, we may note diverse trends. There are *objective observers* like Theophrastus and to a certain extent La Bruyère, and *subjective depictors* like most of the British character writers who took a character as a suitable theme to elaborate epigrammatically, often injecting their own bias into the elaboration. The frequency with which certain characters are painted, such as the prostitute, in her various euphemistic and plainer designations, would form an interesting study in itself as throwing light on the British mind of the sixteenth and seventeenth centuries, but since the literary and occasionally as in Nicholas Breton, the purely didactic impulse are predominant in these sketches, little is offered by them in the way of psychology. The French character writers, on the other hand, are more realistic, but their delineations are composite portraits, and not sufficiently inclusive. While the *British writers relieve themselves in their*

sketches of an animus against a class, La Bruyère squares
himself with certain individuals who had provoked his critical
sense or indignation.

In general, the literary approach to the study of character can provide us only with clues. It lacks most when it lacks the conscious effort to analyse the subject, instead of being guided by random inspiration. In the one case, the investigator is guided by his purpose ; in the other, the products are obtained in a haphazard fashion, and while, in themselves ripe and savory, they cannot contribute towards a wholesome regimen.

Hundreds of characters have been passed in review by these writers, from the most common to the most singular and fantastic, yet if we were to aim at exhaustiveness, that number multiplied by itself would not give a fraction of the possible number of characters, even in our own day, especially if the scope is so broadened as to include considerations of office, circumstances and physical condition, as well as assumed relationships.

The more complicated a civilization grows, the greater the list of characters that would find their place in such collections as Overbury's or Samuel Butler's. Were they to write in our age, they would doubtless satirize the radio fan, the movie theatre frequenter, the cross-word puzzle fiend, and so on *ad libitum.* The truth is that the *character should function as a sort of law under which a large number of individuals might be subsumed as particular instances.* The individualization of character just as the particularization of a law, that is to say, where each case should be governed by a separate law, would be subversive of our entire goal, which is to ensure a modicum of predictability. To be sure, human character presents greater difficulties than all other material, but for that very reason our endeavors must be doubled to obtain a rule of guidance.

As to the rough generalizations of character in the work of Pascal, La Rochefoucauld, La Bruyère, Montesquieu, and other

French writers, it is astonishing to see how many of their maxims and reflections are duplicated in the writings of the psychoanalysts.   Rationalization, the inferiority complex, compensation, projection, and other mechanisms are implied though not discussed by name.   When La Rochefoucauld, for instance, says: " If we had no faults we should not take so much pleasure to notice them in others," the crystallized thought here is of a psychoanalytic stamp as it is also in the further reflection : " Aversion for lies is often an imperceptible ambition to render our testimony of considerable weight and to secure for our words a religious respect."

One cannot afford to dismiss the detached thoughts of these sages from the purview of psychology only because their authors did not put forth any scientific claims.   If they have not worked out their problems, they, at least, have suggested them in the form of stimulating aphorisms.   Despite the fact that there is no train of reasoning in these reflections, they nevertheless give evidence of a consistent position in at least one respect, viz. that *amour-propre* is the spring of all action, good and bad, and that even the virtues of mankind are born of weakness—not an edifying point of view, to be sure, but one which requires examination, and, because of its widespread influence, it must be discussed rather than ignored.

CHAPTER III

We must now come back to see what had happened to the *explanatory* approach to the study of character which had been initiated by Hippocrates and Galen. In one sense it may be said that the original theory is still intact. Our ordinary vocabulary harks back to the assumptions of these Greek physicians. We still make use of such words as *spleen* for rancorous utterances, and *galling* as a synonym for vexing. Indeed, the French have no other word for anger in their everyday parlance than the word *colère*, while I have heard on many occasions foreigners say that a person is without a gall as signifying that he or she is unusually mild-tempered. Similarly the other terms belonging to the ancient doctrine have come to be household words, and no attempts to supplant them in favor of terms of more recent coinage have been of any avail. If the doctrine of humors has now been abandoned, its atmosphere still lingers, as is evident from the very persistence of such expressions as " good humor ", " bad humor ", " ill-humor ", " humorous ", " humoresque ", etc.

Significance of the number four. It is not strange that the number four should suggest a significant range of differences. We must remember the scheme of elements in the philosophy of Empedocles which might have been not without its influence on Hippocrates. It would be a mistake to over-estimate the originality of the great Hippocrates in formulating his famous theory. Before him the Greek hylozoists had already devoted their attention to the causes of illness, and the function of the so-called humors figured greatly in the teachings of Anaxagoras, and even more in those of Democritus, who had written a treatise on the humors, and Alcmeon of Crotona, who attributed disease to the disturbance of the equilibrium of the elementary qualities.[1]

The four directions of the compass, too, might have been a co-operating factor in the establishment of the fourfold temperament doctrine.   The hankering for symmetry and the belief in numerical consistency or, rather, parallelism as a tacit criterion of truth, are to be detected even in the philosophy of Kant, who pointed out that the four temperaments corresponded to the four figures of the syllogism. But, of course, these circumstances alone would not explain the firm hold which the humoral theory has exercised on the minds of great figures in the history of thought.

Aristotle's Modification.   In spite of the vitality of this doctrine, which, because of the celebrity of its originators, had enjoyed for many centuries an un-paralleled security, we must not suppose that it had always remained free from accretions, or that it has advanced untrammelled by the critical demands of modern science.   As far back as Aristotle, the original exposition of Hippocrates appeared in a more scientific cast.   Like Kant many centuries later, Aristotle regarded the blood, because of its general nutrient function, as the basis of all temperamental differences, yet, probably influenced by the teachings of Empedocles, he sought the causes of the fundamental peculiarities in the elemental ingredients of the blood.   Not the other humors were to account for these idiosyncrasies, but the admixtures or components of the blood.   The tendency for blood to clot is due to the earthen element in its composition, and constitutes the fiery or choleric temperament.   Cold-bloodedness is due to watery blood and conduces to fear.   The in-coagulability of the blood is the result of the want of earth material.   In the linking of fear with those individuals

---

[1] P. Malapert : *Le Caractère* (1902), p. 120.

whose blood does not clot, we really have a faint anticipation of the recent work on the adrenal glands.

Medieval Views. For all that, the Hippocratic humoral doctrine survived Aristotle's modification, in the latter form established by the celebrated Galen ; and its truth was not questioned in the Middle Ages, even by the staunchest Aristotelians.

Galen, the medical genius of the second century of our era, had drawn up nine temperaments, of which one was the perfectly normal, while four were simple in which one of four qualities (warm, cold, humid, and dry) was predominant, with the other three qualities in various degrees of equilibrium, and finally four were combinations, such as warm and dry, warm and humid, cold and dry, cold and humid— these constituting the celebrated quartet of temperaments. Among other achievements, Galen has the merit of clearly distinguishing between the melancholic and the choleric types which prior to him were both labelled " bilious ".

Many a subsequent writer draws his support for certain arguments from illustrations based on this theory. Thus, the illustrious Maimonides in the twelfth century, combating the doctrine of fatalism, adduces the following analogy to show how innate dispositions may be either thwarted by lack of exercise or opportunity for development, or else intensified by constant application : " For instance, a man whose natural constitution inclines towards dryness, whose brain matter is clear and not overloaded with fluids, finds it much easier to learn, remember, and understand things than the phlegmatic man whose brain is encumbered with a great deal of humidity. But, if one who inclines constitutionally towards a certain excellence is left entirely without instruction, and if his faculties are not stimulated, he will undoubtedly remain ignorant. On the other hand, if one by nature dull and phlegmatic, possessing an abundance of humidity, is instructed and enlightened, he will, though with difficulty, it is true, gradually succeed in acquiring knowledge and understanding. In exactly the same way, he whose blood is somewhat warmer than is necessary has the requisite quality to make of him a brave man. Another, however, the temperament of whose heart is colder than it should be, is naturally inclined towards cowardice and fear, so that if he should be taught and trained to be a coward he would easily become one. If, however, it be desired to make a brave man of him, he can without doubt become one, provided he receive the proper training, which would require, of course, great exertion." [1]

Literary Conceptions of the Humors. In English literature, Wyclif appears to be the first to allude to the temperaments, or rather, the humors. His sermons, published in 1380, contain the statement that " Blood is most kindly humor, answering to the love of God, three other humors in man answer to three other loves ". Shakespeare has in his plays a number of references to the humors, and Ben Jonson gives us the characteristics of the four temperaments when he describes the true critic in *Cynthia's Revels* as " neither too fantastically melancholy, too slowly phlegmatic, too lightly sanguine, nor too rashly choleric ; but in all so composed and ordered, as it is clear nature went about some full work ". Ben Jonson expresses himself with greater scientific pretensions, if not precision, in his play, " Every Man Out of his Humor," where he writes :—

Why humour, as it is ' ens ', we thus define it,
To be a quality of air or water ;
And in itself holds these two properties
Moisture and fluxure : as, for demonstration
Pour water on this floor.   'Twill wet and run.
Likewise the air forced through a horn or trumpet
Flows instantly away, and leaves behind
A kind of dew ; and hence we do conclude
That whatsoe'er hath fluxure and humidity

[1] Maimonides : *Eight Chapters* (of Ethics).

As wanting power to contain itself
Is humour. So in every human body
The choler, melancholy, phlegm and blood
By reason that they flow continually
In some one part and are not continent
Receive the name of humours. Now thus far
It may, by metaphor, apply itself
Unto the general disposition ;
As when some one peculiar quality
Doth so possess a man that it doth draw
All his effects, his spirits and his powers,
In their confluxion all to run one way,—
This may be truly said to be a humour.

Burton on the Humors. It is, however, in Burton's famed *Anatomy of Melancholy* that we find a detailed and quaint, not to say fantastic, description of the humoral doctrine :—

A humour is a liquid or fluent part of the body comprehended in it, and is either born with us, or is adventitious and acquisite. The first four primary humours are—Blood, a hot, sweet, temperate, red humour, prepared in the meseraic veins, and made of the most temperate parts of the chylus (chyle) in the liver, whose office it is to nourish the whole body, to give it strength and colour, being dispersed through every part of it. And from it spirits are first begotten in the heart, which afterwards in the arteries are communicated to the other parts. Pituita or phlegm is a cold and moist humour, begotten of the colder parts of the chylus (or white juice coming out of the meat digested in the stomach) in the liver. His office is to nourish and moisten the members of the body. Choler is hot and dry, begotten of the hotter parts of the chylus, and gathered to the gall. It helps the natural heat and senses. Melancholy, cold and dry, thick, black and sour, begotten of the more feculent part of nourishment, and purged from the spleen, is a bridle to the other two hot humours, blood and choler, preserving them in the blood, and nourishing the bones. Mention must also be made of serum, and of ' those excrementitious humours of the third concoction, sweat and tears '. An exact balance of the four primary humours makes the justly constituted man, and allows for the undisturbed production of the ' concoctions '—or processes of digestion and assimilation.

The eccentric Burton with his stupendous erudition quotes authority upon authority, citing also conflicting views in his search for the physical causes of melancholy, in this way giving us a glimpse of what was generally thought of the humoral theory in the centuries immediately preceding his.

Taking the next step, the French critic Bouhours, in the seventeenth century traces actual components of literary talent to the functioning of the humors. " The bile gives brilliancy and penetration, the black bile good sense and solidity, the blood engenders grace and delicacy."

Except for slight modifications and extensions, the original theory of the temperaments has in spite of occasional opposition, as notably in the case of Paracelsus, held its own until the modern researches in anatomy and physiology began to expose the fiction of black bile.

PROGRESS OF HUMORAL DOCTRINE MIRRORS HISTORY OF IDEAS

Mysticism. The history of the doctrine which Hippocrates originated is in a sense the history of human ideas, for it mirrors the great scientific interests of the time, even up to our own period.   The temperaments have become almost a symbol of permanence of aspiration changing its form only as a result of the march of progress. The first attempts to modify or at least interpret the ancient table after the time of Aristotle began with the revival of learning when science and fancy were strange bedfellows. Here may be mentioned the allegorical treatment of the temperaments by the sixteenth century mystic Jakob Boehme, who in his *Christosophy* regarded the four compositions as different asylums in which the jewel of man—the soul—is imprisoned.

Alchemy. The age of alchemy also shows its fossil marks on the perpetual theory which was now to be brought into relation with the most important alchemical substances. The basis of the choleric temperament was thought to be the predominance of the sulphuric element. The excess of mercury was supposed to be at the root of the sanguine temperament, and the melancholic temperament was traced to the preponderance of salt in the body.

Impress of Scientific Era. Then came the scientific revolutions of Copernicus, Galilei, and Harvey. Their discoveries gave the cue for further speculations on the temperaments. Toward the beginning of the eighteenth century Andreas Rüdiger in his *Physica Divina* reduced the number of elements responsible for temperamental differences to two, viz. aether as cause of the light qualities, and air as cause of the heavy qualities. Both together, neutralizing each other, they bring about elasticity of the body. Now, since various degrees of lightness and heaviness are possible, the complexions resulting from the fusion of the various grades of contraction and expansion give rise to four different kinds of elasticity :—

(1) Aether and air both rarefed, together with great elasticity—sanguine temperament.
(2) Aether and air both unrefined, together with slight elasticity—phlegmatic temperament.
(3) Aether refined and air unrefined, together with heavy elasticity—choleric temperament.
(4) Aether unrefined and air refined, together with easy contractibility and hard expansibility— melancholic temperament.

Probably one consequence of Harvey's discovery of the circulation of the blood was the shift of emphasis from the composition of the blood to its movement as the determinant of differences in temperament.[1] Anatomists and physiologists were now connecting these differences with the pressure of the blood against the blood vessels, and were looking into the

[1] This as well as several other references in this chapter are taken from J. Henle's " Von den Temperamenten ", in his *Anthropologische Vorträge*, pp. 110 ff.

differences in diameter of these vessels. In a word, the humoral doctrine was beginning to change into a solid theory.

SOLIDS INSTEAD OF HUMORS

Chief among these new investigators was Stahl at Halle, of phlogiston fame, who took into consideration three factors, (a) the constitution of the blood, (b) the porosity of the tissues and (c) the width of the blood vessels. The sanguine temperament he attributed to the thin flow of the blood, loose tissues and moderately wide blood vessels, which conditions produce proper warmth and redness for life's course to proceed smoothly. But where the blood flows thin and the porosity of the solid substance is slight, the choleric temperament will be found ; for the blood will have to be retained more in the blood vessels on account of the inexpansibility of the solid matter. The vessels must then be wide, and the pulse rate must be high because of the resistance to be overcome, and consequently, there is greater heat with this temperament. The conditions of the phlegmatic type are set down as thicker blood, wide pores and narrow vessels, so that the firm tissues are penetrated only by the more fluid, watery parts of the blood, hence the comparatively pale skin and lack of warmth which characterize this type. Finally the melancholic temperament is due to dark thick blood, small pores and considerably wide vessels. A more concise formula incorporating Stahl's theory was brought out by the latter's colleague Hoffmann (1660–1742) as may be seen in this table :—

Temperament	Sanguine	Phlegmatic	Choleric	Melancholic
blood	fluid	thick	fluid	thick
fibres	loose	loose	dense	dense

Haller's Work. It was not until about the middle of the eighteenth century when Haller laid the foundations of modern experimental physiology that the theory of humors received a permanent setback. Haller cited many arguments to show that the connection between the blood and the temperaments is not a necessary one, and on the other hand that the firm parts through which the blood flows, or rather their strength and irritability, are fundamental in accounting for different temperamental constitutions, the choleric being produced by the strength and irritability of these tissues ; the phlegmatic by weakness without irritability ; the melancholic (hypochondriac or hysterical) by weakness with irritability. Haller gave no place to the sanguine temperament in his scheme, but originated the sturdy peasant type, the Bœotian temperament, which he thought differed from the phlegmatic in possessing force, though in common with the general type it lacked sufficient irritability. Haller's disciples included the sanguine temperament in their revision of his great work *Elementa Physiologiae*. The components of this temperament were, according to them, slight irritability with moderate strength.

The Rise of Nerve Physiology. A new era was ushered in with the research work on nerve physiology ; and as heretofore, the doctrine ·of the temperaments took a new turn in harmony with the general scientific outlook of the generation. From humors to solids, and thence to a particular kind of solids—such was the transmigration of the Galenian hypothesis. The nervous system was now to be the seat of the mysterious compositions which of yore were ascribed to the humors alone. The chief of this school was Wrisberg, one of Haller's disciples. His task was to make of the fourfold division a double category, viz., choleric-sanguine and melancholic-phlegmatic. This accomplished, he endowed the former type with a larger brain, with thicker and firmer nerves and with a high sensitivity both of the organism in general and the specific sense organs. Quick perception and keenness of judgment are due to the conditions just mentioned, but in return, there is also an inclination toward pain and anger.

F

The phlegmatic-melancholy type, contrariwise, is marked by a small brain, very fine nerves and duller senses. Such people require strong impressions to actuate them, and are not adapted for scientific achievement, but can bear well the inconveniences of life and its drudgery.

THE NON-MATERIALISTIC CONCEPTIONS

Alchemy, physics, chemistry, pathology, physiology, neurology—all had their contact with the temperaments. It was now high time for philosophy to step in and dismiss all the materialistic theories as either worthless or so highly speculative as to be of little assistance. Platner, a contemporary, and now all but forgotten adversary of Kant, directing his gaze upwards, resorts to an intangible spontaneous (*selbsttätig*) principle of sensation and movement, which to him is definitely connected with the soul. This principle he discovers to be twofold and to reside, in its purer form, in the visual, auditory, and tactual nerves, but in the coarser form, in the olfactory, gustatory and cœnesthetic nerves. The first of these systems gives rise to ideas which refer to abstract concepts and absolute truths; the second system or organ, as Platner calls it, arouses in the soul the vague and hazy feelings pertaining to the animal part of man. It is by virtue of the combination of these two psychic mechanisms that the temperaments are to be explained.

Values Introduced. The departure of Platner from his predecessors is complete in that he invents a fresh table of temperaments and insists on a new centre of gravity in the discussion. He introduces *values* into the erstwhile chemical and physiological constitutions; and his list comprises (*a*) the *Attic* or *mental*, derived from the preponderance of the higher psychic organ (visual, auditory and tactual nervous constellation) over the lower organ (olfactory, gustatory and coenesthetic); (*b*) the *Scythian* or *animal* temperament, resulting from the preponderance of the second organ over the first ; (c) the *Roman* or *heroic*, where both organs or systems are well matched ; and (d) the *Phrygian* or *faint* temperament produced by the lack of energy in either of the two organs. But each of these four temperaments may further be subdivided according as the second psychic organ functions easily and free from inhibition or with difficulty and obstructedly. Consequently the Attic type branches off into the ethereal and melancholic divisions ; the Scythian into the sanguine and the Bœotian temperaments ; the Roman into the fiery and the masculine ; and the Phrygian into the phlegmatic and the hectic (in the sense of wasting).

What makes Platner's obscure view interesting from an historical angle is not only the fact that he had completely broken with the past in seeking out psychological ingredients for the temperaments as well as in localizing the components or, at any rate, assigning them a field of operation, but also the introduction of value denominators for his eight divisions, which was an innovation at this time.[1]

KANT'S DESCRIPTION OF THE TEMPERAMENTS

Kant's treatment of character is more critical. Taking cognizance of the double sense of the term he makes allowance for both meanings (a) character as a mere distinguishing quality, (b) the moral make-up, " if it is a question of possessing

---

[1] In Stern's *Differentielle Psychologie* (Appendix) we meet with a table of temperaments presumably taken from A. J. Dorsch's *Beiträge zum. Studium der Philosophie* (1787), which is the same as Platner's, with whom it must have originated, although Stern does not refer to the latter. Platner's delineations of the eight temperaments, as he conceives them, indicate that he must have mixed considerably with people. In breadth that part of his *Philosophische Aphorismen* (vol. ii, 2nd ed., 1800, pp. 480–514), is superior to Kant's sections in the *Anthropologie* covering the same ground. Kant, however, goes deeper than Platner in search of explanations. Platner's revelation of the type of pleasures which each of the eight types is apt to seek, discloses him as a man of the world as well as a philosopher.

a character at all." Between the two marks of individuality which he calls respectively *characteristic* and character, he inserts the third mark, viz., temperament, which he regards as a mode of sensibility (*Sinnesart*). In keeping with his system of Practical Reason, he predicates of the first two (characteristic and temperament) " what will necessarily become of the individual " ; of the third however—character in the strict sense of the word—he predicates " what the individual is prepared to make of himself, endowed as he is with freedom." Character is for him a mode of thought (*Denkungsart*). The temperaments he considers both as *physiological* facts, such as physical constitution and complexion of the humors, and *psychological* tendencies due to the composition of the blood. Kant, however, is at pains to declare that he is interested rather in the psychological phenomena than in the explanation which may proceed either through the humoral or the neurological channel. Adhering to the ancient nomenclature, he divides the four temperaments into those of feeling (sanguine and melancholic) and those of action (choleric and phlegmatic). Furthermore in his characteristically symmetrical scheme each temperament is subject to two conditions, viz., *tension* and *relaxation*. The sanguine temperament is characterized by rapidity and force but not by depth. On the other hand in the melancholic, the experience takes root with less speed, but lasts a longer time. Similarly the choleric temperament is that of the *hasty* person, while the phlegmatic individual is simply without the affective spur to action, though not necessarily lazy or without life.

Phlegmatic Redeemed. It would take too much space to reproduce here the masterly delineations of the four temperaments as presented by the profound philosopher in his *Anthropologie*—the most readable of Kant's works— and we shall therefore have to content ourselves with the most outstanding features of his exposition. In the first place,

he is one of the first, if not actually the first, to redeem the
nature and prospect of the phlegmatic with whom Kant
must have sympathized not a little.   In our own age we are
beginning to realize that the phlegmatic temperament, while
not socially valuable, is perhaps the most useful to society.
Secondly, though ostensibly unconcerned with the composition of the blood, he still takes his cue from two conditions
of the blood—rate of flow and temperature.   Thus the
sanguine temperament is " light-blooded ", the melancholic
—"heavy-blooded", the choleric—" warm-blooded ", and the
phlegmatic—" cold-blooded ".   In so far then as he retains
elements of the humoral doctrine, it is only in the elaboration
of the rôle of the blood in the temperamental make-up that
he may be said to be a follower of Hippocrates and Galen.

   Disputed Combinations.   Another striking view of Kant's
is his belief that while certain combinations of temperaments
will be opposed to each other (the sanguine-melancholic
and the choleric-phlegmatic), the blend of the sanguine and
choleric as well as of the melancholic and phlegmatic temperaments would result in a chemically induced neutralization.
Accordingly Kant denies the possibility of composite temperaments, e.g., sanguine-choleric, a mixture which he claims is
affected by braggarts who like to appear both gracious and
severe.   There are four and only four simple temperaments, is
Kant's emphatic pronouncement, and he who claims to be of
a mixed type is a perplexing problem to be given up as a
bad job.

   Kant displayed here just as critical judgment as in his
other scientific investigations, but he was handicapped by
the singular unity of his own character and also by the limitations of his age, when psychiatry was yet unborn, and clinical
personality studies were unknown.   The modern concept of
the unconscious not only allows for such compound natures
as are relegated to the world of fiction by the author of the
Critique, but psychoanalysts set great store by the notion of

polarity or duality which they harp on in all their themes. The most direct expression running counter to Kant's position may be found in one of Jung's recent papers where he says : " A man of outspoken sanguine temperament will tell you that taken fundamentally he is deeply melancholic ; ' a choleric ', that his only fault consists in his having always been too ' phlegmatic '. . . . We must therefore find criteria which are accepted as binding not only by the judging subject but also by the judged object," and in another place : " At every step the agreement of the subject must be obtained, and without it nothing can be undertaken or carried out." [1]

PHRENOLOGICAL VIEW OF TEMPERAMENTS

Just about this time the teachings of Gall and Spurzheim were beginning to attract attention throughout Europe. The authority which the former exercised as an anatomist rendered his phrenological doctrine especially influential as a short cut to the diagnosis of character. In conjunction with the advance of physiognomy, revived through the efforts of Lavater, the new so-called science made a move once and for all to discover the elements of character and intellect by correlating the known traits and capacities of noted as well as notorious persons with measurements of their head and palpable characteristics of the skull. Thus Gall could to his own satisfaction draw up a list of capacities and propensities, like order, combativeness, amativeness, language, etc., etc., which taken altogether, constituted the character of the individual. The promoters of phrenology thus hit two birds with one stone ; for not only did they create a new science which purported to give us the most complete localization in the brain of our abilities and disabilities, but what is more important, the science promised to make good its theoretical

---

[1] C. G. Jung : " Psychological Types ", in *Problems of Personality*, pp. 112, 114.

assumptions on the spot. It was as an applied science that phrenology so appealed to the educated man, and its influence which even now is not undermined in certain quarters, can not be over-estimated.

The phrenologists were not content to leave the original division of temperaments unchallenged ; yet while they were approaching the subject from a similar standpoint to Haller's, shifting the emphasis to the constitutional make-up of the individual, they nevertheless clung to the ancient classification of Hippocrates and Galen, with certain reservations, which are of some importance in showing that the founders of phrenology were, unlike their followers, of a thoroughly scientific cast of mind, at least so far as it is a matter of noting fundamental issues.

Spurzheim. "Those who regarded mixtures of elements and bodily constitution, as primary or secondary causes of the mental operations, employed the term temperament sometimes to indicate the bodily constitution and sometimes to designate the mental functions." Spurzheim, from whom this quotation is taken, subscribes to the view that the organic constitution of the brain may be modified by bodily processes such as digestion, circulation, etc., but does not admit that "determinate faculties" and "positive propensities" can be derived from the temperaments. Spurzheim, curious as it may seem, points out the very fact which might invalidate the principles of his science, viz., that "many with a melancholy look are not at all melancholy ; we find sanguine and bilious people, intellectual or stupid, meek or impetuous, whilst phlegmatics are often bold, quarrelsome and imperious ; in many diseases also the humors and organic constitution of the body are much altered, but the faculties of the mind do not suffer a proportionate change". Thus he dismisses the applicability of the doctrine of temperaments as an indication of determinate faculties. "We consider the study of temperaments as the first step in phrenology.

There are some individuals more irritable, more energetic, more fit to be exercised, and more able to contain their mental exercises than others; but the organic constitution of the whole body is not the condition on which the manifestations of the special feelings and intellectual faculties depend. In my work on Characters I speak of four temperaments as of four different kinds of activity." [1]

Flux vs. **Static Properties.** The difficulty so far as it presents itself to me, is that of correlating processes in flux, such as the flow of humors must presuppose, with static facts like the structure of the brain. The one is to a certain extent variable (and Spurzheim himself testifies that his temperament had changed from the lymphatic, i.e., the phlegmatic, to the nervous); the other is practically, if not absolutely, fixed. Spurzheim does not anywhere throw the obstacle in the way of his readers, but a little reflection would bring this troublesome problem to light. As already intimated, however, phrenology has adopted the ancient classification, merely changing the word " phlegmatic " to " lymphatic " and " melancholic " to " nervous ". Both of these temperaments were regarded as pathological or abnormal. But this change in nomenclature led to a further and more serious deviation. Guided by anatomical considerations, the disciples of Gall and Spurzheim looked to the constitutional make-up of the individual for the temperamental index, and thus the temperaments in phrenology began to be known as (a) the motive, based on the muscular system, (b) the vital, indicating the predominance of the alimentary system over the others, and (c) the mental temperament, drawing its strength from the nervous system.   " The first is marked by a superior development of the osseous and muscular systems, forming the locomotive apparatus; in the second, the vital organs, the principal seat of which is in the trunk, give the tone to

---

[1] G. Spurzheim: *Phrenology or the Doctrine of Mental Phenomena,* vol. i, Physiological Part.

the organization, while in the third the brain and nervous system exert the controlling power." [1]

In addition to these phrenological variants of temperament, the characters are listed separately, as appears from the chapter headings in another book of Spurzheim's,[2] in which he dwells on the following six traits : (*a*) morality, (*b*) religious fervour, (*c*) independence of action, (*d*) ambition, (*e*) mirthfulness, and (*f*) courage. The sketches which he furnishes in this book are of historical persons, and illustrated with portraits, they prove naturally what their author has set out to prove, for the obvious reason that the selection of both the traits as well as the illustrative material is purely arbitrary. It is not, however, my concern here to criticize the phrenological doctrines, but to trace the history of the humoral view of temperament.

ORGANIC AND SYSTEMIC VIEWS OF TEMPERAMENT

Probably due to the enlightenment philosophy, the medical writers in France began, toward the middle of the eighteenth century, to connect the temperaments with the functions of general physiological systems and the various degrees of irritability and motility of the organs. Here we find the noted French physician Hallé distinguishing between general temperaments and partial temperaments, and even introducing the notion of acquired temperaments. The first class, numbering three members, he linked up with the vascular, nervous and motor systems, in their relation especially to nervous influences. The two partial temperaments corresponded respectively to the various regions of the body, such as the cephalic, thoracic, abdominal; and the fluids, pituita and

---

[1] Quoted in D. H. Jacques' *The Temperaments*, p. 40. The original source is not given.

[2] G. Spurzheim: *Phrenology in Connexion with the Study of Physiognomy*, Part i : Characters.

bile. The acquired temperaments result from environmental influences on the primary temperaments.

Thomas simply divides people into cranials, thoracics, abdominals and mixed types; and Cabanis, while adhering to the older "solidistic" theory in regard to the density or porosity of the tissues, assigns greater importance to the structure and the relative development of organs like the liver, the lungs, muscles, etc. His table of six temperaments embraces : (a) the sanguine, (b) the bilious, (c) the pituitary, (d) the melancholic, (e) the nervous, and (f) the muscular.

Constitution. It was in accordance with this general trend that the following definition was framed in the *Dictionnaire de Médecine* by Littré and Robin : "Temperament is the general effect on the organism of one organ or system acting predominantly over others." Rostan, following the line of this systemic school to its logical conclusion, substituted the term "constitution" for that of temperament and derived his six kinds of constitutions from the predominance of the various systems in the economy of the organism. The alimentary tract, including the appendages and liver, presided over one constitution. A second comprised the circulatory and respiratory systems. The predominance of the brain and the nervous system was for him the basis of another constitution. The fourth involved the locomotor system, the fifth embraced the reproductive organs and lastly a certain constitution could be marked as consisting in the atony of all the systems—corresponding to the lymphatic temperament.

The phrenological point of view pervaded many of the speculative writings by physicians in the last century, just as to-day psychoanalysis, not to be compared with phrenology, is the gospel of practitioners in the field of nervous and mental diseases. We need not be surprised, therefore, if similar accounts are detected in a number of works pertaining to the subject of temperament, as most of them reveal the influence of Gall's teachings.

On the other hand we must remember that the leading phrenologists were themselves physicians, and were likely to benefit by their acquaintance with the doctrines of their fellow physicians. The constitutional or systemic bias of the French physicians of the eighteenth century was clearly responsible for the form which the phrenological doctrine of the temperaments had taken subsequent to Gall and Spurzheim. The influence seems to have been mutual, and in the last analysis is probably traceable to the progress of the anatomical and physiological sciences.

CHAPTER IV

As we go to the nineteenth century we may note how the main ideas of immediate predecessors are embodied in subsequent theories, and for this reason alone it would be important to supply the missing links in a sketch of this type so as to retain the thread of continuity intact. Just as in music, we may recognize a selection performed as belonging to a certain period, even before we can associate the melody or its elaboration with a particular composer, so each theory of temperament seems to have ingested the nucleus of previous ones before assimilating and applying new ideas that so to speak float in the air.

Dynamic Note. The subjoined passages from Herbart's *Lehrbuch zur Psychologie* (in its English translation) may serve as an illustration of how much Kant's successor at Königsberg was indebted to the famous philosopher as well as to the rise of nerve physiology. As one of the founders of modern psychology and one who has justly exercised a tremendous influence in the whole realm of the mental sciences, Herbart deserves a hearing in the brief historical examination of the temperaments; and it will be noticed that what distinguishes his conception from Kant's is largely the *dynamic* swing which is peculiar to Herbart's system. Like Kant, he sees the double aspect of the subject, the psychological and the physiological, but unlike him, he is not willing to wave the latter aside, but sets it rather down as a " pre-disposition in regard to feelings and emotions ".

" Of the four known temperaments," says Herbart, " the joyous and the sad (sanguine and melancholy) relate to the feelings ; the excitable and the slow (choleric and phlegmatic) to the excitability of the emotions. The rationale of these temperaments is generally easy to perceive ; for the common stage of feeling which the body brings with it, and which accompanies a man through his whole life, can not easily occupy exactly the middle place between the pleasant and the unpleasant ; according as it inclines toward this or that side, a man becomes sanguine or melancholy. He can not be both at the same time, but he has his place somewhere on the line which runs in the two directions. However, a fluctuating temperament is not only conceivable, but is sometimes to be met with in experience, by virtue of which a man is disposed to change from joyousness to sadness without special cause. Furthermore, as the emotions call the physical organism into play, and find in it, as it were, the sounding-board through which they are strengthened and made more lasting, there must be a degree of adaptability in this organism by virtue of which a man is either more choleric or more phlegmatic, so that he may not be both at the same time, but may fluctuate between the two.

" From this arises the possible mingling of temperaments according to the combinations of these two series. The sanguine temperament is either choleric or phlegmatic, and so, too, the melancholy may be choleric or phlegmatic. It is conceivable that one may be neither sanguine nor melancholy, for the zero-point lies just between the two. But it is inconceivable that one should be indifferent in regard to the choleric and phlegmatic temperament. Here the zero-point lies at one of the extremes. The middle is the accustomed excitability—an arithmetical mean, which is to be found by experience, almost like the average stature of the human body.

" *Note.* The names of the temperaments may also be otherwise derived ; and if the expression, choleric temperament be applied to a persistent tendency to anger, then the foregoing does not hold good. As the subject is not purely psychological, a physiological view may be in place here. Of the three systems or factors in animal life, a concealed defect in any one of them may influence the mind. If irritability (i.e., reaction against the environment) and sensibility are uninjured, and if the nutritive system suffers only in so far as to cause a constant discomfort in the general feeling, a choleric bitterness of temperament may arise. This is to be perceived in a few sad cases in children. If the irritability suffers, good-nature, and perhaps, talent may exist, but a sufficiently strong external life will be wanting. If the sensibility suffers generally, the difficulty appears to proceed from a so-called Bœotian or peasant temperament. If only the sensibility of the brain suffers relatively, or, to use a clearer expression, the ganglionic system predominates, this may be the cause of the sanguine temperament. If the nutritive system and irritability are both at the same time weak, we find the phlegmatic temperament. Thus it appears that all temperaments perceptibly prominent imply some defect." [1]

Schelling and Electricity. A different course is taken by another intellectual offspring of Kant, to wit, Schelling. Influenced by the discovery of the powers of electricity, Schelling was ready to graft on to his aesthetic transcendentalism a terminology savoring of polarities and potentials. At the same time such words as irritability and sensibility employed by Herbart in his physiological explanation of the temperaments reveal the fact that they were both imbibing from the same source, as appeared also in the case of Stahl and Hoffmann, mentioned earlier, who though opponents professionally, yet involuntarily met on common ground in their views of the temperaments.

Schelling, in contrast with Herbart, was not satisfied with psychological observations *per se*. He moved in large syntheses, subsuming everything empirical under some universal, or perhaps better, cosmic law. The temperamental differences shared the same fate. Just as nature manifests opposites and polarities as expressions of identity, and just as the real and the ideal are merged in the Absolute, so the organism contains

[1] F. Herbart : *Textbook in Psychology* (Eng. transl.), pp. 100-2.

the two polar principles of gravity and light (substance and movement) which, were it not for the predominance of the one or the other in the individual, would yield total identity, where all differences would be obliterated. The three possibilities reveal themselves through three different dimensions of the organism, viz., reproduction, irritability, referring especially to muscular and cardiac activity, and sensitivity. In normal health, the three dimensions are in equilibrium. As soon, however, as the balance is turned one way or another, temperamental anomalies and pathological conditions ensue.

Influence of Johannes Müller. Schelling's place in a psychological work may perhaps be questioned, but we must not forget that his influence reached farther than that of many full-fledged psychologists ; and text-book writers on pathology and *materia medica* of a century ago went so far as to classify ailments according to these dimensions. Even the celebrated Johannes Müller, whose epoch-making work in physiology did not omit from consideration the subject of the temperaments, discusses the forms of life under the rubrics of reproduction, irritability and sensitivity (*Sensibilität*). Temperaments, according to this author, are the forms of psychic life " conditioned by the permanent relationship of the basic functions ". These three forms are spoken of as " temperatures ", each of which may be further subdivided. The reproductive in relation to the other functions falls into (*a*) the weak-phlegmatic, and (*b*) the enduring phlegmatic types ; the irritable " temperature " into the (*a*) sanguine, and (*b*) choleric temperaments ; and the sensitive form, in accordance with the degree of development of the other " temperatures ", into (*a*) the sensitive, and (*b*) melancholic temperaments.

In more mature years, Müller was content to take a more descriptive and less explanatory point of view. He still talks of an organic basis at the root of these differences, but he is less disposed to speculate on what this basis is. Instead, he takes for his observation posts facts of mental life, viz., the strivings and emotions, in. this way reminding us of Kant's expedient. When these conations and affective States are neither strong nor lasting, the phlegmatic or " moderate " (*gemässigte*) temperament may be looked for. The choleric, the melancholic and the sanguine temperaments are the immoderate temperaments, the first being marked by energetic striving with steadiness of organic action ; the second and third by vehemence of feeling with relatively weak striving and organic action.

Henle and Nervous Tonus. The German-Jewish anatomist, Jakob Henle, co-worker of Müller, bases his theory of the temperaments on the *tonus* of the nervous system, *speed* of the reaction and its *duration*.[1] The approach is a quantitative one, and for this reason he sets the melancholic temperament on a different level as presenting qualitative characteristics. Metaphorically speaking, it seems as if the path between images and the nerves of the voluntary muscles were a rougher and less viable one. The melancholic person resembles the choleric as regards the depth of feeling but appears to be passive like the phlegmatic, though the latter is really unperturbed while the melancholic individual, not yielding to the motor expression of his emotions, suffers inwardly.

Henle sees that people are described by two sorts of words : (1) attributes like " excitable ", " quick ", " vivacious ", " quiet ", " passionate " ; (2) predicates like " cheerful ", " morose ", etc. The first series refers to the individual's stimulability (*Reizempfänglichkeit*) ; the second to his frame of mind or disposition. It is Henle's belief that the second type of qualities is dependent on the first, which for the most part,

---

[1] J. Henle : " Von den Temperamenten " in *Anthropologische Vorträge*.

is due to the tonus of the nervous system. This tonus which is not the same for all persons can be estimated according to the degree of muscular tension in a condition of rest. The degree of excitability of the sensory nerves is to be appreciated partly through the sensations of the stimulated organ, but particularly through the secondary effects of the stimulation, especially what Henle calls nerve sympathies (somewhat akin to what has been later called " complication "), and above all through psycho-motor reactions, whether initiated by ideas or emotions. *Tonus* is presumably responsible for the native keenness of the senses in some people and may be compared with the fine sensitivity of delicate scales. Bound up with this *tonus*, apparently in a causal relationship, is the degree of inertia of the nervous substance which varies with different individuals.

As to the second criterion, viz., the speed of the reaction, this author finds it natural that the *nerve current should not flow at the same rate with all.* Yet he honors Exner's finding that very phlegmatic persons do not on the average react more slowly than others

Erethism. Henle has more to say on the third criterion, viz., the duration of the excitement or, rather more strictly, the relation between the energy of the excitement and its duration. In the sanguine individual, for instance, the ratio is more or less inverse, due to the metabolism of the organic substances. The term *erethism* is suggested to designate this sort of excitability with relatively rapid exhaustion. Such exhaustion often requires a complementary contrast similar to the phenomenon of after images. Hence the inconsistencies of the sanguine temperament where promises are made and not kept, tasks undertaken but not completed. The choleric is steadier in his excitability, for even though he does blaze up only to be soon extinguished, there is something of a hangover in the form of an irritable mood, long after the first spasm of excitement has passed.

G

EMPHASIS TRANSFERRED TO PHILOSOPHY AND PSYCHOLOGY

It was about high time now for the study of temperament to be turned over again to its proper guardians after chemists, physiologists, pathologists and anatomists told their story. Their side was worth listening to, but it must be confessed that they were not conversant with all the facts of the case when they undertook their explanations which, nevertheless, were always interesting and possibly even true, at least in part. These empirical investigators, however, apparently did not realize that the subject was a science in itself, not a lounging place in which to seek diversion after a strenuous search of truth in more businesslike premises. Who but the psychologists and philosophers with psychological interests would be able to devote practically all their attention to this field encumbered with a growing literature of many conflicting views ?

Bahnsen's two-volume *Beiträge zur Charakterologie*, including temperament, is about the first inquiry into the subject on a large scale. Its merit lies rather in the treatment of details than in the systematic presentation of the main problems. Teeming with analogies and poetical quotations, it addresses itself now to the layman and now to the student of the philosophical disciplines, which at this time (1867) were making a show of hospitality to the flourishing physical and biological sciences. Had Bahnsen emancipated himself for the occasion from his metaphysical, even scholastic, method his exposition would have been far more *sachlich* and certainly more lucid. Yet with all its faults, the book deserved to have been better known, especially as some of its conclusions are strikingly sound. For our own purpose now, it is a pity that Bahnsen's work on Characterology is attached to a dialectic bearing the earmarks of both Hegel's and Schopenhauer's systems ; and in consequence of his diffuse, though literary, development of the double topic, we should have to content ourselves with only a paragraph or two on this writer who, nevertheless, gives evidence of having devoted many years of deep contemplation to this study.

Bahnsen's Elements. Proceeding from the thesis that the temperaments are founded on the various degrees of the following qualities : (*a*) spontaneity, (*b*) receptivity, (*c*) impressionability, and (*d*) reactivity, he draws up a table of sixteen temperaments, four main ones and twelve variants. Individuals may be impelled by *their own energy* or remain inert. Some again are attuned to *receive* an arising motive *quickly*. But the impression received may *sink in* and stay in the organism for a considerable, even an indefinite period, or it may be of a fleeting nature. Lastly a man of deep impressionability may react steadily or in a flighty way.

Thus we obtain sixteen combinations, of which these are only samples :

	Spontaneity	receptivity	impressionability	reactivity	temperament
1.	*strong*	*quick*	deep	lasting	*choleric* a
2.	*strong*	*quick*	shallow	lasting	choleric b
3.	*strong*	*quick*	deep	fleeting	choleric c
4.	strong	quick	*shallow*	*fleeting*	*sanguine* a
5.	weak	quick	*shallow*	*fleeting*	sanguine b
6.	strong	slow	*shallow*	*fleeting*	sanguine c
7.	strong	slow	shallow	*lasting*	phlegmatic *a*
..		..			
..		..			
10.	*weak*	quick	*deep*	lasting	*anæmic* a

The italicised words are evidently the typical instances, and the term anæmic (*anämatisch*) presumably stands for the old melancholic temperament. As Bahnsen is inclined to coin neologisms, of which tendency he apparently is aware, it would be a difficult task to follow him in his distinction between temperament and " posodynic " or the capacity for pain and pleasure, of which there are two phases, the *dyskolic* and the *eukolic*, the former to be found in those who have a dark outlook on life, the latter in those who see only the bright side. As an ardent follower of Schopenhauer, Bahnsen would be expected to make much of this capacity for pain and pleasure, which turns up as a fundamental of temperament in the work of Höffding and Meumann several decades later.

Back to Kant. Wundt follows pretty much the outline mapped out by Kant in his *Anthropologie*, but instead of making the blood central in his scheme, he discards the descriptive terms such as "light-blooded" and "warm-blooded", and guides himself solely by the type of reaction a given temperament calls forth. In this way the following table is drawn up of the same four temperaments, however:

	Strong	Weak
Quick	Choleric	sanguine
Slow	melancholic	phlegmatic

The only codicil Wundt added to Kant's formulation is possibly the observation, which in any case is implied in the latter's sketches of the four temperaments, that the quick temperaments, i.e., the sanguine and the choleric, apply themselves more readily to impressions of the present, while the slow temperaments are directed rather to the future. " Not distracted by every chance stimulus, they take more time to develop their own thought." [1]

Wundt is evidently of the opinion that all four temperaments may be made use of at different times by the same person, and throws out the wholesome, though scarcely executable advice, that every person should so order his life as to be sanguine in the minor joys and sorrows of everyday life, melancholic with regard to the more significant events, choleric in matters which claim his profound interest and phlegmatic as to the carrying out of firm resolutions.[2]

Were such a mental regimen possible, it is not safe to say that such chameleon qualities would be an asset in the long run,

---

[1] More recent treatments of this fact resort to the distinction between primary function and secondary function (Otto Gross, G. Heymans). Cf. *infra*, Chapter XIV.

[2] W. Wundt: *Grundzüge der physiologischen Psychologie*, vol. iii, p. 638 (fifth edition).

in other words, it is possible that such extremely opportune changeability would go hand in hand with or indeed call forth a serious personality defect. As a theoretical ideal the view seems rosy enough, but can individuality be so beautifully tractable and at the same time remain unitary and solid, or can it be forced only at the expense of losing its essence ?

OTHER CONTINENTAL THEORIES OF TEMPERAMENT

Let us not linger too much on the efforts of the Germans to elucidate the subject. Other countries, particularly France, have produced equal theorists, and the last decade of the nineteenth century was especially fruitful of attempts. Höffding in Denmark ties up his classification with the fundamental conditions for the preservation of the individual organism—pleasure and pain—and speaks therefore of cheerful and sombre temperaments, each qualified by two pairs of correlatives, viz., strong and weak, and slow and quick, which, through the regular series of combinations, would yield eight kinds of temperaments. The physiological mechanism of these two main types of temperaments—the cheerful and the sombre—is the influence of the vegetative functions on the brain.[1]

Chemical Basis. Pilo, in 1892, looks for the basic differences of man in the chemical composition of the blood and in its thermicity, from which assumption he draws four general temperament-characters, the *plethoric*, the *serous*, the *bilious* and the *lymphatic* with four classes consisting of exaggerations of the former and four attenuated types.[2]

---

[1] H. Höffding : *Psykologi* (omrids), pp. 395–6. The reference is to the Danish third edition (1892) as the English translation, though reprinted six times, is of the first German edition, in which Höffding, not yet oriented, was merely suggesting the addition of the bright and murky temperaments to the well-known four.

[2] M. Pilo : *Nuovi Studi sul Carattere*, cited in the French literature.

Physical Foundation. The most striking theory of this period, however, was advanced by the Russian anthropologist Nicolas Seeland who substituted a *physical* theory for the various anatomical, physiological and chemical explanations. Instead of giving equal weight to each of the temperaments, he conceives a sort of hierarchy.

In the first place there are the strong or positive temperaments, comprising the gay and the phlegmatic. The former again is subdivided into (*a*) the very sanguine, marked by the predominance of the vegetative life and rapid but appropriate reactions (*b*) the sanguine of a lesser order, containing an admixture of the nervous and (*c*) the serene. The phlegmatic temperament never exhibits more than a moderate intensity and displays a remarkable uniformity.

The second main division is the neutral and includes the majority of people. Since there is nothing outstanding in them, science has taken little account of this type.

Finally, the weak or negative temperaments are, whether their type of reaction be quick or slow, characterized by irregularity. Under this rubric appear the melancholic, the nervous with symptoms of alternating activity and depression, and the choleric whose chief mark is high irritability. This last-named temperament is a species of the nervous, and at times may be combined with the sanguine or with the melan- cholic, but is excluded from the serene and the phlegmatic classes.

Temperament Determined by Molecular Vibrations. But the novelty of Seeland's theory is to be seen not so much in the classification as in the physical explanation of the temperamental differences. It is Seeland's belief that what causes a certain temperamental make-up is the kind of molecular vibration in the nervous system, or rather the cerebral substance, while receiving external and internal stimulations. Rapid and harmonious molecular vibrations produce the gay temperament. Less rapid but invariably constant vibrations are to be linked with the phlegmatic temperament. The neutral is due to still less rapid yet constant vibrations, while the negative types are to be traced to either slow and discordant or quick but interrupted vibrations.[1]

Anthropological data. Not the least part of Seeland's paper is the discussion of the anthropological measurements to which he had subjected a number of people with whom he was well acquainted. These anthropometric data should be compared with the much later work of the Italian school of clinical morphology (*q.v. infra*) and particularly the recent observations of Kretschmer on character and physique (mentioned later).

Seeland had worked with different groups of subjects, and the statistical results, even if the number of cases in the various groups is not adequate, would tend to show that there is a drop, with slight fluctuations, in respect of nearly all the measurements, from the gay group to the melancholic. The former excels in visual and auditory acuity, circumference of the neck, and especially in muscular force, where the divergence between the sanguine and the depressed is unmistakably wide. But more important still is the result that the formation of the head is irregular among the melancholic, less so among the neutral group, while the gay and to a less extent the phlegmatic show the greatest regularity (cf. the hypoplastic type of Kretschmer).

It is evident that Seeland takes a view of temperament which favors the gay or sanguine individual, and incidentally in this class he places, to our surprise, the Great-Russian (though he tells us in a footnote on page 101 that only the

[1] N. Seeland : " Le tempérament au point de vue psychologique et anthropologique," *Congrès International d'archéol. et d'anthrop. préhist.* Moscow, 1893.

Ribot has inaccurately given the place and date of this publication as St. Petersburg, 1892, and this slip has been perpetuated by the French writers on character and temperament who mention Seeland's work.

rural population counts for this estimation, as the urban
inhabitants, the members of civilized society, have had their
nerves already fairly spoilt). The Little Russians, or as they
are now called, the Ukrainians, he classes among the
phlegmatic, together with the Dutch, English, Norwegians,
and Finns.

Not an environmentalist. Lest this author's standpoint
lend itself to misunderstanding, it ought to be stated that
although he provides a physical basis for the difference in
temperaments, viz., the rapidity and constancy of the
molecular vibrations in the nervous substance of the brain,
he does not believe, in accordance with the evidence of his
dietetic experiments, that there is a noticeable change in
temperament due to metabolic changes in consequence of
different kinds of nutrition, except in the case of the choleric
who is stimulated to irritability on taking alcoholic beverages
or drugs. The physical basis of temperament is not of an
environmental or assimilative nature, but is already more
or less fixed in the nervous dispositions.

BRITISH NOT INTERESTED IN TEMPERAMENT STUDIES

British writers made no systematic effort to study the
temperaments. In fact Alexander Stewart, who wrote his
popular presentation in 1887, claims that he found no books
in English on temperament in any of the Cambridge University
libraries. Finally he was able to trace the whereabouts of a
collection of sermons on the temperaments, a second edition
of which appeared in 1874, and he was able to obtain a copy
of this book from the author, William Clark.[1]

On the whole, it is true that the British took little pains to
develop this subject. Occasionally a physician would lecture
on temperament and publish his address. A few pamphlets
and one or two books were thus brought out in England

---

[1] A Stewart : *Our Temperaments*, p. 5.

and the United States, which evidently were not listed in the library consulted by Stewart, who, however, now made it his business to cite almost every passage in the contemporary literature, including newspapers, which referred to temperament. His work, therefore, bears the character of a concordance; and where he does not indulge in quotations, the phrenological flavor is quite perceptible.

In Great Britain the subject was always under the sway of medical men, and these, like Hutchinson, were either too cautious to commit themselves, except to say that if we knew more about temperament the diagnosis of disease would be facilitated, or else, like Stewart himself, were prepared to march under the banner of phrenology and spin out, by the aid of material contained in French medical treatises, relationships between physical and mental characteristics much after the fashion of present-day character analysis.

Temperament from a Religious Angle. Since Stewart's book, the British have been content to keep the study of temperament in the background and nothing of an extensive order can be reported on until the comparatively recent volume by Stevenson,[1] which is a popular study of the temperaments as seen through a religious bias. The work is by no means a scientific essay, but it is wholesome, displays good common sense, and is charged with what the newspapers would call "human interest", belonging to that class of literature of which Smiles's books are shining examples. Here we find an abundance of illustrations from biography, mainly of religious-minded people, for each of the traditional four temperaments, but to these Stevenson has added two more temperaments, the artistic and the practical, which are probably cross divisions of the stereotyped quartet.

The missionary spirit of the book is fairly evident, and the last chapter on the temperament of Jesus is merely a

---

[1] J. G. Stevenson: *Religion and Temperament*, 1913.

mystic interpretation of the dreamer of Nazareth who was supposed to have been the embodiment of all the six temperaments. Indeed, in order to sanction the cultivation of mirth and the sense of humor, the author must find humor in Jesus; for was He not " more than once found at weddings and feasts where laughter and jest and song were part of the order of the happy hours " ? [1] And furthermore argues the advocate of fun, " If Jesus had no sense of humor, how could He so patiently have borne with Peter, who repeatedly must have been either amusing or intolerable ? "

This inconsequental reasoning, however, does not detract from the value of the illustrations. The point ought to be made that when an author has an " axe to grind ", and one which is not commonly employed, as in this case, his illustrations will be even more useful than when the exposition is not emotionally colored. We may discount his conclusions, take them *cum grano salis*. Yet the instances selected are apt to make us see another side, or only a nook perhaps, which otherwise would have remained concealed. We may readily make allowance for such implications as that the phlegmatic have no sense of humor (because Herbert Spencer lacked it) or that the British are regarded as a sanguine people, but we cannot afford to overlook the dominant note in the book, viz., that character can triumph over temperament ; and whatever the spirit which prompted the development of this theme, it is for us to take its claim under advisement.

FRENCH ATTEMPTS

Before continuing the German trend which began to take definite shape in the hands of Kant, we shall pause a while to mention the work of the French psychologists, who, however, concerned themselves mainly with what they considered to be the study of character ; that is to say, their territory was ostensibly character, but they traversed it in such a way

[1] Op. cit., pp. 293 ff.

as to suggest the influence of the humoral approach. Owing to this cross bias the subject-matter of the French investigators is not clearly demarcated ; and consequently it would seem best to defer the French main contribution to this field until we come to the discussion of character classifications. To confine ourselves only to representative writers on temperament in France, we should have to reckon with the views of Fouillée, and in a less degree with those of Manouvrier and Ribéry, one of Ribot's disciples.

Bio-physiological Theory. Fouillée invokes a biological principle to explain differences in temperament. Redintegration and disintegration he observes is the vital rhythm in nature. Integration takes a centripetal direction, while disintegration is centrifugal. With the former he connects the idea of concentration, with the latter the idea of expansion. The one is a female element, the other a masculine principle. Upon this he builds his two-fold division of temperaments into the saving temperaments and the spending temperaments, the one being sensory, the other motor. If the general direction of the temperament is that of redintegration, i.e., the sensory type, the reaction will be along the lines where no sustained effort is demanded. Reaction will take the form of expression, words, gestures, facial movements—in a word the reaction will be emotional. In the active or motor type on the other hand, the organism will seek an outlet in muscular work.

What happens is this : the very rapid repair which takes place in the sensory nerves prevents the motor tendency from being propagated adequately to the motor fibres and the agitated nerve cells quickly resume their equilibrium as a result of the prompt restoration of the *status quo*. Naturally whatever emotions are brought into play by the shock would not last in consequence of the rapidity of the changes. Hence the slight intensity which goes with this sort of temperament, in this case the sanguine. The necessary attributes of such rapidity and mobility are superficiality and slightness. On the other hand, a disintegrative temperament, whether the process, and hence the reaction, be rapid and intense (choleric) or slow and weak (phlegmatic), is out of gear with the inhibitive mechanism in the brain, which depends on the molecular reparation of the nerve cells in order to function properly.[1] Of course it is evident that the problem Hering had to cope with in his theory of vision, viz., how any excitation can ever be anabolic, must arise here with regard to Fouillée's correspondence between feeling and redintegration.

Fouillée expands his two divisions into four, in order to satisfy the ancient classification, by dividing each class into two groups, hence we obtain four types : (a) the sensory reacting quickly and corresponding to the sanguine temperament ; (b) the sensory with intense reaction or the nervous ; (c) the active with a quick and intense reaction, i.e., choleric ; (d) the active with a slow and weak reaction, to wit, the phlegmatic.

Potential Energy. Manouvrier's theory [2] is not far different from the above, except that it appeals to the concept of potential energy for the key to the situation. Starting from the point that anatomical variations should be the determinants of temperament, he realizes that these are too complex for consideration, and therefore proceeds to examine whether there may not be something in the physiological make-up of man that one could bring to light in this connection. The individual mark he finally finds in the amount of *potential energy* possessed by different individuals. In other words, the general metabolism of the organism realizes a potential which may be theoretically raised or

---

[1] A. Fouillée : *Tempérament et Caractère.*

[2] Manouvrier : " Le Tempérament," *Revue Mensuelle de L'Ecole d'Anthropologie de Paris*, 1896. " Caractérisation physiologique des tempéraments et homologation, des tempéraments classiques," ibid., 1898, cited in P. Malapert's *Le Caractère*, pp. 150 ff.

lowered, although we may well assume that each organism originally possesses a disposition for a certain potential, which possibly is a product of the nutritive functions.

Three clearly demarcated stages of variations in potential are next distinguished, the sthenic or superior, the mesosthenic or average and the hyposthenic or inferior. Each of these may be viewed under the catabolic and the anabolic aspect, the former involving a disintegrative process, the latter an integrative process. In addition, these temperaments may be subdivided under each of these two phases according as the processes are slow or rapid, though these are by no means fixed or definable. The asthenic and hypersthenic temperaments are found only in pathological or otherwise very exceptional cases, such as the record breakers in the various sports. The sthenic class is made up of the leaders of thought and politics, while the lazy shiftless individuals are recruited from the asthenic class.

Instance of French Formalism. Ribéry gives scope for more combinations. His division runs like this : (1) amorphous; (2) sensitive, comprising the sanguine and the nervous ; (3) the sensitive-active, made up of (*a*) the sanguine-choleric and (*b*) the nervous-choleric ; (4) the active, composed of the choleric and the phlegmatic, and lastly the balanced temperament. Ribéry's classification will come up again under the French Schools of Character.

CHAPTER V

Psychiatric Observations on the Temperaments. As might have been expected, the mental and nervous disorders could not be studied without offering some suggestions in regard to the temperaments. The contact, however, did not become definitely established until Kraepelin's comprehensive systematization of the prime disorders. Since the beginning of the twentieth century, when the psychological conception of insanity became ingrained in the fundamentals of psychiatry, a number of monographs appeared dealing with various phases of the adjacent territories, which naturally were to culminate in the joint scrutiny of personality on the part of psychology and psychiatry. Some of these investigators like Hirt and Hoffmann singled out the temperaments for special study, while others like Koch, Kollarits, Kronfeld, and Kretschmer (the opposition here between the H's and the K's is quite fortuitous) put all the weight on the concept of character, and for this reason we shall reserve their treatment for their proper rubric.

Institutional Approach. Many of the older monographs, coming for the most part from the pen of institutional directors, are popular in character and not marked by scholarship. One of these writers, for instance, in order to confirm his standpoint by an apparent reference to Hume, says : " An old English philosopher, if I am not mistaken, said that man is nothing but a bundle of feelings." The psychological literature on which they draw is of a restricted scope, and their citations betray a mere *dilettante* acquaintance with the more theoretical problems. For all that, the observations by these practitioners are truly valuable because of their contact with the many types of people who make up the world ; and their descriptions of the outstanding milder psychopathic cases may be read with profit by the psychologist who is interested in any phase of personality.

Representative of this order of writing is Hirt's *Die Temperamente*, etc., in which he regards the determinants of temperament as variations of the speed, quantity and energy of certain psychophysiological processes, largely the feelings. But even the reflex reaction, according to this author, exhibits traces of temperament. At least he knows of a " lively (nervous) and a phlegmatic course of reflexes ".[1] The reflex arc, he thinks, displays differences in tempo and energy due probably to the metabolism of the organism, especially of the nervous system, rather than to the influence of anatomical relations.

A Detailed Description of Types. On the strength of his professional experience, he divides the temperaments as follows : First there is the *average* type belonging to the man in the street, who in his mediocrity jogs along day in day out, discharging his duties mechanically and never bothering to undertake anything out of the usual. A step lower down the scale is the *phlegmatic*, cold and indifferent even in regard to his own prospects, and in the accentuated form approaching the well-known *morbid apathy* so commonly seen in hospitals. A composite of the phlegmatic and the melancholic often appears in which a gloomy mood is superimposed upon the indifference, but aside from this class, the phlegmatic-*blasé* type, with a disposition to *dementia praecox* must be mentioned. Persons of this sort are not only inert but lack insight. They either refuse to answer questions or give irrelevant replies, and are even too lazy to complain of their plight.

---

[1] E. Hirt : " Die Temperamente, ihr Wesen, ihre Bedeutung für das Seelische Erleben und Ihre Besondere Gestaltungen," in *Grenzfr. des Nerven = und = Seelenlebens*, 1905, no. 40, p. 62.

The sanguine type bears something in common with other temperaments which will be presently described, but in itself it scarcely needs an introduction, as its marks of excitability, enthusiasm and unreliability are common knowledge. " With all these peculiarities of his psychic life " asserts Hirt, " the sanguine man has acquired something immature, something of the *Backfisch*." His constant adolescence is due to the lability of his movements, his suggestibility and shift of attention. What may be considered as sub-classes of this temperament are the nervous and the hysterical temperaments. The animation and euphoria of the nervous temperaments are readily noticeable at a very early age. The hysterical person is afflicted with lack of control. He will build castles in the air and cannot realize the impossibility of his plans. Vanity, a craving for applause, and a craze for enjoyment are the mainsprings of his actions.

The choleric type is subdivided into (a) the suspicious, who are forever detecting treachery, envy, avarice and ill-will, and (b) the grumblers, who are continually criticizing the work of others in the belief that they could do better if only given the opportunity. The choleric individual is close to the manic-depressive patient.

Among the melancholic people, Hirt points out those who, while filled with pessimism and embitterment, are yet endowed with strength of will and sometimes break out with unwonted vehemence, resembling in this instance the choleric with whom they are at times confused. These are the persons who show a manic disposition, in contradistinction to those who are depressed, slow in their resolutions, never certain about the outcome, always embarrassed with scruples, and ever on the lookout for difficulties and obstacles of their own making. The manic type constitutes the men of action ; the depressive type represents the speculative individuals, the dreamers and brooders.

Hirt furthermore distinguishes other temperaments—the

man of moods and the emotional person (*Gefühlsmensch*), the difference being largely one of duration. The moody individual does not change so rapidly as the emotional person, and, moreover, is not affected by external reactions to the same degree as by his own lingering mental states.

RECENT GERMAN STUDIES

One of the most thorough attempts to deal with temperament is that of Meumann. Meumann's treatment is complex yet not diffuse. Building on his voluntaristic framework, he finds room for the temperaments in the affective forms of the will, which in turn are grounded in the innate affective dispositions of man. Temperaments he defines as affective forms of action which depend on the co-operation of innate affective and volitional dispositions. But how can we get at these affective dispositions ? Meumann answers the question by directing us to the fundamental qualities of the feelings, which suggests the following approaches : (1) As regards quality, they are either pleasant or unpleasant. (2) They may be graded according to intensity, strength or vividness. (3) Their duration may be of different degrees. (4) They may be called forth by stimuli in various degrees of ease or difficulty. (5) They may reverberate in consciousness in different ways, or produce a lasting effect. (6) They may have various kinds of genesis, being produced more readily by external or internal stimuli or being conditioned more by the content of thought than by its form or *vice versa*. (7) They may fuse with other contents of consciousness, forming in some cases an organic complex. Sometimes they may be transferred by means of association to certain objects. Meumann would have in mind here the conditioned reflex. (8) Our feelings may be *objectified* as in speaking of a cheerful day or a pleasant neighbourhood, or *subjectified* when we recognize them only as " affections " of ourselves.

Affective Expression in Temperament. The numerous

H

combinations resulting from such a list of qualities would be sufficient to discourage us from the task of tabulating all the possible classes, but Meumann adds another important consideration, viz., the mode of expression of our feelings in all its detail. These expressive tendencies affect the central nervous system, the motor apparatus, and the vaso-motor mechanisms differently for pleasantness and unpleasantness. For the most part, pleasantness increases activity and irradiates (active), while unpleasantness diminishes the activity of the organism and is restrictive (passive), but different people will display different reactions. In anger one might turn red while another will pale. Hence an adequate table of temperamental forms would be no more than an ideal.

A simplified scheme of the affective dispositions could at least give one an idea of the method in general, and the appended combined and modified table may be of some orientative aid.

TABLE OF AFFECTIVE DISPOSITIONS (TEMPERAMENTS) ACCORDING TO MEUMANN

Quality of feeling	Ease or difficulty of excitability		Intensity and persistence		Active excitative or passive (depressive character of the feelings as increasing or decreasing:				
pleasure	easy *phleg.*	difficult *sanguine*	slight *sang.*	great *phleg.*	active *sang.*	1. muscle tonus & motor activity. 2. vaso-motor activity 3. (central) nervous activity	passive *phleg.*	1. 2. 3.	as in act
displeasure	easy *choler.*	difficult *melan.*	slight ?	great *melanch. choler.*	active *choler.*	1. 2. 3. as above.	passive *melan.*	1. 2. 3.	as above.

In his fundamental qualities, pleasure and displeasure, Meumann's position is aligned with that of Höffding, but Meumann is clearer and more to the point in his deduction. He opposes the sanguine and the phlegmatic to the choleric and the melancholic on the basis of feeling-tone; the shallow to the deep natures on the basis of persistence alone. Both may react promptly or with difficulty, both may be pleasantly or unpleasantly attuned, yet the reaction in the one is fleeting;

in the other it is lasting. Hence we may have frivolous as well as morose, and joyous as well as speculative or brooding temperaments. As regards the active-passive avenue, we may have, on the pleasant side, the energetic worker full of vitality or the mere enjoyer without the brimming energy, while on the unpleasant side there are both the active men whose work is carried on amidst permanent sadness (of whom Michelangelo is an example) and the depressed individuals wallowing in pessimism and never sufficiently active to accomplish anything.

A Neo-Kantian Scheme. In his solid little book *Charakterbildung* published in the same year as the preceding account of Meumann, Elsenhans rounds out Kant's scheme far more neatly than Wundt. Conformably with the prevailing German view, he looks upon temperament as the formal or attributive aspect of character. Character in itself is marked by a content. Differing somewhat with Kant, Elsenhans restricts temperament to the feelings entirely, claiming that Kant's temperaments of action, in the last analysis, go back to a type of affective constitution which determines the activity associated with the volitional life. His table of temperaments which follows is, if not altogether acceptable, at least clear and consistent.

TABLE OF TEMPERAMENTS ACCORDING TO ELSENHANS

| Temperament | Excitability of affective life | Form of the affective course | | Motivation force of the feelings |
		Mobility	Strength	
Sanguine	light	alternating	weak	*Slight* the man of moods *Considerable* the fickle person
Melancholic	deep	persistent	strong	*Slight* the visionary hypochondriac *Considerable* the idealist of action
Choleric	light	alternating	strong	*Considerable* the vehement man of will *Slight* the excited man of feeling
Phlegmatic	deep	persistent	weak	*Considerable* the cold-blooded, tough minded *Slight* the indifferent, apathetic

From this table we may see that Elsenhans has coupled the degree of motility and the strength of the feelings with the ease of the transition from a given stimulus to a feeling, and thence to a will impulse (motivation force).

TEMPERAMENT AS DRAINAGE OF ENERGY

In a piquant book [1] exhibiting the mental agility of its Viennese author, we meet with an unexpected simple solution of the problem. The key is to be found in the *mode of drainage* of the individual's psychic energy, which corresponds to the libido of psychoanalysis. The most natural way in which this energy is worked off is that which is also the most favourable and economical for the individual, viz., through the channel of pleasure. Here we have the basis of the sanguine temperament.

It is, however, not given to everybody to let his affective life take this direct course. There may be scruples against it. The libido will then seek other ways of relief ; and two alternatives are possible. Either the pent up energy will express itself in a melancholy indisposition, or else it will take the form of an expansive excitement. In the former we recognize the melancholic temperament ; in the latter we note the choleric. All three represent the hyperemotional type, the individual with a rich affective life. But so far the phlegmatic person has not been mentioned, and he too must be accommodated in the scheme, which is not difficult on the supposition that phlegmatic people possess only a small supply of psychic energy and thus constitute the class of hyperemotional individuals. The further information is ventured by the same author that a sadistic disposition is favorable for the development of the sanguine and the choleric temperaments, while the melancholic temperament usually runs in those of the masochistic disposition. Since the distinction between these

[1] H. Apfelbach : *Der Aufbau des Charakters*, 1924.

dispositions will be reverted to in a later chapter as forming the central idea of Apfelbach's classification of characters, no more need be said about it just at present.

A SOCIOLOGICAL COLORING

In Jastrow's *Character and Temperament*, we may note the influence of the modern sociological development. Temperament is here brought into relation with all the factors of an over-civilized world. On account of the *causerie* style of the book, it is difficult to pick out the core of the chapter on temperament. But from all appearances it would seem that the author is influenced in his classification of the temperaments by the French school, more particularly by Ribot, as may be seen from the following divisions :—

(1) *Sensitive*-ACTIVE, corresponding to the sanguine type.

(2) SENSITIVE-*active*, representing the melancholic temperament.

(3) SENSITIVE-ACTIVE, answering to the choleric temperament.

(4) *Sensitive-active*, generally spoken of as the phlegmatic.[1]

The above scheme seems a bit oversimplified in comparison with the many views which have taken into consideration not merely one attribute, like strength or intensity, which is clearly indicated in Jastrow's classification, but several, like depth, duration, rapidity, etc. Certainly one might justly transpose (1) and (3) and argue that the choleric has a greater urge to expression than the sanguine. Our uncertainty is to be imputed to the lack of discursive exposition in Jastrow's book.

CLINICAL MORPHOLOGY AND TEMPERAMENT

One of the latest outgrowths of the *rapprochement* between anatomy, anthropology, and psychiatry is the experimental move to correlate temperament with bodily proportions. The

[1] J. Jastrow : *Character and Temperament*, pp. 255–6.

school seems to have originated in Italy with De–Giovanni about 1890,[1] whence it branched out afterwards with an endocrinological accretion. More recently, Ernst Kretschmer in Germany has come to somewhat similar conclusions on the strength of his own clinical experiences; and in spite of his disinclination to employ the word "temperament", which to him does not connote a sufficiently definite fact, Kretschmer speaks of the two main temperaments as the cyclothymic, producing the manic depressive type, and the schizothymic or split-up personalities (*dementia praecox*).[2] Since Kretschmer's contribution will be taken up under the head of character, we shall in this section try to catch a glimpse of the Italian work in this field, represented in the United States by Naccarati who appears to be a disciple of Viola, Ravà, and Pende, synthesizing the evidence from the ductless glands and the results from bodily measurements.

De-Giovanni had formulated a "law of deformation" to the effect that "Individuals having a small trunk tend to assume a longilinear body which corresponds to the phthisic habitus; individuals having a large trunk tend to assume a short body which corresponds to the apoplectic habitus; individuals having a normal trunk tend to maintain normal proportions of the body." [3]

Bodily Proportions. Taking up the thread of De-Giovanni's investigations, Viola has in a series of works developed a tritypal classification of forms, viz., (1) the *microsplanchnic*, where the vertical diameters are overdeveloped in comparison with the horizontal diameters, so that the body presents an elongated appearance, (2) the *macrosplanchnic*, showing a predominance of the trunk over the extremities, and giving the impression of stoutness, and (c) the *normo-*

---

[1] A. De-Giovanni : *Morfologia del Corpo Umano.*
[2] E. Kretschmer : *Körperbau und Charakter.*
[3] S. Naccarati : "The Morphologic Aspect of Intelligence," in *Archives of Psychology,* 1921, vol. vi, p. 3.

splanchnic, with a constant proportionateness between the vertical and the horizontal diameters of the body.

That there is a harking back in part to the constitutional and systemic views of the French medical men of the last century may be seen from this quotation which I take again from Naccarati's monograph. " The trunk, as Viola observes, contains the organs of the vegetative life which represent the nutritional system. These organs fulfil a task different from the muscular and nervous systems and skeleton, which constitute the animal system or a system that mediates contact with the external world. These two systems show a certain degree of independence and even antagonism during the development in the sense that they do not grow simultaneously but in alternate phases ; and the more an organism develops the animal system, the less it develops the vegetative system, when considered in relation of their reciprocal dependence." Apparently this reference to the antagonism between the two systems is a corollary from Pende, who, we are told in another article by Naccarati, " has made a further distinction of hormones promoting the development of the animal system (constituted by organs and apparatus which mediate contact with the external world) and hormones which promote the growth of the vegetative system," and later he traces Pende's division back to Viola (and even farther back to Bichat) who saw an antagonism between the animal and the visceral systems with an alternate predominance of the one over the other.[1]

Clinical Observations. From yet another article by the same writer, one more passage is culled presenting some recent findings by the Italian morphological school. " Ravà in a recent study has found that neurasthenics and psychasthenics are mostly found among the microsplanchnics and that manic-depressives are mostly macrosplanchnic types.

[1] S. Naccarati : " Hormones and Intelligence," *Journ. of Applied Psychol.*, 1922, vol. vi, p. 223.

Ravà thinks that emotional and instinctive individuals are opposite types and considers the neurasthenics as emotional, the manic-depressives as instinctive. Therefore, for this author, microsplanchnics are mostly emotional types while the macrosplanchnics are instinctive types." [1]

In another study, the same author has examined 100 patients with a view to their morphological index which he obtained by dividing the length of one arm plus the length of one leg by the volume of the trunk. He found that the extreme types (micro-and-macrosplanchnic) yielded a larger number of psychoneurotics than the normosplanchnic, also that the asthenic patients more frequently came from the micro-splanchnic and the emotional psychoneurotics from the macrosplanchnic class. [2]

Applying the same measuring methods to 54 students who were given several of the better known emotional tests and questionnaires (Woodworth Personal Data Sheet) supplemented by a rating scheme consisting of the composite of a self-estimate by each individual, and a double rating (one at the beginning and another at the close of the session) by the instructor in psychology, Naccarati and Garrett tentatively drew the conclusion from the results that " temperamental disturbances of an emotional nature are found in those of low morphological index (relatively large trunk and short extremities) more often than in those of high morphological index (relatively small trunk and long extremities)." [3]

CONSTITUTIONAL MORPHOLOGY

The French School. While the Italians, under the leadership of De-Giovanni, were making notable contributions to that

[1] S. Naccarati and H. E. Garrett : " The Influence of Constitutional Factors on Behavior," *Journ. of Exper. Psychol.*, 1923, vol. vi, p. 457.

[2] S. Naccarati : " The Morphologic Basis of the Psychoneuroses," *Amer. Journ. of Psychiatry*, 1924, vol. iii.

[3] S. Naccarati and H. E. Garrett : " The Relation of Morphology to Temperament," *Journ. of Abnormal and Social Psychol.*, 1924, vol. xix, p. 263.

branch of science which has received the name of human morphology, a group of French physicians with Sigaud as the central figure penetrated into the subject through a somewhat different path. Indeed, Sigaud, in apparent ignorance of the work of De-Giovanni, claims to have laid the foundations of this " *science nouvelle, La Morphologie humaine* ", through a series of researches begun in the nineties of last century.

In emphasizing the predominance of some one physiological system in the development of the organism as a basis of classification of types, Sigaud of course made no departure from his predecessors in France who had even adopted the term " constitution " to replace the word " temperament ", but he was more systematic in his observations, and fostered the experimental method among his pupils, so that it was possible to quantify the data instead of merely hazarding conjectures.

Sigaud's starting point was the methodical exploration of the abdomen, the results of which form the backbone of his classical work *Traité clinique de la Digestion*, etc. (1900 and 1908). Like the contemporary *Gestalt* psychologist who holds that the total configuration must be studied in the light of both the figure and the background, Sigaud taught that the human organism and its pathology are functions of both the milieu and the original disposition. The surgical and experimental methods, he complains in opposition to the medical spirit, deal with the part and not with the whole organism (ensemble) and " analyze the reactions evoked by an accidental or artificial determination ".[1]

Interplay of Environment and Organic System. To each of these systems, there corresponds a milieu which plays on the organism and which affects the system directly connected with it. There is the atmospheric environment, the source of respiratory reactions, the alimentary system

[1] C. Sigaud and L. Vincent, *Les Origines de la Maladie*, 2nd ed., 1912, p. 44.

giving rise to the digestive reactions, the physical environment in which the muscular reactions are grounded, and the social milieu eliciting the cerebral reactions.

In consequence of this correspondence, the French pathologist sets up his four types of man, viz., the respiratory, the digestive, the muscular, and the cerebral, a classification which is redolent of Kretschmer's fourfold division (see Chapter XV). Each of these types demands special activities along its predominant characteristic. Practically every individual, because of the marked development of a particular system necessitating the underdevelopment of another system, is morphologically asymmetrical and will react to environmental variations in a different way than would another individual. Adaptation does not proceed in the one case as it does in another, and lack of adaptation brings in its wake a cellular disturbance, especially as cellular irritability—and this is a proposition by which Sigaud's school sets great store—diminishes from birth till death.

Variation of Form Due to Adjustment of Organism. "Varieties and variability of form are in the last analysis but morphological imprints engraved as a result of the efforts of the organism to adapt itself to the environment"[1] is the rather significant inference drawn by Sigaud, whose ideas are often in accord with the findings of contemporaries in other countries with whose researches he seems to have been unfamiliar.

It is not necessary to dwell on the physical marks of Sigaud's four types. They are almost self-evident from their names. Besides, his pupils, Tricolet, Chaillou, and Mac-Auliffe have treated this phase in greater detail, the former in a dissertation at Lyon (*La Différenciation des quatre types morphologiques individuels, correspondant aux quatre variétés de l'ambiance cosmique*, 1909) and the two latter in a work called *Morphologie Médicale : Étude des quartre types humains* (1912). The data

[1] Loc. cit., p. 74.

here are discussed minutely and in such a way as to link the Bertillon measurement scheme with the whole morphological problem.

Physical Marks of Four Types. For each type, the face is divided into several parts. In the respiratory man, for instance, whose thorax and neck are larger than in other types, the part of the face which is especially developed seems to be that between the bridge and the tip of the nose. In the *typus digestivus*, on the other hand, the lower part of the face, particularly the jaw, is most prominent ; the eyes are small and supplied with fleshy eyelids, the neck is short, the thorax also short but wide, while the abdomen is very capacious.

The face of the muscular man is well formed, lending a somewhat square aspect to the countenance ; the eyebrows are deep and not arched, the hair grows down on the forehead almost to a straight line, the organs are fairly proportioned, and the bodily musculature is highly developed. Finally the cerebral type is marked by a frontal prominence which is usually divided by a tuft of hair in the centre. The eyes are bright and the ears large, the arms and especially the legs are small.

True to their countrymen's tradition of exploiting combinations, Chaillou and Mac-Auliffe allow for a number of fusional forms (cerebro-muscular, musculo-digestive, etc.).

A Tinge of Historical Materialism. In *La Vie Humaine* (1923), which is appearing in a series of monographs, Mac-Auliffe has gone into elaborate measurements of individuals at different stages in life to show how differently the four constitutional types develop under the influence of both heredity and environment. Heredity is represented as the theme to which are added later the variations, supplied by the milieu.[1] In fact the environment is supposed to have been instrumental in differentiating the types in the first place.

[1] L. Mac-Auliffe, " Devéloppement, Croissance " : *La Vie Humaine* (Études Morphologiques), 1923, p. 27.

In luxuriant country, the digestive type is prevalent. The respiratory man thrives in mountain regions or in arid lands. The muscular system becomes highly developed in places where great physical exertion is required, while the " cerebral " is a product of city life. As the third and fourth monographs of *La Vie Humaine* deal with personality, we may infer that the four constitutional types have been made the basis of differentiation in personality.

Colloidal Properties at the Root of Type Differences. In his third monograph on *Human Life* [1] Mac-Auliffe deviates from the track beaten out by Sigaud and starts anew on a purely physico-chemical groundwork. He now aligns himself with the bio-chemists and appears to centre his discussion of personality about the various colloidal states of the human organism. Human beings are to him " walking lumps of jelly " with all the semi-liquid and coagulating properties of gelatine. Their aggregates of molecules are in constant oscillation between compression and dispersion—solidification and liquefaction, either of which states, if actually reached, would mean death.

Now among the chief properties which differentiate human beings is the greater or less craving of the tissues for water. Some individuals are composed of colloidal cells which are extremely hydrophilic. Their tissues are easily filled with liquid and tend to stay in that condition. Their flesh offers a resistance to the hand like a rubber-ball filled with water. This class of people constitutes the " round " type. In these people, there is great surface tension and osmotic pressure, and a considerable expenditure of energy with a corresponding dynamic sweep.

The " flat " type on the other hand is determined by the slight craving of the tissues for water. The cells, not having

[1] L. Mac-Auliffe, " Les mécanismes intimes de la vie—Introduction a l'étude de la personnalité," 3rd Monog. of *La Vie Humaine* (Études Morphologiques), 1925.

imbibed much, do not swell, and because of this fact, there is little surface tension. The flesh is flabby or elastic, the figure slight and elongated, the lines angular and the movements somewhat awkward. Since the solubility of a gas in a liquid is in the inverse ratio of its surface tension, we can deduce the principle that in the " flat " individuals the metabolic processes will take place rapidly, the general reactions will be quicker, and the cellular irritability more marked than in the " round " type ; yet the chemical processes are to a degree retarded, which brings about an economy of energy expenditure ; and an inherent general sobriety usually characterizes individuals of this type. The " flat " person should not be confused with the merely thin person ; for the one is a morphologic type while the other is possibly reduced through circumstances.

In these lectures delivered at the Sorbonne, the author has gone extensively into the physical and chemical properties of the human body, in order to furnish us with a simple dichotomy which scarcely required such a tremendous scaffolding, but from some of the legends under the figures it may be gathered that in the forthcoming monograph entitled *La Personnalité*, Mac-Auliffe will deal at length with the problem of typology. It is in one of these notes (p. 78) that he refers to the different phases of the sympathetic nervous system which predominate in each of the two types. In another of these legends he mentions the name of Pende and reveals an acquaintance with the " *typus picnicus* des Allemands " (p. 74), alluding of course to the work of Kretschmer [1] and his followers. We must therefore wait patiently for the sequel of this colloidal treatment of personality.

Constitutional Morphology in Germany. Bauer, referring to his own statistical data,[2] corroborates in his thorough

---

[1] See Chapter XV.

[2] J. Bauer, *Konstitutionelle Disposition zu innere Krankheiten*, 3rd ed., 1924, pp. 48–9.

textbook of constitutional pathology the general division of types, as drawn up by the Lyon School, but remarks that Zweig, who undertook at his instance a similar investigation, discovered that Sigaud's types were not permanent throughout life, although they held good up to a certain period. The French authors far from denying this result, I believe, tend to make allowance for it.

In Germany, the problem of constitutional types was broached long before Kretschmer. Even Beneke nearly a hundred years ago distinguished between the type with " relatively small heart, narrow arteries, long legs, small liver and short intestinal tube and the *habitus quadratus (apoplecticus, arthriticus)* in which the characteristics are reversed ; and Bauer affirms that the basis of Beneke's doctrine still holds good to-day.[1]

If Beneke recognized only two constitutional types, his contemporary, C. G. Carus, one of the outstanding figures of his day in comparative anatomy, drew up a list of sixteen forms, one of which, the plethoric, is subdivided into the arterial and the venous.[2] Here we find the cerebral, the athletic, the asthenic, the pneumatic (which would correspond to the French " respiratoire "), and the bœotian, which answers the description of the digestive or alimentary type of Sigaud and his school (pyknik in Kretschmer's terminology).[3] In Carus's table there are to be seen traces of Platner's approach and even some of his terms, but the former had at his command a mass of anatomical data obtained at first hand, which of course were lacking in the case of Platner.

Measurements and Meanings. It was Carus's ambition to construct an interpretative chart of man's physique and motor expression, and in his *Symbolik der menschlichen Gestalt,*

---

[1] J. Bauer: *Vorlesungen über allgemeine Konstitutions-und Vererbungslehre,* 1921, p. 144.

[2] H. Kern, " Die Charakterologie des Carl Gustav Carus " : *Jahrbuch d. Charakterol.,* vol. i, 1924.

[3] See Chapter XV.

which first appeared in 1853 and has been, thanks to Klages, reprinted in 1925, he makes an heroic attempt to assign symbolic values to each of the human organs, so that variations from the ideal or standard can be dealt with accordingly.

Since each of the organs has its own significance, it certainly must make a difference whether the head is more prominent than the abdomen or vice versa, whether the extremities are large or small in comparison with the trunk, etc. Carus, while possibly lapsing at times into the pitfalls of phrenology, vehemently combated Gall's teachings, maintaining that it was the function and not the faculty with which he was concerned. (The renewed interest in Carus is shown by the reprinting of his more important works with illuminating introductions.)

Kretschmer's much discussed four types, which we may call less technically and therefore perhaps somewhat inaccurately, *the plump*, *the athletic*, *the slight*, and *the disproportionate*, are not as we can see for ourselves, a new discovery ; but the very fact that there is so much in common among investigators whose conclusions have been independently arrived at is in no small degree encouraging.

There is a good deal of evidence indicating that the pathologist and the psychiatrist have come to realize that they can meet on common ground in studying the constitution of their patients, and from their observations construct a correlational scheme which may be applied subsequently not only in diagnosis but in prophylaxis.

MOTOR EXPRESSION AND TYPE

In relating physique and constitution to temperament and character types, it is perhaps natural that the motor expression of the organism is omitted from the picture. As Gurevitch [1] points out, the more serious motor disturbances, akinesis,

---

[1] M. Gurevitch, " Motorik, Körperbau und Charakter " : *Arch. f. Psychiat. u. Nerv'ten*, 1926, vol. lxxvi.

hyperkinesis, and the various catatonic manifestations constitute the only phase of this whole sphere which is not neglected. The "motorique" of man in general, e.g., the intensity of movement, tempo, muscle tonus, automatic movements, gracefulness, coördination, ambidexterity, manual skill of adjustment, rhythm, formation of movement formulae, etc.—all this is not usually included in such treatments.

Lewy [1] has found, for instance, that from the motor point of view there are three types, (a) the skilled people, with good motor co-ordination due to the predominance of the sub-cortical mechanisms, and correlating with the fleshy (pyknik) type of Kretschmer ; (b) the clumsy type with a preponderant development of cortical mechanisms answering to the schizoid (split-off disposition) of Kretschmer's table, and (c) the asthenic, whose characteristics are rapid fatigability and lack of strength. Lewy's asthenic type in reality belongs with the schizoid class in Kretschmer's scheme.

In a later report, Lewy [2] adds the tetanoid type with its disposition to cramps and spasms. He distinguishes also between the individual's fundamental tempo and the partial tempo of organs either singly or in groups which bears the same relation to the fundamental tempo as does the overtone to its fundamental tone. Owing to wide differences in tempo, it is sometimes next to impossible for persons to get along with each other in social intercourse (walking, dancing, etc.).

In the Moscow psycho-neurological children's clinic, under the direction of Gurevitch, a number of experimental researches are being conducted with the purpose in view of linking motor characteristics with physique on the one hand

---

[1] F. H. Lewy, *Die Lehre vom Tonus und der Bewegung*, 1923.
[2] F. H. Lewy, "Ausdrucksbewegungen und Charaktertypen." *Jahresvers d. Südwestdeutsch. Psychiat., Vereinig.* 1924 (Frankfort A. M.)

and character on the other. Four motor types are thus recognized by Gurevitch : (1) those with fluent, balanced, dexterous, and exact movements, plump in physique and belonging to Kretschmer's cycloid class ; (2) those with crude, angular movements, more or less nimble and coördinated as regards the rougher acts, but less dexterous in the finer processes involving the fingers especially—the athletic type ; (3) those whose movements are feeble and awkward, although their manual dexterity is of a high order—the asthenic in physique and schizoid in character according to Kretschmer ; and finally, Gurevitch introduces a type which he designates as the " childish-graceful ", characterized by insufficiently exact although esthetically agreeable movements, corresponding apparently to a species of the hypoplastic physique in Kretschmer's classification. This type, found especially among women, is susceptible to hysteroid reactions and is endowed with dramatic and rhythmic talent.

The investigations of other workers in this Russian Institute detail a number of differences among the various types with reference to the motor system. Ozeretzky, e.g. found that the individuals of slight build, as compared with the plump or thick-set, were deficient in the capacity of prompt innervation and denervation, in rhythmic capacity, in speedy adjustment, automatic action and defensive reactions, but especially in energy. On the other hand, the former, i.e. the asthenic, excel in forming new complexes of movement and in their purposive and consequential application. The motor divergence between the plump and the slight is explained physiologically as due to the greater equipment of the extrapyramidal nervous centres in the heavier type.

Yizlin [1] discovered marked differences in the handwriting of the pyknik and asthenic types. In the one case, the letters

---

[1] S. G. Yizlin (Jislin), " Körperbau, Motorik, Handschrift " : *Zt. f.d. ges. Neurol. u. Psychiat.*, 1925, vol. xcviii.

are well rounded and uniformly made, the handwriting is fluent and marked by ease of execution and the elements are connected. Again, the pyknik script shows greater homogeneity. The asthenic group, on the other hand, present such characteristics as micrography, split words and even letters, irregularity in the formation of letters, and sharp angles instead of rounded curves.

Much graphic and tabular material is offered by Sukhareva and Ossipova [1] to prove tentatively the relation between constitutional types (from the diagnostic standpoint) physique, motor capacity and talent.

EIDETIC IMAGERY AND PSYCHOLOGICAL TYPES

We can scarcely afford to leave the section on constitutional disposition without referring to the work of the Marburg Institute which has stimulated a large number of researches on what has been termed eidetic imagery. The discovery that many young children are able to describe objects in detail after removal, has led to the further revelation, according to investigators, that many individuals have lingering after-images, in other words, exhibit the *eidetic* phenomenon. But two types of *eidetic* people are possible, according as the images resemble more nearly the visual after-image or the memory image. In the one case we have the tetanoid (" T ") type ; in the other the Basedowoid (" B ") type.

If it were all a matter of imagery types, we should not naturally devote so much as a line to this phenomenon which of course belongs in the cognitive field ; but it is claimed by the brothers E. R. and W. Jaensch who have for the last

---

[1] G. E. Sukhareva and S. W. Ossipova, " Materialien Zur Erforschung der Korrelation zwischen den Typen der Konstitution " : *Zt. f.d. ges. Neurol. u. Psychiat.*, 1926, vol. c.

NOTE.—The names of Russian writers mentioned in this section have all been transliterated into phonetic English, instead of being left in their Germanized form (Gurewitsch, Ssucharewa, Jislin, etc.).

ten years studied this phenomenon, that the two different eidetic types are marked by an altogether different set of characteristics. Famous representatives of each of the types are Johannes Müller with his rigid features, reminding one of the tetanic picture, and Goethe whose features and expression presented signs which in their exaggerated form would be taken as symptoms of the Basedow disease ; bulging eyes, extreme excitability, soft velvety skin, etc. : but the chief difference between the two classes is that the " B " type develops images of the flexible and variable sort. Individuals of this type are endowed with an inner psychic life independent of their everyday experiences ; and the persistence of their imagery, moreover, is unaffected by the supply of calcium, which in the case of the " T " type serves as a strongly inhibitive factor. It is the contention of E. R. Jaensch and his associates that " just as the senses react to almost immeasurable quantities of energy, so is our psychic life in the sphere of the senses (*Sinnesseelenleben*) where naturally the eidetic phenomena belong, a very fine indicator for inner relationships in the personality, for its physical and psycho-physical make-up ".[1] The " B " type of imagery which is found among those artistically inclined, and most frequently among women and children, often goes with a slightly enlarged thyroid and with an intense reaction to psychic stimuli, especially in the sympathetic nervous system, while the " T " type is found in individuals who react rather to the environment than to their inner stimuli. It would seem that the " B " type would correspond with the circular cyclothymic disposition in psychopathic individuals, and the " T " type with the split-off (schizothymic) make-up.

The constitutional connection of these types has been worked out further by introducing the microscope to observe the formation in the capillaries of the skin. The results, it is

[1] E. R. Jaensch, *Deut. Zt. f. Nervenheilkunde*, 1925, vol. lxxxviii, p. 200.

claimed, yielded a third type, differing from the normal in the malformation of the capillaries, and on the mental side, in a low intelligence. In these individuals who may be vastly improved by calcium treatment and other prepared substances, the capillaries remain in their infantile form instead of developing the regular hair-pin shape (neo-capillary).

Although the eidetic phenomenon has been established by a number of investigators, it is not so certain that there is a direct relation between the type of imagery and the psycho-physical constitution. The effect of calcium on many individuals has been referred to by several writers, but the fact is not sufficient to warrant a classification of people on this basis, although it may serve as one of the links in the chain of constitutional differences.

REVERSIBILITY OF REACTION

The general trend of the work done on temperament in its relation to bodily constitution has been to make the psychological fact dependent on the physiological. Hammett,[1] however, believes that his experiments on the albino rat warrant the conclusion that the reaction is reversible, thus bearing out Osler's [2] conception of the modifiability of temperamental tone and with it the constitutional relationship through voluntary effort. The endocrine system would still in a large measure direct the reciprocal relation. The way in which different people are subject to their intermediate metabolism usually determines the state of emotional or temperamental excitability. Now it has been shown that when the " temperament of an albino rat is changed by gentling from the condition where excitability and irritability are expressed by flight and pugnacity to a state where the

---

[1] F. S. Hammett, " Observations on the Relation between Emotional and Metabolic Stability " : *Am. Journ. Physiol.*, 1926, vol. liii.
[2] W. Osler, *Aequinimitas*, etc., 1904.

degree of expression of these instincts is reduced almost to insignificance, then the animal becomes markedly more resistant to the loss of the parathyroid secretion ". Furthermore in more recent experiments, the wild Norway rat, a still more excitable animal, has proven itself to be far more dependent on the parathyroid glands for its existence than the albino rat.

It is worth noting the fact that the parathyroids are regarded as the regulators of the calcium supply in the system, and that the " B " type of eidetic " imagers " which, as we shall remember is the excitable type as compared with the " T " type, does not show any susceptibility to calcium. The effect of added or diminished calcium supply is seen by W. Jaensch and his co-workers in the case of the tetanoid type.

The interaction between the temperamental tone and the constitutional make-up naturally would find support in the investigations of Cannon and his students as summarized in *Bodily Changes in Pain, Hunger, Fear and Rage.*

FROM HUMORS TO HORMONES

It is one of these curios of cultural destiny that after so many migrations and transformations, the doctrine of humors should, like a colossal ballad or rondo extending over twenty-five centuries, hark back to the beginning when all explanations centred around the fluids of the body. The original theory, now concluding its cycle in the almost universally received opinion of to-day that the secretions of the endocrine glands, injecting into the blood hormones of various sorts, are of vital importance in the organization of a given temperament, provides at present much food for thought, even if the thinking, without the indispensable experiments back of it, must necessarily remain of the groping kind.

What if the old terms are no longer used in discussions of the effects of the ductless secretions, the *manes* of Hippocrates and Galen can still point with triumph to their speculative child and say their " I told you so ". On the other hand let us not underestimate the progress of science, and the achievements of those whose explanations seemed so fanciful and empty as to be discarded. They all have a share in whatever we know of the subject to-day. Connections that are seemingly remote must be examined to throw some light on the possible causal relationships between temperamental constitution and bodily organization. As in philology, we need our comparative grammarians, our Grimms, Bopps and Brugmanns.

Comparative Treatment Necessary. To take an instance or two, can we disregard the fact that a synonym of phlegm is pituita, used especially by Kant and his successors, and that the so-called pituitary personalities are the intellectuals of the world ? Furthermore, is it not striking that these persons are given more to chest troubles (tuberculosis, bronchitis, etc.) and in general manifest weaknesses that are more apt to produce phlegm in the ordinary sense of the word, than people of other types ? Again, supposing that after close investigation it were established that the choleric person had a gallstone and liver diathesis, and that such a one revealed also a hyperadrenal functioning, should we not be justified in bestowing greater attention on " stones which the builders rejected " if we wish to secure an advantageous observation point ?

Beginnings have already been made in this territory which, if followed up, may yield a valuable harvest. Lévi and Rothschild have even gone so far as to claim to have changed the temperament of a patient, whom they diagnosed as suffering from the underfunctioning of the thyroid gland, by administering to her thyroid extract which transformed her from a depressed and weary girl into a vivacious person.[1]

[1] Léopold-Lévi and H. de Rothschild : *Études sur la Physio-pathologie du corps thyroïde et de l'hypophyse*, pp. 54 ff.

Even the highly speculative and vociferous claims of Berman,[1] should not be discarded *in toto*. Desultory suggestions in his book may lead to the formulation of new problems.

Glands and Personality. In Italy, much work has been done bearing on the relationship between the endocrines and conditions of mind and body. To quote Naccarati again, " Pende has made an attempt to study body development from the point of view of endocrinology. Of the hyperthyroid constitution, which corresponds to the microsplanchnic type of Viola, he says: ' From the morphologic point of view, in clean-cut cases, the subjects show . . . precocious and pronounced morphologic differentiation, longitudinal diameters of the body in excess over the horizontal diameters . . . habitual thinness hardly overcome by hypernutrition . . . diminished carbohydrate tolerance ; accelerated basal metabolism, great irritability of the vegetative nervous system, especially of the sympathetic subdivision, marked psychic irritability, hypermotivity, cerebral restlessness . . . precocious and often pronounced intelligence development.' In opposition to this type which he calls microsplanchnic, Viola has recognized another type, the macrosplanchnic or megalosplanchnic, which he considers an infantile type because it shows poor morphologic differentiation. This type possesses a large and very active visceral system, a large cutaneous surface in relation to body volume, anabolic processes in excess over catabolic." [2]

The authors say further in the same article : " When due allowance is given to race, sex, age, and diseases suffered by the individuals whose morphologic characteristics we want to study, we can, with a fair degree of probability, determine which are the hormones that have acted on the soma before birth."

[1] L. Berman : *The Glands Regulating Personality.*

[2] S. Naccarati and H. E. Garrett : " The Influence of Constitutional Factors on Behaviour," *Journ. of Exper. Psychol.*, 1923, vol. vi, p. 257.

On the basis of their measurements and other applications, the authors are inclined to the belief that " those endocrines which affect the morphology and the mentality of a given individual very probably influence his emotional life also ". [1] We see then what an interesting vista has been opened up by the Italian school in conjunction with the newer investigations on the ductless glands. Whether we are within our rights, in the present state of affairs, to argue for the responsibility of this or that gland as conducive to a given temperamental condition is disputable. There can, however, be no question but that some day, with the increasing progress of isolated experiments, the connection between the over- or under-functioning of certain glands and striking temperamental make-ups will be just as manifest as the relation between the thyroid gland and intelligence.

EXPERIMENTAL INVESTIGATIONS

The sore need of experiments on temperament has already been alluded to. Lest, however, it be supposed that no one had thought of such a possibility, let us be reminded that already Haller, in the eighteenth century, had subjected himself to a dietary control, taking alternately wine and meat, or abstaining from both, in order to prove that the quality of the blood had nothing to do with the type of temperament one possessed ; for as a result of different food elements, entirely new blood could be produced without there being a noticeable effect on the temperament, as he claimed to have shown through his own experiments. [2]

Temperature and Temperament. Further experiments were carried on about a century ago by the young French anatomist Béclard, who recognized only two temperaments : the sanguine or alimentary and the nervous, attributing the one

[1] S. Naccarati and H. E. Garrett : " The Relation of Morphology to Temperament," loc. cit., p. 263.

[2] J. Henle : *Anthropologische Vorträge*, p. 112.

to the Northern peoples and the other to the Southern races. The sanguine temperament again could be subdivided according as it tended to produce more flesh or more fat. To prove that the temperature of a country exercised a determining influence in the development of a constitutional type, he had accelerated the hatching of chicks at a high temperature and also at a lower temperature. Those that broke the shell at a high temperature had large heads and small hearts. With those born at a lower temperature the converse was true.[1] From this Béclard inferred that his assumption of linking the large physique with the lower temperature was well-founded. Such naïve attempts were of course inadequate to prove anything. We know nothing of how the chicks developed and what other factors might have entered to account for the results.

Metabolism and Temperament. Another circumscribed series of experiments with a negative purpose similar to Haller's was conducted by Seeland. Since it was his contention that the metabolism of the body bore no relation to the temperaments, he studied the variation in weight, secretions, and excretions of sanguine and choleric individuals placed under an identical diet, and found no differences between the two classes.[2]

Psychological Experiments. It is only recently that a psychologist took a hand in the experimental investigations of temperament, after the physiologist, the anatomist and the anthropologist (Seeland) took their turns. On the basis of a large number of carefully conducted experiments in which the strength of the will was tested by having the subjects respond with a syllable other than the one that they had learnt in previous experiments, Ach has presented a number [3] of results that bear on the problem before us. The play between determination and motivation in the diagnosis of tempera-

---

[1] *Loc. cit.*, p. 118.
[2] N. Seeland : " Le Tempérament," etc., *loc. cit.*, p. 121 ff.
[3] N. Ach : *Über den Willensakt und das Temperament.*

ment is a feature which takes on a decided coloring with the steady advance of dynamic psychology. The distinction between motivation and determination is one which would have been slurred in orthodox psychology but a decade ago, only to receive special emphasis at the present time, and from various quarters.

Ach too deems it proper to retain the usual nomenclature, but he has added a fifth temperament, viz., the deliberative (*besonnene*) manifesting itself in a tendency to obviate all the obstacles that interfere with a prompt reaction and to avoid slips. The affective reaction becomes less intense as the determination toward an accurate and rapid reaction becomes stronger. With these subjects, success was accompanied by the awareness of " I am able ", while failure brought on a state of self irony with the awareness " if I only seriously want to ". Great associability of ideas is also a mark of this temperament.

The sanguine temperament is coupled with carelessness and a light-hearted attitude, also a decrease in the intensity of the determination in the course of the experimentation period.

The choleric temperament is characterized by a weak determination which calls for greater effort on the part of the subject in order to realize the act, but the intensive set which is the result of increased excitability in order to attain success leads to a neglect of the means by which the goal might be attained. It also is accompanied by an unpleasant feeling-tone.

If the individual is characterized by weak determining dispositions and also by a reduced state of sensory and motor excitability, as well as by weak motivation, then the chances are that we are dealing with a melancholic type of temperament.

When reduced motivation, following decreased general excitability, comes simultaneously with an intense determining disposition, we have before us the foundation for the phlegmatic temperament.

Motivation and Determination. The play between feelings, motivation, and determination for the five temperaments is described as follows : In the *deliberative* individual there is an intensive feeling of expression, as well as an intense determination ; and all the circumstances and conditions are considered in the *Vorsatz* or undertaking period. The *sanguine* person is distinguished by a very pronounced but gradually decreasing determination. The result is often failure, but this very failure becomes the motive for a more energetic impulse that finally meets with success. Hence the outer signs of inconstancy and unreliability that go together with a certain optimistic carelessness. The *choleric* is marked by increase of motivation with heightened motor and sensory excitability, where only a slight determining disposition is present. Owing to the slight determination, a stronger will act is needed ; but owing to the heightened excitability, failure is often the result. An intensity of effort out of proportion to the degree of success goes with a strong feeling reaction which leads to renewed effort and finally success. The *melancholic* is characterized by a weak determining tendency and low sensory and motor excitability with a negative feeling-tone. The *phlegmatic* shows slight motivation, but great determining disposition, which drops very slowly.

Somatotypology. The constitutional approach, often criticized because of its typological presuppositions, has, thanks to W. H. Sheldon,[1] found a technique which, to a large extent, obviates the difficulty, in that each individual is regarded as a synthesis of three components, in various proportions. Instead of a very limited number of types,

[1] W. H. Sheldon, S. S. Stevens, and W. B. Tucker : *The Varieties of Human Physique*, 1940. W. H. Sheldon and S. S. Stevens : *The Varieties of Temperament*, 1942. W. H. Sheldon : *Varieties of Delinquent Youth*, 1949.

there will be innumerable patterns, classifiable on a quantitative basis.

Four thousand photographs were used for the purpose of discovering some features that might serve as basic differences in form or build ; and thus there came into being the somato-typing of an individual according to (a) endomorphy, (b) mesomorphy, and (c) ectomorphy. In the first class, the viscera, i.e., the inside of the trunk, largely derived from the embryonic inner layer (endoderm) predominate ; in the second, the bones and muscles receive chief prominence, while the third class is made up of those whose nervous system and the skin, derived from the outer embryonic layer, and there-fore more exposed and less protected, are chiefly involved. Although we can find extremes on rare occasions, the large majority falls into the three classes, so that if each component were given seven values, we might have, 1, 1, 7 ; 4, 2, 4 ; 7, 1, 1, etc., designating the proportion of the components.

The somatotype is only the physical designation corre-sponding to a psychical counterpart. Thus the endomorph (*viscerotonic*) who is fleshy, pyknic, as Kretschmer would call him, will be easy to get along with, self-indulgent, sociable, cheerful, and earthy. The mesomorph (*somatotonic*) with his muscular frame will seek power and show aggressiveness and daring, while the ectomorph (*cerebrotonic*) with his highly developed and sensitive nervous system will be the reflective type, seclusive, self-conscious, a poor mixer, no organizer, and averse to routine.

The fact that an individual is not put into a definite category but is given a number even to a decimal point is naturally an advantage, but the numbers themselves unless they represent a fine balance, like 333 or 343, reveal the predominance of one type as against another.

The question before us is : to what extent does somato-typing help to recognize character ? From scattered investiga-tion it would appear that character, in the ethical sense, will be found mostly in the ectomorph, i.e., the cerebrotonic, while the mesomorph or somatotonic because of his aggressive qualities and craving for domination will, despite his courage, persistence, and occasional good turns, yield the largest percentage of criminals.

Sheldon supposes that if we had taken into consideration the somatotonic character of the German people, we might have been able to avert the cataclysm of 1939. Whether or not this yardstick could apply to whole nations is a moot point. The German menace perhaps lies more in the *submissiveness of the majority to a few* somatotonic individuals ; and the submissiveness would argue for a viscerotonic predominance, which is more in conformity with the general idea of the average German entertained by the world at large.

To what extent old classifications crop up anew in a different framework may be seen from the fact that Sheldon's main types are the exact counterpart of the vital, motive, and nervous temperaments about which the phrenologists of a century ago would make much ado.

It is perhaps well to add that the somatotyping of individuals has, in some investigations, acquired an accessory of late, in that the masculine or feminine component is added in each case as a special morphological criterion. Thus a woman whose anthropological measurements and physiological signs show a departure from the general norms in the direction of masculine proportions and characteristics would be said to have a weak feminine component, and vice versa with the man whose measurements and other indications fall within norms regarded as feminine.

CONCLUDING NOTE

We have now come to the end of our fairly comprehensive historical survey of temperament ; and the sanguine person who started out with the fond hope of finding the puzzle solved in this age of radio and telephotography will likely betray some evidence of disappointment at this bewildering labyrinth of theory. The truth of the matter is that there is no cause for mortification at the seemingly slow progress of the bi-millenary inquiry. *E pur si muove.* Our knowledge of the temperaments has advanced, even if we do not appreciate the gain. Before the psychological attack, armed with the munition of endo-crinology, could be successful—and this seems to be the destiny of the study from present indications—it was necessary for the other theories to serve as scientific fodder. Some of these have gone to become the flesh and bone of more vigorous doctrines ; others have once for all been cast off as refuse, but even these latter have their historical value. It is interest-ing in this historical light to note how a certain theory keeps cropping up again and again throughout the ages in an increasingly modern form. The common element in many theories is of even greater significance. *A central tendency* in all the listed theories could be discovered, although it would be far from reasonable to affirm that this central tendency represents more nearly the truth than some isolated point of view latterly held.

In general, more agreement is evinced in the writings on temperament than appears at first blush. The study of character, as Wundt has remarked, is a more complex subject ; and it may be added, offers difficulties from the very outset, even in its subject-matter. The temperaments, at least, exhibit a definite locus which is the same for the majority of writers ; and the divergence of opinion enters largely in the explanations and correlations.

The time is now ripe for further experimentation on tempera-mental dispositions, and by the further aid of tests and questionnaires and the co-operation of public institutions, we may anticipate in the not distant future a body of data which would be of incalculable value not only theoretically *per se*, but practically in the reduction of the amount of unhappiness caused so frequently by the following factors : (1) the entering into relationships without sufficient insight into one another's natures, (2) misunderstandings due to unfamiliarity with temperaments other than our own, (3) obstacles in the way of terminating fundamentally incompatible relationships, (4) temperamental adjustment in the industrial system, (5) the effects of various foods, drugs, alcoholic beverages, etc., on one's temperamental disposition.

But this leads us to touch on the applied psychology of temperament which should not be overlooked in a general survey of human types.

CHAPTER VI

THE APPLIED PSYCHOLOGY OF TEMPERAMENT

Most of the emphasis in applying the knowledge we have about the temperaments to everyday life has been hitherto laid on the diagnostic stage. Even a book like Hollingworth's *Judging Human Character* is primarily occupied with the question of how we shall be able to read character or temperament from the features, in the meantime having to content ourselves with other methods.

In my opinion, the problem of reading a person's temperamental make-up is not so significant. An intelligent and experienced person has no difficulty in classifying many people he meets, and he who is without that gift of estimating strangers will never learn the art in spite of amassing all the particulars contained in books on character analysis.

Surely we are not going to subject our newly introduced acquaintances to measurements of the head ; and even if we could so impose on them, how much allowance ought we to make for compensatory data ? As I asked elsewhere " Granted that a snub-nose, high forehead, somewhat square chin, etc., denote indecision may there not be present some other characteristic to offset this defect, or at least to modify it ? " [1]

Since every individual is a case by himself, our rules will become annoyingly encumbered with exceptions, until they will become of no practical value whatever. And yet in a measure, without resorting to rules, we intuitively, or rather through associating our experience in the past, grasp that one person is sanguine, another depressed, still another inclined to be irritable. We say such a man looks grumpy

[1] A. A. Roback : *Psychology with Chapters on Character Analysis and Mental Measurement*, p. 112.

or grouchy; this woman behind her agreeable exterior hides a nagging disposition, etc. And only a few minutes' conversation on topics of personal interest would serve as a further guide to put us on the right track.

Recognizing Temperaments. The outstanding temperamental characteristics leave their impress on the features and movements. The tense expression and the jerky gait of the nervous, high-strung person; the cool and calculative mien of the bovine phlegmatic individual; the jolly and often ruddy appearance of the sanguine hale and hearty fellow; the depressed attitude of the melancholic are usually unmistakable indications to the man of the world. Those who do not possess detectable outward signs of their temperamental make-up usually are not well marked cases, but constitute combinations of types which, for applied purposes, are not important to single out, since they can be adapted almost to any line of endeavour.

The Choleric Waiter. It is the clear-cut choleric or sanguine individual who provides for us a problem in applied psychology; and part of this problem is to be shouldered by the personnel division of applied psychology; for the temperamental element in some cases is more important than the ability element in the individual. In all employments where agreeableness is a prerequisite, it would be incongruous for a choleric person to hold a job which would necessitate his coming in contact with the people served. No matter how efficient a waiter may be in other respects, if his anger is easily aroused, he will be more of a liability than an asset to the establishment which engages him.

The porter whose credo during working hours was that the patron or customer must always be right had the proper attitude for that type of a job. If his principle militated against this attitude, then either he should have taken on some other kind of employment, or else bear the consequences of the incompatibility between his personal dignity and the require-

K

ments of his employment. There is no room for a morose servitor under any circumstances. Since it is possible in our vastly ramified industrial system to fit in somewhere almost with any disposition, unless it is so striking as to need medical treatment, there is no reason why we should not take account of temperamental idiosyncrasies in the " hiring and firing " of men.

Salesmen are Sanguine. The average salesman, as every employer knows, would be out of place with a morose, depressed temperamental make-up ; and the more difficult it is to make the sales, and the less expert the prospective buyers, the more sanguine will as a rule the successful salesman turn out to be. How to recognize the sanguine salesman, who is not made ineligible through defects more serious than the sanguine quality is advantageous, falls beyond the scope of our present discussion, which is not psychotechnical. We are content merely to show the bearing of temperament on applied psychology, not to point out how to obtain certain practical results.

The choleric person can scarcely be happy in any environment, but there are places in which he can assert his independence. These places are few because they are at the top of a given calling, but any one who reaches the highest rung of his profession can exercise his authority without being required to temper his irritability. The unusually skilful surgeon, the expert engineer, the very adroit advocate can hold his own in spite of the outbursts to which he would subject friends and acquaintances. Those, however, who are dealing with superiors can hardly advance unless they curb their irritable temper at least in their relations with these superiors, who would have to be extraordinarily detached in order to place ability above temperamental qualities, especially in matters affecting themselves.

Assets of the Choleric. The disadvantages of the choleric temperament can be counterbalanced, then, only by ability of a high order, especially in a sphere where personal contact is not an element in the vocation, or where the contact is with many individuals who do not form an organized body (patients, clients, customers). On the other hand the choleric temperament is an asset in military affairs, where discipline counts, and especially in war where it generates a doggedness useful in combating the enemy. Most great generals seem to have been possessed of the choleric temperament, which partly accounts for their effectiveness under trying conditions. A warrior with a regularly depressed mental attitude would be an anomaly; and the wavering behaviour of " Cunctator " is stigmatized by that very sobriquet which was applied to Quintus Fabius Maximus.

It would not be far from the truth to affirm that even in intellectual battles such as those waged by great reformers, whether religious, political, social or educational, a considerable dose of the irritable disposition would be required, else the propaganda work which is so essential in undermining the old system would never be begun, and the resistance which a new idea always meets with could never be overcome.

Adaptations. Not only are certain temperaments suited for certain vocations, but often the type of employment will draw out a particular trait from among the others for cultivation, in keeping with the process of selective adaptation. The man in a commanding office, while it is true that he must have been somewhat choleric to begin with, although possibly meek towards his superiors, will develop a brusqueness about him which will at once cow his subordinates. Similarly the prima donna temperament is partly acquired after securing a solid footing in artistic circles. The flightiness is no doubt inherent in all histrionic natures, but the super-imposed choleric quality is not given free rein before a measure of success is achieved.

Seeming Anomalies. That there are exceptions goes without saying. Who can fit into the narrow compass of a generalization all the manifold cases of striking anomalies due to the conjuncture of diverse circumstances ? And who can interpret a tendency so unmistakably as to make allowance for all possible slants ? Tolstoi becomes an apostle of peace at all costs, and yet, viewed from another angle, such inexorable propaganda cannot issue but from a warlike make-up. Most of the spiritual leaders in history come under this category. The antinomy is only superficial, yet the combative spirit with a peaceful ideal will appear to the unenlightened as an inconsistency.

Our considerations in this chapter are intended for the type only, which includes of course the vast majority of individuals who are definitely recognized both as to their temperamental status and vocational standing. Various historical and political turns may bring about unexpected appointments which would tend to discredit the rules noted ; but for our purpose these exceptions do not count. That there is a correspondence between temperamental organization and vocational success is one of the facts which need no further demonstration. The task for psychotechnicians is to ascertain the particulars of the correspondence and to apply the data in individual cases.

We need not enter into all the departments of applied psychology which may benefit by the contact with the study of character and temperament. What is difficult to understand is that with all the interest apparently evinced in the subject, the ground has scarcely been more than broken. Even such a relatively simple question as the mutual attraction or repulsion of temperamental types has not been scientifically answered.

There is a universal belief that opposites attract, and common observation bears this out. Friendships are usually formed on this basis ; and the best place to study the formation of such bonds is the psychopathic hospital, because it is there that extremes meet. There is nothing more common than to find a strong tie of friendship between the manic and the depressed inmates, the cyclic and the schizoid types. A statistical study of such attachments would be of great service in helping to settle a mooted point.

Attachment of Unlikes. The saying that like attracts unlike is most strikingly illustrated in the sphere of sexual attachment. It is unusual for two of a kind temperamentally to become fond of each other. Biological reasons (natural selection) have been advanced to account for this circumstance, but the more momentous question that awaits a reply is whether the hetero-temperamental attraction lasts just as long as a homo-temperamental union, if established, would endure. Offhand one would answer this in the affirmative, since each one generally requires the complement in the opposite temperament either as a regulative agency or else as an expansive influence, but a designedly permanent relationship such as the state of marriage, and one which entails such a complexity of interrelations, obligations, etc., might not be subject to the considerations that bear on the more disinterested forms of association which, though they may last a lifetime, do not offer the same troublesome problems or involve the obligations of modern married life. Like everything else, I suppose, it is a matter of degree ; and while opposites attract, it may well be that in situations requiring judgment, tolerance, and even patience, the stable and the unstable temperaments are bound to clash more frequently than temperaments which are both more alike. The seriousness of the conflict naturally is another issue. With different combinations one may expect to find different consequences. The intensity of the disagreement, its compass and duration are all affected by the degree of incompatibility between the two temperamental natures.

Science of " Eugamics." Here, then, is another cue for an investigation which may help to bring relief in certain quarters of suffering humanity, if its results should turn out to be decisive. True, it is questionable whether the many cases of domestic incompatibility would have proved more successful, if one of the incompatible partners, or both, had been wedded to any one else. The fact, however, remains that there is an important phase in the most vital part of civilized life which is as yet unexplored, and whether one likes it or not, the examination of temperamental kinks and quirks in relation to marriage is one of the foundations which underlie the hitherto unknown science of what I should call *eugamics*.

For this reason, the anchorage on the recognition of a certain temperament by features or gestures becomes a scientific luxury which may never be attained as compared with the application of our knowledge about the various temperamental relations. I say it is a luxury because the man in the street, as well as the psychologist who panders to him, simply wishes to learn the trick of reading character, either for its entertainment, or, as is more commonly the case, because he is too impatient to employ the methods furnished him by painstaking observers ; or again he may be incapable of making judgments on the basis of his experience, i.e., applying his art in such matters. At any rate such a person cannot be guided by science ; for though he have all the rules at his finger tips, he will not be able to make proper use of them in classifying a given individual, unless the case is so pronounced as to make rules unnecessary in the diagnosis.

Room for Change. The necessities of life should claim our attention first. Granted that we have patiently gathered our information, that we can label our individual as irritable, sanguine, phlegmatic or depressed, we should do well to find out how the particular knowledge could be exploited to the advantage of all concerned.

In former days, when social conditions were pre-determined, when vocations were limited in number, when the needs and demands of the barons were the ruling forces of the industrial arts, when conventions were iron-clad, it would be next to impossible to benefit by such results as could be obtained by a practical study of temperament and its social and economic consequences. To-day we are adopting more and more the point of view that the whole texture of society is subject to a gradual change in accord with the findings of science.

CHAPTER VII

THE PROVERBIAL LORE AND INSPIRATIONAL LITERATURE

I. POPULAR REACTIONS

There is a well-grounded suspicion of proverbs in scientific circles. The reasons are not far to seek. A proverb at best is a generalization and that in a vague or loose way. Proverbs can be found to satisfy almost every point of view; and different peoples will be able to produce divergent sayings to corroborate their beliefs.

The proverbial lore on physical and chemical subjects is not extensive. It is when we come to the realm of human nature that we meet with a harvest which, perhaps after proper sifting, will yield only a small proportion of wheat, as Münsterberg contended in his readable essay, *The Popular Mind*.[1] Nevertheless the onus is on the psychologists to disprove the thoughts accumulated during centuries of sad experiences.[2] The transmission of a proverb from generation to generation is of course not to be taken as an indication of its validity. It is, however, a challenge, a fact to be grappled with; and even if the saw should contain a half truth only, the question of its origin and its influence may furnish a clue for scientific investigation.

Proverbs Common Ground of Genius and Philistine. In many cases too, the line between popular proverbs and epigrams uttered by illustrious men of letters is not, and cannot be, sharply drawn. Many of our everyday expressions, employed even by the illiterate, expressions such as " hitting

[1] H. Münsterberg : *Psychology and Social Sanity.*
[2] Pessimistic as this may sound, nearly all proverbs tell the story of disillusionment in their pithy way, or else when apparently gay, they introduce a cynical note.

118

the nail on the head " or " Fear has many eyes " are credited to great individuals like Rabelais and Cervantes ; and yet we can never tell how much these writers have been indebted to people in the lower strata of culture, how much they have assimilated from those in a humble station, their servants perhaps.

The vast epigrammatic literature must be taken more seriously than in the past. For the present, I am not referring to the inspirational literature of an essay nature, embracing addresses and sermons. It is the crystallized thought intelligible to the man in the street which is to form the subject matter of this section ; and to say that there are thousands of aphorisms, maxims, thoughts and sayings coming under the caption of character is to repeat something which practically every one knows. Each of these utterances may be expanded into an essay, just as the quintessence of most of Montaigne's essays can be compressed into a single thought. When Montaigne, in his essay on " cruelty ", speaking of virtue (for which may be substituted the concept of character), says " She requires a rough and stony passage, she will have either external difficulties to wrestle with . . . or internal difficulties . . . ", does he not express the same idea as Goethe in his couplet about the formation of a character in the swift current of the world ? And when we reflect upon the dictum " every sore-eyed person is an oculist ", do we not see in it the germ of the inferiority theory, which Adler has been expounding in his several books ? A similar thought is conveyed by Cicero's comment, according to Plutarch, that " loud bawling orators are driven to noise by their weakness as lame men to horse ".

Sometimes the analogies between human character and qualities in inanimate nature are indeed apt because there is a common basis underlying both. The adage " Still waters run deep " or " Empty vessels make most noise " will scarcely need revising after statistical treatment.

The picturesqueness of a given proverb is not to be con sidered in our discussion. We are concerned solely with its content; for instance in the saying "A character, like a kettle, once mended, always wants mending ", the analogy is weak, and there is no reason for likening a character to a kettle in any respect, except perhaps to suggest something else, very concrete and universally known, to which the same property is applicable. The inquiry, nevertheless, remains an inquiry, viz., whether a character once it begins to show a defect will constantly need setting right ; but the reason for this, provided the supposition is borne out by fact, offers even more material for our whole investigation, for it knocks at the inner door of the problem of character.

Method of Inquiry. It may be that some epigrams on character come into being through the union of a hankering for cleverness with a flair for paradox. Wherever significant words are transposed or contrasts flaunted, the validity of the saying is less likely to be acceptable, but even in such instances, the content of the apophthegm is independent of its form ; and our decisions should be guided by empirical observation even in examining such remarks as that credited by Plutarch to Cato the elder : " They that were serious in ridiculous matters would be ridiculous in serious affairs " or the Rabelaisian saw " A young monk makes an old devil ". We must ask ourselves, namely, whether the same lack of judgment, the same want of insight which makes people behave incongruously in one event is also responsible for their mistuned conduct under the reverse circumstances. In the second utterance, we have before us evidently the problem of compensation. Does it mean, as Anatole France in his refined cynicism has on more than one occasion (e.g., in *Thaïs, The Human Tragedy*, etc.) implied that some time during life the craving for the sensuous will be keenly experienced, and if favored by opportunity will cause the bridle to be loosened ? Or does it refer to the retarded maturity in worldly affairs of the introvert, whose inhibitions have left him gradually as he was becoming a part of the world around him, and whose desires have remained young while those of the once "regular fellow" had played themselves "out" in the "settling" period? The Dutch proverb "A man at sixteen will prove a child at sixty" offers the same alternative explanation.

FIXITY OF CHARACTER IN POPULAR LORE

At the same time, and seemingly in disagreement with the former, though not necessarily so, we note the numerous sayings relative to the fixity of human character. "Can the Ethiopian change his skin?" is the metaphor given in the Bible to designate this immutability of psychological law, or, as we have it more quaintly in the couplet

> "The ape though clothed in silk it be
> Is ape to all eternity,"

and in the somewhat inelegant saying which is represented by variants in other languages, "You can't make a silk purse out of a sow's ear."

The volcanic Robespierre expressed it more sententiously in the words "No man can climb out of his own character", and someone else has said "To a bad character good doctrine avails nothing". The Spanish saying "*Genio y hechura hasta sepultura*" (Natures and features last till the grave), and our own "Crooked sapling, crooked oak" and "At seventy as at seven"[1] express the same thought. A similar interpretation may be put on the proverb "He who is born to be hanged

---

[1] The thought of second childhood, I believe, is foreign to this proverb ; for with the Jews, who are responsible for this saw, the septuagenarian is respected as a man of wisdom. The etymology of our word *senator* too suggests that the aged were respected for their anything but childish behavior. Another Yiddish proverb bringing out the same idea is "*Vee azoi men vert geborn, azoi, vert men farlorn*" (As you come into the world, so you leave it).

will not be drowned ".[1] Scores of such proverbs could be quoted from different languages, showing that the common people—for even if the proverbs originated through men of parts, they could not take hold of the masses, unless they were in accord with the experiences of the man in the street—believed character to be essentially an immutable quality.

This immutability has received its most poetical crystallization in Goethe's *Faust* :—

> *Du bist am Ende . . . was du bist,*
> *Setz' dir Perücken auf von millionen Locken*
> *Setz' deinen Fuss auf ellenhohe Socken*
> *Du bleibst doch immer was du bist.*

DEEPER MEANINGS OF CERTAIN PROVERBS

The superficiality with which we treat our everyday proverbs and the contempt that the scientifically trained man has cultivated for them have prevented us from penetrating the apparent mystery of certain proverbs. Even if a saying is palpably untrue or exaggerated, there must surely be some reason for its wide vogue, not to mention its origination. We have often heard it said " Lucky in love, unlucky in cards " or " in business ". Is it possible that the exceptions will be noticed and the generalization based on these ? This is hardly tenable. It is more probable that the observations were correct, but the cause attributed to luck is really to be sought in the fact that he who is busy making love and conquering hearts is not likely to attend to business, and also that the " ladies' man " is usually not the one to be blessed with a marked purpose in life. As a Spanish proverb runs : " They that are bold with women are never bold with men." And now it is for psychology to discover the " why " of

---

[1] This proverb may be regarded as illustrating the law of predestination, but in that case all its subtlety would be lost. The contrast between hanging and drowning (an accidental death) is, it seems to me, significant.

this fact, or if it should challenge its truth, undertake to correlate man's aggressiveness with the opposite sex and his aggressiveness with men.

Compensation Recognized. Similarly one of Pascal's *Pensées*, " *Diseur de bons mots, mauvais caractère* " must be examined in the light of psychology, quite apart from the possible prejudice which the reclusive philosopher had for the social wit, especially as there are several proverbs conveying the same thought. On the other hand, Burton in his *Anatomy of Melancholy* takes Aristotle as his authority for the surprising statement that "melancholy men of all others are most witty ", and we may remember the story of the famous Italian comedian who, when consulting a noted physician about his spells of despondency, was advised to witness the performances of Carlini, who was standing there unknown before him in utter despair. If, then, there is a positive correlation between melancholy and wit (not in the sense of continually cracking jokes) can we look upon it as due to a compensatory factor in the make-up of the individual ?

One of these puzzling *dicta*, frequently found among the French, is the expression " It belongs to great men to have great defects ". Are we to understand that great defects are to be condoned in great men, or that the source of the greatness is at the same time a source of great failing in a particular direction—a view resembling that of Lombroso's school ?

" How " and " Why " in Sayings. A popular saying can never have true psychological value until the reason for the generalization is known. In fact it is more important to become cognizant of the explanation than of the universality, were such possible, of the fact described by the proverb. Thus in Addison's quotation of the lines :

When a man talks of love, with caution trust him!
But if he swears, he'll certainly deceive thee,

it is possible to ascribe this relationship between strong asseveration and deception either to a conscious motive or to an unconscious cause. The interpretation in the first event would be that having gone through these protestations of love more than once, the tendency is to add impetus to the process by increasing vociferation. But the other explanation is just as plausible, viz., that the sanguine person is relatively inconstant and unreliable, and the certain deception is likely to be the consequence of the sanguine person's ardent declarations.[1] The first explanation refers to the " why ", the motive; the second answers rather the " how ".

Enough has been said to illustrate the Delphic qualities of many proverbs. Granted, however, that one must occasionally ponder over the equivocal sense of a popular saying, there is still something to be gained by looking into the cases which the proverb purports to cover; and in this we are aided by our empirical observations, experiences and reflections on them. The ancients have given evidence of almost uncanny insight in many of their scattered thoughts on both character and temperament, though we must remember that the concept of character was often enveloped in other concepts such as wisdom or virtue.[2]

CRITERIA OF CHARACTER IN ANCIENT LORE

One of the most clear-cut expressions with reference to character, a striking epigram that might well have been uttered by one of the modern literary lights, occurs in that treasure of law and lore, the Talmud, which contains numerous passages dealing with human nature. This epigram, in the form of a pun, ascribed to Rabbi Ilaï, reads, " By three

[1] This is borne out by the proverb : " A man apt to promise is apt to forget."

[2] A Burmese proverb runs : " One should judge a horse by its speed, an ox by its burden, a cow by milking, and a wise man by his speech." It is evident that wisdom is meant here to denote the quintessence of man, the chief desirable characteristic.

things is a man recognized : by his cup, by his purse, and by his temper (literally anger)." [1] In a non-canonical minor tract of the Talmud, called *Derekh Eretz* (Comportment), the observation is repeated that the scholar—and in those days the scholar was first of all a gentleman—could be recognized chiefly by his cup (b'khoso), by his pocket-book (b'khiso), and by his anger (b'khaaso).

These three words, in which only a change of one vowel has taken place, need perhaps a bit of interpretation ; but it will not be difficult to see the connection between the pocket-book and the acquisitive instinct (and if I were a psychoanalyst, especially of Freud's school, I might find room for the sex instinct here too, for the word *kis* in Hebrew has a double meaning ; [2] and Freudians would surely regard this double meaning as significant on the basis of a psychoanalytic determinism). The second criterion of character, according to the obscure Jewish sage of antiquity, refers to the whole situation of drinking and includes doubtless not only the power of control and habits of temperance, but the manner of drinking, the quantity imbibed, and most important of all probably, the verbal consequences. The third mark, the anger response, again taps an instinctive source.

In this apparent pun there is revealed then the psychological approach to the study of character, and one which forms the groundwork of this essay. It matters little that the abstract word for character is wanting in the Talmudic dictum. The concept of character is implied in the circumlocution " Man is known ".

The German criteria of character are much like those of

---

[1] *Erubin* 65, column 2. It is worth mentioning that fear was never looked upon as an evil among the Jews. On the contrary, it was regarded as a desirable frame of mind in alliance with obedience. " The rudiment of wisdom is the fear of the Lord," every Jewish child would repeat every morning.

[2] A. A. Roback : " Character and Inhibition," in *Problems of Personality*, p. 180.

the ancient Talmudic scholar. " By three things we learn men : love, play and wine," reads the German proverb which, it would seem, does not display the same comprehensiveness and earnestness (in spite of the pun) as the Hebrew. The Dutch say, " A man is not known till he cometh to honor."

II. CHARACTER IN THE INSPIRATIONAL LITERATURE

Thousands of sermons have been preached on character, and hundreds of books and essays have been written on this subject. They may all have imparted some inspiration to the listeners or readers for the time being ; but as a rule, an address or an essay which is nothing but inspirational, though its author may have been inspired at the time of its presentation or composition, is of no consequence after the ephemeral use to which it has been put. Most of the allusions to character by orators of all descriptions are either platitudes, such as " Character is a great word, one of the greatest " (Hitchcock), or " Character is the governing element in life and is above genius " (Saunders), or else cryptic expressions dressed in metaphors that becloud the issue. An example of this is the following: "Character is impulse that has been reined down into steady continuance " (Parkhurst). The eloquence of some of these well-turned phrases is undoubted, and the value of powerful exhortations from the pulpit or rostrum cannot be questioned ; but for the purpose of discovering the *differentiae* of our term, they are worthless, except perhaps for fanning an interest in the subject.

Emerson's Crystals. Again it must be pointed out that one should not object to the figurative language, provided there is an idea lying concealed amidst the shining metaphors and similes. The chief complaint is to be lodged against the application to character of phraseology which may well fit anything at all that we deem important. There need not be any decrying of the literary treatment of character, provided the writer can rise above the commonplace. In Emerson's superb essays on character, conduct, manners, heroism, and representative men, there are enough truisms, and not a few statements that will fail to pass a strictly philosophical scrutiny, but then with all the chaff there is still enough wheat to feed a world of critical minds. When he says that character is " a reserved force which acts directly by presence and without means ", it is true he lays himself open to the charge of surrounding character with a halo of mysticism, but at any rate, the crystal which he framed compels our attention. The question is whether the same quasi-definition could be applied to " genius " or " intelligence ". If not, then Emerson has won his point ; his intuition has burst through a new channel. Similarly when he places character above " the purest literary talent " because the latter " appears at one time great, at another time small, but character is of a stellar and undiminishable greatness ", he gains our most attentive and respectful hearing, only, however, to draw a sceptical knit of the brow ; for is not character known only through actions just as talent or genius through actual production ; and is not a man of noble character apt to make a slip just as a man of genius may sometimes err ?

What Emerson does is to expose different facets of the gem which he is handling. Sometimes we receive a good enlightened view ; at other times, the angle of exposure gives us a distorted vision. As he turns the stone, the light is reflected differently, but always so as to give a striking effect, as for instance when we are told that character is the " moral order seen through the medium of an individual nature ". It is of little consequence whether you believe or not in a moral order other than that made by man. You may substitute Comte's term "humanity" or some other concept which entails uniformity, system, sequence, or what-not to express the opposite of chaos.

Stress on Principle. Emerson's scintillations really embody in a germinal way the main ideas of the constructive part of this volume. The cementing of course is lacking. Instead we

L

have picturesque metaphors and analogies to saturate the beautiful hues of the sparks. " A healthy soul stands united with the just and the true, as the magnet arranges itself with the pole, so that he stands to all beholders like a transparent object betwixt them and the sun, and whoso journeys toward the sun journeys toward that person. He is thus the medium of the highest influence to all who are not on the same level. Thus men of character are the conscience of the society to which they belong."

It is questionable whether the last conclusion holds, whether after all, it is not the society which comes after them, rather than that to which they belong, that looks back with reverence to those heroes of action who were possibly despised by their fellow-men when alive. Emerson's first emphasis, however, manifestly is on the *existence* and *immutability of principles.* The next stress is on the *resistance of circumstances* which to him is the natural measure of the power of the man possessing character. Herein we have the popular counterpart of the psychological concept of inhibition which will be discussed more fully in chapter XXX.

Character and Resistance. One of these pregnant ideas which are so plentiful in the works of the great American transcendentalist is that " Character is centrality, the impossibility of being displaced or overset ", and he goes on to explain that " a man should give us a sense of mass. Society is frivolous and shreds its day into scraps, its conversation into ceremonies and escapes. But if I go to see an ingenious man, I shall think myself poorly entertained if he give me nimble pieces of benevolence and etiquette ; rather he shall stand stoutly in his place and let me apprehend, if it were only his resistance ".

Smiles's Message. As an equally, if not more, inspiring essay may be cited the book *Character* by Samuel Smiles. If Emerson soared above the clouds, fulminating figures of speech and colorful generalizations, Smiles, with both feet on the ground, armed with hundreds of picked illustrations, fought his point with the ammunition supplied by the men who made history. If Emerson was exhibiting a precious opal which he masterfully turned slowly at all angles so as to disclose all its variegated shades, Smiles may be said to have with deft hand gathered together on a string a beautiful array of multicolored beads. As a treatise on character Smiles's book would not take precedence over the many scores of similar exhortative works on the subject. It is the fact that its author had been able to live in spirit with great characters, which renders his message so inspiring; although, shorn of its illustrative material, it could scarcely have the power to command a careful reading beyond a narrow circle. Smiles preaches self-control, forbearance, truthfulness, and the rest of the catalogue of virtues so well-known and so ill-practised, but he gives no enlightenment on the crux of the subject, that is to say, no delimitation of the concept, no particularized treatment.

The best way to illustrate my meaning in denying Smiles scientific status or the gift of searching analysis, and at the same time crediting his contribution with a superior quality not discoverable in other works of this kind, is to cite two typical passages from the book in question, which will also serve to throw into relief his conception of character :

" Character exhibits itself in conduct, guided and inspired by principle, integrity, and practical wisdom. In its highest form, it is the individual will acting energetically under the influence of religion, morality, and reason. It chooses its way considerately, and pursues it steadfastly; esteeming duty above reputation, and the approval of conscience more than the world's praise. While respecting the personality of others, it preserves its own individuality and independence; and has the courage to be morally honest, though it may be unpopular, trusting tranquilly to time and experience for recognition.

" Although the force of example will always exercise great influence upon the formation of character, the self-originating and sustaining force of one's own spirit must be the mainstay. This alone can hold up the life, and give individual independence and energy. ' Unless man can erect himself above himself,' said Daniel, a poet of the Elizabethan era, ' how poor a thing is man ! ' Without a certain degree of practical efficient force—compounded of will, which is the root, and wisdom, which is the stem of character—life will be indefinite and purposeless—like a body of stagnant water, instead of a running stream doing useful work and keeping the machinery of a district in motion.

" When the elements of character are brought into action by determinate will, and, influenced by high purpose, man enters upon and courageously perseveres in the path of duty; at whatever cost of worldly interest, he may be said to approach the summit of his being. He then exhibits character in its most intrepid form, and embodies the highest idea of manliness. The acts of such a man become repeated in the life and action of others. His very words live and become actions."

The second passage accentuates even more markedly the nucleus of independence, spontaneity and steadfastness. " Energy of will—self-originating force—is the soul of every great character. Where it is, there is life ; where it is not, there is faintness, helplessness, and despondency. ' The strong man and the waterfall,' says the proverb, ' channel their own path.' The energetic leader of noble spirit not only wins a way for himself, but carries others with him. His every act has a personal significance, indicating vigor, independence, and self-reliance, and unconsciously commands respect, admiration, and homage. Such intrepidity of character characterized Luther, Cromwell, Washington, Pitt, Wellington, and all great leaders of men."

Concept not Delimited. For all that, one feels that

character, as here described, still remains a transcendental something which, curiously enough, is fraught with meaning for the well-bred layman but lacks the psychological background or antecedents. We fail to see how it emerged as a whole, what it includes, and what it may dispense with. Writers of Smiles's type build character up out of virtues, but if the concept is to have any application at all we must look for its genesis in instincts, emotions, sentiments, and ideas. To induce striving in the individual, the inspirational method is useful, but it will not bear examination when our aim is to make evaluations that demand objectivity.

Is there then no centre of gravity discoverable in the inspirational accounts of character ? one may ask in disappointment. The answer is that much will depend on the author, but if we were to pool the weighty particles of each of these treatments, we should probably find that the main emphasis is laid on what would now be called " carrying on " in spite of external obstacles. Perseverance and courage might be regarded as the boundary lines of this essential.

Whipple as Protagonist of Perseverance. This is a dominant idea of Whipple's *Character and Characteristic Men*, which both in thought and style may easily be mistaken for some of Emerson's essays. Though Whipple seldom rose to the conceptual heights of his greater contemporary, this undeservedly forgotten author has said many things more eloquently, if less dispassionately, than the Concord sage. " Character," writes Whipple, " whether it be small or great, evil or good, thus always represents a positive and persisting force and can therefore like other forces be *calculated*, and the issues of its action be predicted. There is nothing really capricious in character to a man gifted with the true piercing insight into it." In an earlier passage, the emphasis on persistence appears even in bolder form. " Character, in its intrinsic nature, being thus the embodiment of things in persons, the quality which most distinguishes

men of character from men of passions and opinions is
persistency, tenacity of hold upon their work and power to
continue in it. This quality is the measure of the force inherent
in character and is the secret of the confidence men place in
it—soldiers in generals, parties in leaders, people in statesmen.
Indeed if we sharply scrutinize the lives of persons eminent
in any department of action or meditation, we shall find
that it is not so much brilliancy and fertility as constancy and
continuousness of effort which make a man great. . . . The
universal line of distinction between the strong and the weak
is that one persists, the other hesitates, falters, trifles, and at
last collapses or ' caves in ' ".

Foster's Emphasis on Decision. *Determination* is the
Leitmotif of John Foster's *Essay on Decision of Character*,
written more than a century ago ; and it is noteworthy that
this pulpit preacher has offered some suggestions on the
constitutional requirements of a decisive character which
were hardly to be expected from his quarter. In the second
letter of his essay, he remarks, " The action of strong character
seems to demand something firm in its corporeal basis, as
massive engines require, for their weight and for their working,
to be fixed on a solid foundation. Accordingly I believe it
would be found that a majority of the persons most remarkable
for decisive character have possessed great constitutional
firmness." Introducing the analogy of the lion in comparison
with other beasts as to determination of action, Foster concludes that " A very decisive man has probably more of the
physical quality of a *lion* in his composition than other men ".
The less inflexibility of character in women the author ascribes
to the less firm " corporeal texture " of their physique, and
the individual differences in the determination of men are
similarly explained on the strength of this physical quality,
which, however, may be compensated for in the case of
" resolute spirits asserting themselves in feeble vehicles "
by a combination of other requisites.

It would be paradoxical to mention Schopenhauer's several essays on character and allied topics under the head of inspirational literature. Yet his maxims and views on life contain much more that is to the point than many of the exhortative commonplaces with which the inspirational literature teems. But more of Schopenhauer in its proper place.

III. CASUAL OBSERVATIONS ON CHARACTER

Aside from the direct discussions of character in their own right, there are countless incidental expressions with some bearing on our topic. To list even a small fraction of these utterances would be setting ourselves a preposterous task. At most then only a few samples could be cited so as to show how literary men of all ages and countries have at one time or another ruminated on character and character differentiation, and how the results of their excogitations might offer a foothold for further inquiry.

Bacon's Remarkable Aperçus. Francis Bacon was not only the first to broach the critical study of character but has bequeathed to the world some exquisite ideas expressed in his characteristically felicitous style. That his counsel was more salutary than his actions were consistent with his own precepts should not detract from the value of his extraordinary insight into the nature of man.

It would hardly be an exaggeration to place this versatile genius in the forefront of sages of all time, as a perusal of the *Advancement of Learning* would go far to prove. This work bristles with keen observations on human characteristics, wreathed in the florilegia of ancient authors both classical and biblical. It is, however, not my purpose to list them all, but rather to select a few of the more important dicta which may profitably be ruminated by students of character. It is among the aphorisms which Bacon culls from Proverbs and Ecclesiastes and illustrates by way of commentary that some of these interesting gleanings are to be found. Here is stated, for instance, that men may be known in six different ways, viz., by (1) their countenances; (2) their words; (3) their actions; (4) their tempers; (5) their ends; and (6) their relation to others. The surest key for unravelling the secrets of others, he holds, is to search either their tempers or their designs; the former he recommends when dealing with the weak and simple, and the latter, if probing the more prudent and close.

" It is surprising yet very true," says this author in another place, " that many have the logical part of their mind set right and the mathematical [1] wrong, and judge truly of the consequences of things but very unskilfully of their value." Here he approaches tangentially the territory later to be traversed by the school of Dilthey and other representatives of the *Geisteswissenchaften* who look upon character as essentially an expression of one's *Lebensverfassung* (life-plan), one's value-emphasis in life. Thus Bacon explains his profound utterance in the following words : " Hence some men are fond of access to and familiarity with princes ; others of popular fame, and fancy these to be great enjoyments. Others again measure things according to the labor bestowed in procuring them, imaging themselves to have advanced as far as they have moved." And further he warns those who, by misapprehending the true order of their ambitions, " frequently err and hasten to the end when they should only have consulted the beginning and, suddenly flying at the greatest things of all, rashly skip over those in the middle. . . ." [2]

Character of Kings. Let us now cite his commentary on the verse from Proverbs which reads " A man diligent in his business shall stand before kings, and not be ranked among the vulgar ". I shall not enter into the Chancellor's exegetical

---

[1] He might rather have used the word " ethical " here, but Bacon moved in a sphere of expediency and hardly in an ethical universe of discourse.

[2] F. Bacon : *Advancement of Learning*, Book VIII, chap. II.

ability to invest an ordinary exhortation with undue significance. This interpretation, however, is the occasion for revealing a bit of human nature, and by reason of Bacon's situation, bears the authority of an expert. The aphorism, as our author styles it, is represented as intimating that of all virtues which kings appreciate in their servitors, that of expedition and resolution in the despatch of business is the most readily appreciated. Men of depth are suspected of scrutinizing them too closely, and of " being able by their strength of capacity . . . to turn and wind them against their will and without their knowledge. Popular men are hated as standing in the light of kings. . . . Men of courage are generally esteemed turbulent and too enterprising. Honest and just men are accounted morose and not compliable enough to the will of their masters." So that no virtue is so acceptable as that of despatch in executing orders. " Besides," adds Bacon, " the motions of the minds of kings are swift and impatient of delay ; for they think themselves able to effect anything and imagine that nothing more is wanting but to have it done instantly."

Lastly, attention may be directed to the same author's epigram that " grave, solemn and unchangeable natures generally meet with more respect than felicity ". This attribute he regards as a defect often innate, but sometimes acquired by habit or " from an opinion which steals into men's minds, that they should never change the method of acting they had once found good and prosperous ".

Goethe's Pronouncements. Enough has been said about character shaping destiny and rising above circumstance ; so that we can afford to overlook such preachments, even when coming from such a mind as Carlyle's. But when Goethe says " We cannot escape a contradiction in ourselves ; we must try to resolve it ", it is our business to study his meaning and bring it in harmony with the modern doctrines of conflict. Again we must ask ourselves whether he is justified in his belief that

" men's prejudices rest upon their character for the time being and cannot be overcome, as being part and parcel of themselves. Neither evidence nor common sense nor reason has the slightest influence upon them." Sometimes Goethe manifests himself in the light of a pure-dyed idealist as when he eloquently declares : " To live in a great idea means to treat the impossible as though it were possible. It is just the same with a strong character ; and when an idea and a character meet, things arise which fill the world with wonder for thousands of years ", and in the motto " Character calls forth character ". Like a true individualist, he makes a sharp qualitative distinction between the masses and the towering *élite*. " It is failings that show human nature and merits that distinguish the individual ; faults and misfortunes we have in common, virtues belong to each one separately "— a notion which in some form or another has been entertained by more than one writer both before the great German poet and after him.

We need not, however, accept Goethe as an oracle. It is for instance an impression of his that " rough warriors . . . remain true to their character, and as great strength is usually the cover for good nature, we get on with them at need ". At this generalization we can simply shrug our shoulders. Similarly his view that a man does not mind being blamed for his faults, so long as he is not required to give them up, is one of these questionable rules which our present-day methods would not countenance. In one place, Goethe implies that there is an incompatibility between character and good manners, and in another he contends that " characters often make a law of their failings. The weak often have revolutionary sentiments ; they think they would be well off if they were not ruled, and fail to perceive that they can rule neither themselves nor others ".

British Essayists on Character. Similar disputable comments on life and character are met with in Jean Paul and

Lichtenberg, in many of Schiller's dramas, and other German works, but for informal utterances bordering on modern psychology we have to search far to excel the common sense and perspicacious observations interspersed among the British essayists from Samuel Johnson to Macaulay, who often would draw on a text from the classics. Thus the former cites Cicero (" Tully ") as the author of the remark that " every man has two characters ; one which he partakes with all mankind, and by which he is distinguished from brute animals ; another which discriminates him from the rest of his own species and impresses on him a manner and temper peculiar to himself ", and Cicero enjoins us to cultivate and preserve this character provided it is not repugnant to society. On this text Johnson in the *Rambler* (No. CLXXIX) develops the view that " scarce any man becomes eminently disagreeable but by a departure from his real character, and an attempt at something for which nature or education have left him unqualified ".

Macaulay Adumbrates Most Recent Psychological Doctrine. One would hardly expect to find psychological material in Macaulay's essays, his scientific inclinations being altogether absorbed by his literary and historical interests ; yet how much food for thought is contained in this passage from his *Madame D'Arblay*, and how close to the concept of integration he comes in the last sentence. Indeed the two paragraphs read as if they might have been quoted from Galton's works.

" There is in one respect a remarkable analogy between the faces and the minds of men. No two faces are alike ; and yet very few faces deviate very widely from the common standard. . . . An infinite number of varieties lies between limits which are not very far asunder. The specimens which pass those limits on either side form a very small minority.

" It is the same with the characters of men. Here too the variety passes all enumeration. But the cases in which the deviation from the common standard is striking and grotesque are very few. In one mind avarice predominates ; in another pride, in a third love of pleasure, just as in one countenance the nose is the most marked feature while in others the chief expression lies in the brow or in the lines of the mouth.   But there are very few countenances in which nose, brow and mouth do not contribute, though in unequal degrees, to the general effect ;   and so there are very few characters in which one overgrown propensity makes all others utterly insignificant."

The keenness of the famous English man of letters in this somewhat foreign sphere is extraordinary, for not only has he anticipated Shand's discussion on the influence of one exaggerated sentiment on all the rest, but in some measure he foreshadows the fundamental doctrine of the *Gestalt* school, which is all the more remarkable because his countrymen are given to atomizing qualities and elements, and associating them without taking into account sufficiently the dominant influence of some one on the rest so as to change the complexion of the whole.

We need not draw out this chapter any longer, fascinating as the material may be.   Enough has been quoted to show that both in the popular mind and in the estimation of inspirational writers, the qualities of fixity, persistence and independence are most closely connected with the concept of character. There is no disagreement between such a view and the more technical treatment.   The difference consists rather in the fact that while the latter at least makes an attempt at analysis, the former is content to emphasize now one trait, now another, without telling us how the fundamental traits of character are related, and on what ground they are held to be fundamental, except that they lead to success in life.

CHAPTER VIII

CRITICAL APPROACH TO THE STUDY OF CHARACTER

The first, at any rate modern, writer to direct attention to the baneful neglect of the study of character appears to be the Chancellor philosopher, who for a long time held such an exalted place in the history of philosophy on account of his progressive ideas. After all, it takes a practical mind to discern that there is such a problem as cataloguing individuals, though as in his other innovations, he was able to suggest new lines of thought without actually possessing the genius necessary for making genuine discoveries, or even following up a single method to its fruitful completion. That Bacon's plea should have remained in his generation and century a *vox clamantis in deserto* is not in the least surprising, but that it should have had no echo till the middle of the last century, when his intellectual descendant, the younger Mill, mapped out the field anew, is indeed a matter for astonishment.

Bacon's First Scientific Project. "So then the first article of this knowledge," writes Bacon, "is to set down sound and true distributions, and descriptions of the several characters and tempers of men's natures and dispositions, specially having regard to those differences which are most radical, in being the fountains and causes of the rest, or most frequent in concurrence or commixture, wherein it is not the handling of a few of them in passage, the better to describe the mediocrities of virtue, that can satisfy this intention ; for if it deserve to be considered, ' that there are minds which are proportioned to great matters, and others to small,' which Aristotle handleth or ought to have handled by the name of magnanimity, doth it not deserve as well to be considered, ' that there are minds proportioned to intend many matters, and others to few ? ' So that some can divide themselves, others can perchance do exactly well, but it must be but a few things at once ; and so there cometh to be a narrowness of mind, as well as a pusillanimity. And again, ' That some minds are proportioned to that which may be dispatched at once, or within a short return of time ; others to that which begins afar off, and is to be won with length of pursuit.' . . . So that there may be fitly said to be a longanimity, which is commonly ascribed to God, as a magnanimity. So farther deserved it to be considered by Aristotle, ' That there is a disposition in conversation, supposing it in things which do in no sort touch or concern a man's self, to sooth and please ; and a disposition contrary to contradict and cross' ; and deserveth it not much better to be considered, ' that there is a disposition, not in conversation or talk, but in matter of more serious nature, and supposing it still in things merely indifferent, to take pleasure in the good of another, and a disposition contrariwise, to take distaste at the good of another ' ; which is that properly which we call good-nature or ill-nature, benignity or malignity. And therefore I cannot sufficiently marvel, that this part of knowledge, touching the several characters of natures and dispositions, should be omitted both in morality and policy, considering it is of so great ministry and suppeditation to them both. A man shall find in the traditions of astrology some pretty and apt divisions of men's natures, according to the predominances of the planets ; lovers of quiet, lovers of action, lovers of victory, lovers of honour, lovers of pleasure, lovers of art, lovers of change and so forth. A man shall find in the wisest sort of these relations, which the Italians make touching conclaves, the natures of the several cardinals handsomely and lively painted forth ; man shall meet with, in every day's conference, the denominations of sensitive, dry, formal, real, humourous, certain, ' huomo di prima impressione, huomo di ultima impressione,' and the like : and yet nevertheless this kind of observations wandereth in words, but is not fixed in inquiry. For the distinctions are found, many of them, but we conclude no precepts upon them : wherein our fault is the greater, because both history poesy and daily experience, are as goodly fields where these observations grow : whereof we make a few poesies to hold in our hands but no man bringeth them to the confectionary, that receipts might be made of them for the use of life." [1]

But Bacon is keen not only in realizing the possibilities of inborn character but in anticipating also the many influences which are at work in altering the original nature of man such as : " those impressions of nature, which are imposed upon the mind by the sex, by the age, by the region, by health and sickness, by beauty and deformity, and the like, which are inherent, and not extern ; and again, those which are caused by extern fortune ; as sovereignty, nobility, obscure birth, riches, want, magistracy, privateness, prosperity, adversity, constant fortune, variable fortune, rising *per saltum per gradus*, and the like."

Rousseau. Among the early inquirers into the subject of differences in the mental and moral make-up of man from a modern angle is Jean Jacques Rousseau who, through his *Émile* and *La Nouvelle Héloise*, opened up new vistas for pedagogy and has led the way to the numerous educational reforms which have been subsequently inaugurated. Rousseau, as is well-known, was one of the staunchest supporters of the " environmentalist " view. " All characters," he makes Madame de Wolmar say in his *La Nouvelle Héloise*, " are in themselves good and sound." It was this thinker's belief that temperament is a quality we are born with, and that it determines genius and character. Like Fourier, a century later, who made application of the same principle on a gigantic scale, Rousseau thought that in the better order of things,

---

[1] F. Bacon : *Advancement of Learning*, Book VII, chap. 3.

every man would have his assigned place, and that it was only a question of finding this place. None so bad in this world that his talents and traits could not be put to good use. We shall see presently how Fourier is more articulate on this question.

For the most part, however, the issue which Rousseau argues back and forth is that of the changeability of character ; and the burden of his discussion seems to be this : that we must treat each individual separately in order to bring out all the good that is in him. Rousseau's object is to mould public opinion in the interests of individual differences, and his particular slant is pedagogic and moral.

Mill's Ethology. It was not really till J. S. Mill wrote his *Logic* (1843) that an attempt was made to find a place for a science of character in the scheme of sciences and subject to the principles of methodology. It was Mill who, like Kant, with regard to metaphysics, asked the question : How is a science of character possible ? But it cannot be said that he contributed much in the way of furthering our knowledge about character, thus reminding us in this respect of Francis Bacon, who, with all his programmes for discoveries, was not able to bring out a single new scientific result.

Nevertheless it remains true that Mill gave the proper direction to the inquiry and has raised the subject from a dogmatic side issue to a critical study, even if he has surrounded it with an ethical rather than a psychological atmosphere.

In the Sixth Book of his *Logic*, Mill asks : " Are the laws of the formation of character susceptible of a satisfactory investigation by the method of experimentation ? " And he answers this in the negative. Still less weight does he lay on the method of observation in this connection, for, says he, " There is hardly any person living concerning some essential part of whose character there are not differences of opinion even among his intimate acquaintances."

Yet these various drawbacks do not prevent Mill from

outlining the plan of his new science of character which he calls "Ethology". "The progress of this important but most imperfect science," says Mill towards the end of the chapter, "will depend on a double process : first, that of deducing theoretically the ethological consequences of particular circumstances of position and comparing them with recognized results of common experience and secondly the reverse operation : increased study of the various types of human nature that are to be found in the world ; conducted by persons not only capable of analyzing and recording the circumstances in which these types prevail, but also sufficiently acquainted with psychological laws to be able to explain and account for the characteristics of the type, by the peculiarities of the circumstances, the residuum alone, when there proves to be any, being set down to the account of congenital dispositions." [1]

This passage is cited not merely to provide an historical background, but to show in what way the so-called science of characterology has sprung up, and how its motive force was primarily ethical.

Galton's Anthropological Method. An anthropological impulse was lent the proposed science when Galton, several decades later, addressed the British Association for the Advancement of Science (Biological Section, Department of Anthropology) submitting this message :

" I propose to speak of the study of these groups of men who are sufficiently similar in their mental characters or in their physiognomy or in both to admit of classification ; and I especially desire to show that many methods exist of pursuing the inquiry in a strictly scientific manner, although it has hitherto been too often conducted with extreme laxity.

" The types of character of which I speak are such as those described by Theophrastus, La Bruyère, and others, or such as may be read of in ordinary literature and are universally

---

[1] J. S. Mill : *A System of Logic*, Book VI, chap. v.

M

recognized as being exceedingly true to nature. There are no worthier professors of this branch of anthropology than the writers of the higher works of fiction who are ever on the watch to discriminate varieties of character, and who have the art of describing them." [1]

But in developing his main idea in this presidential address, he strayed from the subject, as we understand it to-day, and instead, spoke of the personal equation in reaction time, of the traits of criminals, of the desirability of employing "photography to obtain careful studies of the head and features" and of certain phases of what was afterwards to be called eugenics. Galton certainly pushed ahead until the various inquiries which he mentioned were established on a firm footing. The individual measurements which he refers to again and again, in this paper, were to form afterwards the branch of differential psychology which Stern had done so much to systematize, but the study of character received little benefit from Galton's gigantic labors. In fact it is doubtful whether this pioneer had fully grasped Mill's problem, which by the way he does not allude to. It seems as if he did not take the trouble to differentiate between intelligence and character, lumping under the latter head everything with regard to which individuals might differ from one another—intelligence, reactive functions, temperament, and even physical qualities.

Le Bon Stresses the Unconscious. It was at this time that the polyhistoric Le Bon also took a hand in the attempt to consolidate our knowledge about character.[2] True, he came to his task inadequately prepared, hinting that he would some day publish his work on this subject, in which his count-less observations would be incorporated—an unredeemed promise by the way—nevertheless it would not be out of

---

[1] F. Galton : *Nature*, 1877, vol. xvi, pp. 344–5.

[2] G. Le Bon : " Notes sur l'étude du caractère " : *Revue Philos.*, 1877, vol. iv, p. 509.

place to summarize here the contents of Le Bon's article. Any one who is at all acquainted with this author's general outlook would naturally expect to find Le Bon's stress on the non-rational factors of man reflected in this short study. Character to him is the result of association of feelings and ideas; and the changeability of one's character is explained by the variability of the elements which go to make up the self.

Le Bon, I believe, takes his place as a forerunner of the psychoanalytic movement in the weight which he has attached to the unconscious; and in that very article, he dwells on the tendency to rationalize. "When such individuals as the one I have just cited are intelligent— as is frequently the case—they generally imagine that they possess fine judgment, good logic, and always end by finding reasons for justifying in their own eyes their constant changes, which furthermore they take the greatest pains to dissimulate, and are pretty soon convinced that these changes are the result of their reflections and will."

Since, however, he admits that with all the chance possible, there is still a permanent core, he would have us look for this nucleus of stability by noting the forms of expression as well as the physiognomical and physiological details which distinguish one person from another. Phrenology he discards, yet his remarks on the significance of the shape of the head, with specifications of certain prominences correlating with particular traits and abilities, place him almost in a class with those he repudiates.

Le Bon's paper is not a contribution, but it represents a link in the chain of French writers who usually have underestimated the vastness of the field. And does not the fact that we miss among his numerous works an extensive study of character, suggest that Le Bon bethought himself of the enormous task, and turned his attention to more promising labors?

Mill's Influence. Mill's advocacy of ethology has, besides influencing such men as Bain and Shand, occasioned a number of writers to make enthusiastic claims for the subject. It goes almost without saying that not a single one of these writers has advanced the projected science beyond the stage where Mill has left it, viz. the embryonic stage. T. J. Bailey, to take one instance, under the promising title " *Ethology*: *Standpoint, Method, Tentative Results*", makes an attempt to link certain traits and qualities in a rather complicated manner, which is not simplified by the accompanying diagram, and finally has to admit that his sketch is " hopelessly incomplete and the most valuable technical features of the work have not even been mentioned ".[1]

One may readily anticipate that Mill's view would receive a rebuff in certain quarters, and this quotation from Ward is representative of the negative position which many British philosophers and psychologists took up toward Mill's scheme. " We may safely count it as one of the curiosities of speculation that an empiricist of so extreme a type as Mill, who cannot be sure that there is not a world somewhere where two plus two equals five, and a world, if so we may call it, somewhere else, in which causes have no place, should yet believe in the possibility of an *a priori* science of character that can deduce universal laws from the truths of psychology, originally ascertained, as he insists they must be, from observation and experiment." [2]

Study Helped by Individual Psychology. It is perhaps the growth of individual and variational psychology that has given the final turn to the study as we have it to-day. The positivistic tendency of the eighteenth and partly of the nineteenth century has been to slur over individual differences

---

[1] T. J. Bailey : " University Chronicles," *University of California Publications*, 1899, vol. ii, p. 31.

[2] J. Ward : " J. S. Mill's Science of Ethology," *International Journal of Ethics*, 1890–91, vol. i, p. 458.

either as anomalies or as contingent and irrelevant matter. The *principles* of human nature constituted the desideratum of the positivists. It was the *genus homo* with which they were concerned, and not particular men.

But even in its most recent stage the subject has still its drawbacks. In the first place, as Mill has observed, it is a field where experimentation is footless. Even Ach's conclusions with regard to temperament are not derived in strict empirical fashion, and it is only by courtesy that that part of his book *Über den Willensakt und das Temperament* can be called experimental.

In the second place, character and temperament have been so interlocked in their ordinary usage and more popular treatment in literature that confusion of the two terms is almost invariably the result. It is easy to mistake the one for the other, as in either case a particular combination of traits is referred to, and sometimes, indeed, it is difficult to draw a demarcation line between the one and the other. In ordinary life we know what is meant by either of the words, but when we come to pick out the principle of the difference, we are at a loss.

Popular Distinction. In the language of the street, character is often applied when speaking of more or less distinguished men, while temperament of one sort or another is something everybody is supposed to have without exception. Temperament is used in a more democratic sense and serves a social purpose, whereas character sets off the individual as a force by himself.

It is temperament which affects one's close relatives. The influence of character has a farther reach, and is appreciated not so much by brothers or sisters, parents or wife, when a man is great, as by associates, subordinates and the world at large. The value of an individual's character does not depreciate with the lapse of ages ; his temperament is merely a matter of interest. Little is known of Giordano

Bruno's temperament or disposition except that he was melancholic ; his character stands out in bold relief on the pages of history. That Carlyle was bilious, choleric, or grouchy is certainly deplorable, but Carlyle's temperament, which counted so much with those he came in contact with, does not determine our estimate of the man from the point of view of character.

Possibly the German view of associating temperament with the affective side of man and character with the volitional aspect will account for the ordinary usage of the two terms. We may remember how Kant made the will fundamental in ethics when he said " There is nothing in the world unconditionally good except a good will ". Although the method of approaching our problem has changed considerably since antiquity, there is but little difference in our conception of what really character or temperament is. Many writers still go on pointing out that character etymologically means " an engraven mark ", and that temperament is merely a technical term for a mixture or blend. This suggests, at least, that the general notion of character and temperament is the same as it was two thousand years ago. Even in the most recent works, the classification of temperaments is brought in accord with the time-honoured table of Galen, who conceived his scheme on a metaphysiological basis.

Character as Characteristic. But let us here confine ourselves to the examination of character. It is precisely because character originally meant a distinguishing mark that it has been regarded by some writers as synonymous with characteristic in the biological sense. Galton in his *Inquiries into Human Faculty* treats of character in this rather miscellaneous sense [1] in a brief and but superficial

---

[1] Klages in his *Prinzipien der Charakterologie* (third edition, p. 17) points out that there are at least three senses in which the word is used, the broadest of which practically coincides with the word " quality or property ", the other two answering practically to the English words

essay which concludes with the injunction that schoolmasters, since they have a splendid opportunity of studying the character of school children, should not neglect making such observations.   Otto Weininger's somewhat distorted account of character in his book *Sex and Character* may be cited as an exaggerated form of this tendency.   According to this book, which both through its sensational claims and the morbid life and dramatic death of its youthful author has received a wide circulation, there are two principles in life, the male and the female,[1] or, what is to him practically the same division, the Aryan and the Jewish.   All characters partake of the two principles in varying proportions, there being very few individuals who are entirely masculine or entirely Aryan, or who, starting out as ordinary mortals, contaminated with the other principle, have been able to conquer their femininity and rise to the pure stage of masculinity and Aryanism.

Dichotomies Galore.   The dichotomous division, which is the simplest form of classification, serves a useful purpose in science as a starting point.   In this way it has a heuristic value.

" personality " and " moral character ".   He supposes that the circumstance is due to an animistic tendency hanging over from prehistoric days.   It seems, however, just as likely that the concept " character " originally connoting a distinguishing mark, was deepened in the course of time so as to designate the individual stamp of a person.   The savage's notion of character differs very much from that of an educated person.

[1] The doctrine of bi-sexuality which afterwards was incorporated in psychoanalysis, particularly in Stekel's system, had really germinated in the mind of Fliess, who published his important work, *Der Ablauf des Lebens*, in 1906.   As Wittels relates in his *Sigmund Freud* (pp. 102–103), the master of psychoanalysis " must have divulged various things which Fliess had told him in confidence ", among these being the theory of cellular bi-sexuality, of which Weininger had learned, through a friend who was a patient of Freud's.   Whether Weininger actually profited by Freud's loquaciousness or not, the latter's indiscretion, according to Wittels, led to the subsequent rupture between Freud and Fliess.

In our particular instance, it is not difficult to see its origin. We are constantly seeing things in light and shade, we think in contrasts, and we recognize other people as different from ourselves, or what amounts to the same thing, we know ourselves through other people. And so we eventually come to learn of the two different types of people under various headings. You may call them the men of thought and the men of action, or spiritual and worldly, or you may talk of them as the intellectual type and the "red-blood"; all these divisions are only another way of observing the fact that there are differences between men, that are recognized by the common people as well as by the special students along this line.

In the picturesque language of Jastrow: "The contrast persists: aristocrat and philistine, gentleman and vulgarian, Bromide and Sulphite, Athenian and Bœotian, are but different portrait titles for the same sitters, portrayed by different artists, with distinctive expressions and properties." [1]

In addition to the cognate categories which Jastrow has brought together, we may even accept the further divisions of H. G. Wells into poietic and kinetic, of James into tender-minded and tough-minded, of Jung into introverted and extraverted, or still further, the more technical classification of J. M. Baldwin into sensory and motor types, although here we are approaching the intelligence range rather than the field of character and temperament.

Yet in spite of this first clue that we got through experience and race intuition, we are still at sea as to a satisfactory basis for a classification of characters. In the course of this essay we shall see how most classifications are either arbitrary or simply logical; at any rate, not psychological; and, upon closer examination, the main obstacle seems to be that we have reached no agreement as to the essentials of character.

[1] J. Jastrow: *Qualities of Men*, p. 59.

Indefiniteness of Term. " It is a disposition of the will,"
says Wundt ; and this is the note struck by the German
school in general, with Meumann as one of its foremost
exponents. " It is the power to keep the selected motive
dominant throughout life," is the view of Münsterberg
(*Psychology General and Applied*). " Character is the system
of directed conative tendencies," says McDougall (*Outline
of Psychology*). " Character is life in action," according to
Jastrow, which is a good metaphor but not a practical guide.

Life *versus* Abstractions. Shall we accept the statement
that " Character is the power to keep the selected motive
dominant ? " Münsterberg is careful enough to add that the
motives may be egoistic as well as altruistic, and that they
may serve an ignoble as well as a noble end. But does such
a view of character tell the whole story, and, above all,
can it satisfy our inmost and firmest convictions ? We
shall remember that, in an earlier part of this book, the plea
was to the effect that character is a subject taken from
life and is to be handled in life. In cases of doubt, then,
our life attitude must be the judge and decide, or else our whole
problem will be artificially decked out with borrowed
ornaments. Is it not, after all, the character of our daily
social intercourse that we are studying and not an abstraction
that has no place in the universe of our daily conduct ?

Character and principle must by all means go together.
since we regard them as inseparable in our everyday
judgments. The burglar and the mountebank have dominant
motives ; yet we should not ascribe to them that quality
called character. If we do call them disreputable characters
or if we *do* say that a certain criminal is quite a character
in the underworld, it is evident that we are using the word
in a derived sense.

Caligula and Nero and, indeed, anybody who is obsessed
by some *idée fixe* all through his life, can certainly keep his
selected motive dominant if he is powerful enough, but we do

not as a rule think of them as possessing character. A dog may be said to have as his dominant motive in life bone-gnawing in much the same way, and yet we should be chary of endowing the dog with character in its significant sense.

The contention in this presentation is that the predominance of a certain motive is inadequate. A substantial modification or amendment is suggested, viz., that the impulses of the *will must be controlled and checked by certain inhibitions* that are evoked by the intellectual and moral make-up of man. Character thus arises from an interplay between the disposition of the will and that of the intellect.

Dominant Motive Inessential. The case of the great Italian statesman Cavour happens to occur to us and will furnish us a happy illustration of the view expressed here. Although Cavour was no more scrupulous a man than his vocation allowed, we do admire the firmness of his character not merely because he succeeded in keeping his selected motive uppermost, but because he was *actually guided by certain principles that he never flinched from*, though sometimes his resoluteness brought him into sharp conflict with higher authority. The strength of such characters lies in the fact that, even though they may realize themselves to be on the brink of downfall, they would not save the situation for themselves by doing something they thought was not in accordance with their sense of dignity.

That is why the character of a *Tartuffe* is so repulsive, although he of all persons is bent upon carrying out his conceived plans. Were it not for the fact that he is capable of causing so much mischief, the attitude toward him would be that we take toward a jelly fish. Nor does his whole outlook on life differ essentially from that of the lower animals. There is only this difference : the purpose of the former is explicit, articulate, while that of the latter is implicit, organic.

Far from the pursuit of any one fixed motive, *character*

rather presupposes the possibility of change as our range of experience grows wider and richer. A blind " will ", heedless of a controlling intelligence, would be as devoid of character as Schopenhauer's universal principle.

When we begin to examine the implications of such a view, it is perhaps possible for objectors to detect a *petitio principii* in it, since it might be said that the occurrence of scruples or inhibitions to the agent already presupposes character. In answer to this, it may be pointed out that the " pure will " theory fares no better, since one can easily urge that a person's will-power depends to some extent on his character, but, as is usually the case in such apparent circular procedures, the influence develops on a mutual basis as soon as the first impetus is given, and the same holds true of the inhibitions that lead to the establishment of a character, and that in their turn are engendered by the reaction of the personality to the environment. There are certain facts in life that take shape gradually in spite of the " either-or " method in logic, else no one should ever have learnt to swim, else instruments should never have come into being and the construction of tunnels should have been a physical impossibility.

Is Character a Reaction or the Cause of Reaction ? Friedmann [1] contends that we must have a scientific definition of " character " before we proceed any further, and he proposes the following one : " Character is a form-complex of reaction which keeps on recurring again and again and cannot be grasped as something general or inter-individual, but, nevertheless, appears as something typical among the most widely different constitutions."

Yet, curiously enough, toward the end of the article he tells us that we can *understand* those individuals only whose characters bear some quantitative relation to our own, but the question is : If character is merely a recurrent reaction,

[1] R. Friedmann: "Vorwort zur Charakterologie," *Arch. für die gesamte Psychol.*, 1913, vol. xxvii, p. 198.

then why need we understand the reagent any more than we need understand the earthworm ?   It seems that there is the confusion here of two points of view.   Either character is not merely a type of reaction, but is something more than that, viz. the outer aspect of personality, and thus the fountain-head of reactions, or else if it *is* a reaction complex, then it ought to be possible for us to study characters without having to live them as Friedmann requires.   Friedmann is evidently immersed in the same dilemma which confronts the behaviourists to-day, who eject introspection through the front door and take it in stealthily through the rear.

CHAPTER IX

It is not taking too much for granted to assume that every intelligent person knows what is meant by the terms character and temperament. In truth, however, there is a certain measure of latitude in the treatment at least of character, as had already been intimated. Before we proceed further then it seems necessary to discuss the various acceptations of the words, so as to avoid confusion in names.

Definition of Temperament. Since there is much less disagreement as regards temperament, we shall do well to begin with this concept. I think that one is safe in taking temperament to be the *sum total of one's affective qualities as they impress others.* If we cling to the traditional four temperaments, we may say that the melancholic person will react to the world with a sad undercurrent that perhaps, in the last analysis, takes its root in worry, which in turn is a species of fear. The connection between fear and mild depression is one which ought to be further examined.

The sanguine person, on the other hand, is dominated by affective states like hope, enthusiasm—not that he is immune from fits of depression in consequence of his having soared too high, but these are of short duration and less frequent than his buoyant states. The emotional stream of the sanguine person may be thought of as interrupted by depression only at the nodes, while the waves themselves are suffused with enthusiasm, expansiveness, self-elation.

The choleric temperament is clearly an affective constitution in which the anger response is touched off very easily. We may regard then the emotion of anger in various stages

155

and degrees as ruling the affective stream of the choleric by its frequent occurrence which is made possible through its instinctive mechanism, aggravated sometimes by acquired factors and environmental circumstances.

In the phlegmatic temperament, the emotional flow is regularly weak with no predominance of any one affective state. In other words, here it takes a stimulus of greater intensity to touch off fear, anger, grief, and joy; and when called forth, their expression is not very pronounced.

Neither intelligence nor volitional qualities enter into the temperamental make-up of a person; and on this point it is my impression that all are agreed. As to the number of temperaments, their physical or chemical basis, etc., we have seen what a labyrinth of theories has evolved in the course of centuries. But that need not detain us here.

Concept of Character Differently Understood. It is altogether different with the twin concept character. Here there are at least three divergent views. First of all, character may be understood in the broad sense comprising all qualities in regard to which human beings differ, intelligence traits included. Few writers take this extreme connotation. The next sense is that which makes character equivalent to personality minus the intelligence component. For most of the French psychologists character was synonymous with personality, and the tendency in the United States is to follow the same course. Hollingworth, who is representative of the American school, defines character as a "characteristic mode of human behaviour".[1]

Morton Prince has given expression to a similar view. To him character is the manifest or overt personality while "personality is the sum total of all the biological innate dispositions, impulses, tendencies, appetites, and instincts of the individual and of all the *acquired* dispositions and tendencies. It would seem then that the personality is the

[1] H. L. Hollingworth: *Judging Human Character*, p. 2.

reservoir of elements the integration of which, with emphasis on some or others, constitutes the formation of character. Hence the character of the one is said to be ' good-tempered ', the other ' bad-tempered '. Yet every normal personality will manifest anger in some situation." [1]

Latent and Overt Qualities in Personality. The objection to this view is that since people differ little as to the raw material or potential qualities, we should be led to suppose that differences in personality do not exist, or at least, are negligible. But, and here we might interpose our second objection at the same time, common sense tells us that personality counts a great deal, and we feel it to be just as much actual and overt as character, if not more so. Prince's distinction between the inscrutable, potential personality and its actual and observable phase is valid, but why call the latter character and reserve the term personality for that which furnishes only the raw material for personality, when the derivation of the word personality is clearly to be connected with the word which means a mask ? And certainly no one in conversation referring to personality has in mind the dormant or latent qualities, whose existence cannot be proven except through inference or in cases of pathological dissociation, as in the Beauchamp tangle. Again if the traits are knowable, then why relegate them to the potential level any more than other traits which are observable only under certain conditions ?

Characteristic in Sense of Significant. I find it difficult to subscribe to the definition of character as the characteristic mode of human behaviour on another ground. *Many are the modes of human behaviour which, though characteristic, are not significant.* Under character we should understand reactions or traits of paramount importance. The various idiosyncrasies, peculiarities and habits that are associated with different individuals while forming an integral part of the personality

[1] M. Prince : *The Unconscious*, p. 532.

are not generally regarded as entering into that complex which we call character. The manner in which a person holds his pen or pencil, his individual gait, his tendency to lisp, are characteristic, but what have they to do with character ?

Difference Between Man and Beast. Rather should we modify the definition so as to read that character is a *characteristic mode of human behaviour in that sphere which distinguishes man from animal.* In other words, it is a mode of behaviour in regard to that which is characteristically human. There is no psychological function which can be denied the lower animals, at least the primates, in some rudimentary form—not even thinking—save the ability to perform acts or refrain from them in accordance with rational principles, so as to come within the class of responsible beings. Animals have no doubt certain traits which may be adjudged desirable or not. The dog is faithful ; the fox is sly ; the elephant and the horse are said to be vindictive [1] and so on, but their traits partake more of fixed mechanisms and show very little variation. Character as applied to human beings permits of modification in keeping with the situation. But a better line of cleavage is to be seen in the fact that animals of one species are pretty much alike in their characteristic reactions. Human beings differ widely in any trait mentionable. It is for this reason that the signification of character should apply to that behavior sphere which chiefly divides man and beast. It is not intelligence, not the speech function, but the ability to be guided in action by a standard in the form of what will be later referred to as the principle of consistency. It is this possibility which bestows upon man alone the attribute of worth. The noblest animal does not possess it, and is no more a subject for the appraisal of character than a labor-saving machine.

This conclusion does not rest on religious or ethical considera-

[1] Azam begins his book *Le caractère dans la santé et dans la maladie,* with a chapter on the character of animals.

tions. Underlying it is rather a foundation of comparative psychology. No doubt it may serve the cause of ethics, but it is by no means dependent on this discipline.

Double Phase of Personality. In this book, I am taking the position that personality is the sum total of all our cognitive, affective, conative and even physical tendencies. The sum total here does not mean a simple addition but an integration. Now there are two modes of appraising personality, and we may therefore speak of two levels or phases of personality. As I have had occasion to write elsewhere " Most people are inclined to pay too much attention to the external manifestations of personality, such as charm, bearing, carriage and presence. In the long run, however, it is the invisible which counts. In biography, personality is represented, it seems to me, mainly by character and temperament traits. The principle governing our estimates of personality appears to be that the farther we are removed from an individual, the more do we concern ourselves with his internal personality and the less with his external qualities." [1]

What is usually referred to as personal magnetism is nothing more than an exceptionally pleasing externality, including a certain genial expression both of the countenance and the voice and perhaps even of gesture (grace, motor co-ordination, adroitness). It is evident that in due course the charm of these physical qualities wears off for the friend of long standing and the deeper or inner personality begins to stand out. It is therefore this phase of personality which should claim our attention rather than its superficial aspect.

Of course it ought to be recognized, too, that there are certain personality factors which, though dynamically effective, are not intuitively observable. They must be inferred after an elaborate analysis of the phenomena, as Morton Prince has done in his multiple personality studies. These latent yet

[1] A. A. Roback: *Psychology with Chapters on Character Analysis and Mental Measurement*, p. 19.

N

operative factors may be labelled the latent personality, and the study of the personality in its entirety would have to include these more or less hypothetical tendencies in its programme.

The terms temperament and personality having been disposed of, we shall now turn to the delimitation of the term character as required by our exposition, by way of supplementing what has already been said on this head earlier.

Character is that part of the personality which remains after the cognitive, affective, and physical qualities have been abstracted. Character, then, covers the volitional and inhibitory phases of behaviour ; and yet it is dependent on intelligence to a large extent, and is affected by temperament in some measure, or at least it bears some relationship to it.

Gauging an individual personality is no easy task because of the different standards involved, depending on the estimater. Sometimes a high abstract intelligence compensates for poor social sense or objectionable temperamental traits. At other times the so-called personal magnetism conceals an inferior character. But it is the whole picture, and not a stroke here and there which counts in our judgment of personality ; and as our judgment changes, we shall note that the character component is the most lasting and most significant determinant of the composite and cumulative judgment.

Significance of Character not in Morality. Yet character need not be envisaged in a moral sense. We do not prize the man of character because he is ethical, or because he conforms to conventions, or obeys the laws, or follows a code of honor, but because in order to carry out the law of nature as intended for man (not through Divine prearrangement but through the steady evolution of reason) he possesses the strength of inhibiting his individual tendencies ; without such inhibition that law which is embodied in evolution cannot be effective, but is broken, thereby contradicting the fact that man has reached the human level.

The possession of character, then, is the declaration that man has reached not only the reflective stage but the stage of control in co-ordination with this reflection. Differently expressed, the man of a high type or level of character is respected because he has overcome the average man's resistance—a difficult feat—in order to achieve a desirable result, not desirable perhaps for him individually but on general principle, and only through this channel desirable for him, and the more so the greater self-denial his act or restraint entails. As to what is desirable, this is a question of intelligence or rather intellect ; and no one can be dictated to in this respect, so long as he is consistent with himself and others at the same time, i.e., so long as he does not make one rule for himself and another for others, or, what is more apt to happen, act from desire, whether to the disadvantage of his fellows or not.

A Fundamental Thesis. Another point which may be anticipated in this chapter on fundamental concepts is the simple polarity of character which I hold against the general consensus that character is bi-modal, that is to say, that it permits of two varieties of categories, viz., good and bad on the one hand, and strong and weak on the other. It is supposed by all writers on the subject that a bandit or cruel ruler must necessarily have a strong yet mean character, while a man of good character may be weak-willed. This practically universal fallacy rests on inadequate analysis, and on the confusion between character and will on one side, and between character and morality on the other.

As for me, I can admit but one bi-furcation in character, call it good and bad, high and low, noble and base, or fine and poor. Character like intelligence proceeds in a linear direction ; and there is no reason why we should be able to apply the twofold series of attributes to character any more than to intelligence. High intelligence means strong intelligence also and low intelligence means in its more extreme stage feeblemindedness. Why should it be otherwise with character? The common belief that a bandit has a strong character reduces simply to the fact that he is more *reckless and apparently, therefore, inhibits the most vital instinctive tendency.* The so-called weak character cannot readily inhibit his instinctive mechanism, which touches off the fear emotion. It is all a matter of the *number and type of instinctive urges* which are inhibited. What seems to be responsible for the idea that some characters are strong but bad, while others are good but weak is the fact that certain combinations of qualities are apt to mislead the uncritical mind, The man of high character cannot be a weakling, for it is only by acting his part that his character co-efficient manifests itself, not through desiring or wishing or feeling benevolently inclined.

A Fallacy Exposed. There is a popular notion that strength of character is indicated by impetuosity, dash, mere stubbornness, recklessness, and lastly success. That is one reason why character has been invested with the attributes "strong-weak". As a matter of fact a gentle person who merely resists an unjust measure, even though seemingly without effectiveness, will show a higher character co-efficient than a Machiavellian politician.

In fine, then, the "strong character" either is a character of high type, what ordinarily might be called a good character, if this sense were not mixed up with morality and altruism, or else it is merely a superficial halo cast around a low type of character as a result of insufficient insight on the part of the judges, who mistake bullying, forceful behaviour, enterprise and allied traits for strength.

The more detailed treatment of this important question is deferred to a later chapter because of the material which must be first introduced as the basis of our doctrine of character.

PART II

CLASSIFICATION OF CHARACTERS

INTRODUCTORY

THE PROBLEM OF CLASSIFYING CLASSIFICATIONS

If every writer on character has had to cope with his special problem of how to classify human types, then the person wishing to present a survey of the different classifications is doubly at a loss ; for the possibilities of classification multiply as the subject is carefully gone into. So many methodological rules come forth with their claims that it is difficult to accept any one principle. Certainly the chronological method cannot appeal to us, although it is worth keeping in mind that chronological remoteness will of necessity result in essential differences of viewpoint. On the other hand, it would seem the proper thing to untangle the psychological issues involved in the various classifications and to group them accordingly, but the complexity of the process is too obvious to make this method practicable.

I have therefore decided to treat these classifications as national conceptions, not that they constitute ethnic points of view, but because it is more convenient to group them in this manner, and also for the reason that there is a convergence along national lines. All the French writers adopt a similar method. The Germans do not stick together so closely in their views, yet there are common ideas on the relation between character and temperament in most of their writings, for instance that temperament is the formal phase, and character is the content phase of the same thing, that temperament answers the question *how*, while character corresponds to the *quale* and points to the direction of an individual's inner nature. The French are *formalists* in that they seek to *combine* types by using simple formulae. The German writers on character are, on the whole, more analytic and endeavor to deduce *principles* which often, however, are too much encumbered by secondary considerations. The British, on the other hand, are inclined to develop character out of *affective atoms* with special emphasis on the *sentiments*. This legacy appears to have been handed down to the American investigators, who are interested more in individual traits than in character.

Whether we can speak of a French School or a German School of character is a question that need not seriously engage our attention. Let us speak of schools rather than of a school, and accept even this device as a fiction which is necessary for methodological reasons, though it may turn out to be sound on the strength of the presuppositions of ethnic psychology.

CHAPTER X

If I begin the part on classifications with the French schools, it is because more than a century ago, a Frenchman who was not primarily a psychologist, but is known rather for his endeavors to reform the social order, has given us the most original, and at the same time the most detailed, scheme of characterology that we have yet had. Charles Fourier's grasp of human relations and destinies was stupendous, almost cosmic in its reach, and the development of his thought most systematic; yet probably because of his erratic tendencies, which are evident in his writings at every turn, his name finds no place in psychological discussions, except for two pages devoted to him in Bain's book on character. It is true that Fourier's number-complex and fanciful analogies often make us wonder whether the man is not a reincarnation of some mediaeval mystic pottering with the Apocalypse, a cabalist of the fifth century. Nevertheless, when allowance is made for this fantastic streak in his make-up, and when his work *The Passions of the Human Soul* is read as a whole and not merely in snatches, one cannot help deciding that this genius, whose combination of uncritical dogmatizing and rare insight reminds us very much of his greater compatriot Pascal, was in many respects ahead of his time.

In order to do justice to Fourier's theory of character, one would first. have to define hundreds of terms which sound like gibberish. Of course it would be out of the question to do this, yet it is possible to present some idea of his views by mentioning only the salient points.

Chief Premise of His System. Fourier's psychological work is only a tool in his hands for the exposition of his social system, his thesis being that our civilization is corrupt, perverted and wicked.   In order to regain our original status and live as happy beings, we must enter the stage of harmony, which Fourier is outlining for us with all the eloquence and (sometimes inaccurate) erudition at his command.   For him the unit of harmony is not the individual or even the family. It is the *characterial community* ;   and herein he reveals himself the social psychologist of a high order.

Fourier combines in his writing the acumen to see through things—a quality which distinguishes most of the French social thinkers—with an extraordinary faculty for relating his observations under a tremendously ramified organization of ideas.   His utopian plans must often evoke a smile ;   for both his number obsessions and the fundamental thesis of his system, viz., that civilization has only perverted the works of God and defeated His purpose, are peculiar twists of his original mind which also seems to have been possessed of an extraordinary degree of synaesthesia.[1]

One might suppose that on account of his mystic and scholastic tendencies, this French philosopher is abstract to the point of being unintelligible.   The reverse is true. Once we grasp his terminology and follow his illustrations, only one or two of which are here reproduced owing to lack of space, his classifications, though faulty from the modern psychological viewpoint, appear anything but artificial, and social psychologists of to-day would do well to examine some of Fourier's contentions, born of his strictures against society.

---

[1] Fourier makes all sorts of parallels, analogies and correspondences between colors, tones, odors, and numbers in his search of identities in the universe.   The emblem of justice, for instance, is the tulip, that of truth is the lily.   Both justice and truth are the two elements of honor ; here Fourier shows himself true to the gallantry of his race.   The tulip excludes the two blues, azure, which is the color of the supremely unjust passion, viz., love, and indigo, the color of the cabalistic (i.e. the intriguing) spirit which in *our civilized order* is the enemy of justice.

Characterial Community. What then is Fourier's doctrine of the characterial community which is so bound up with the salvation of man ?

" Man in his bodily nature," remarks Fourier, " is composed of two individuals only, the one male, the other female," but that is not true of the passional sphere where there are all sorts of heterogeneity. " In some avarice predominates, in others prodigality ; one man is inclined to openness, to gentleness ; another to cheating, to cruelty, from which it is evident that the passional man or soul is by no means complete in a single couple like the material man, or the male and female body.

" It has already appeared, in the treatise on the industrial series, that a great number of individuals and inequalities, graduated in all directions, is required to form a harmony of passions. Let us admit provisionally that this necessary number consists of 810 different souls or characters, assembled in a proportion of about twenty-one males for twenty females, and distributed into sixteen tribes and thirty-two choirs ; the necessity of this distribution will be seen farther on.

Dominants and Tonics. " Each of the 810 characters is provided with the twelve radical passions, but more or less subject to the influence of one or of several : I call *dominant* the one that holds the rudder of a character. The dominant of the miser Harpagon is ambition, of which avarice is a shade or specific development. Therefore we shall say of Harpagon, that he has ambition for his dominant, that *ambition steers him*, that is to say, that it holds the rudder of his character.

" In the same way that there are a host of shades in each of the primary colors, red, blue, green, etc., so also each of the twelve radical passions has several shades or subdivisions. Ambition furnishes distinct branches, such as self-love and meanness, pride, suppleness, cupidity, the love of glory and of power, etc., etc. You may consequently assign to each radical passion a gamut of shades or of species that will, moreover, be subdivisible into varieties, whereof each presides over a character. It is not sufficient to say that such a character has for his dominant ambition, is a slave to his ambition; you must define what shade governs him, and this shade is the *tonic* passion. Thus Harpagon has for dominant, ambition; for tonic, avarice, which is a branch of ambition.

Monogynes Steered by One Dominant. " The gamuts of tonics are not regularly divided into twelve degrees. One passion may only furnish ten degrees to the gamut, another fifteen. Amongst the monogynes of taste, one man is for a special kind of good cheer, another for a particular kind of drink; thus two men may have taste for their dominant, and have very different tonics, like the gastronomer and the tippler. . . . A character may have several dominants; it may be steered at the same time by ambition and by love, so that in different junctures these two passions share the empire of his soul without a perceptible superiority, and without one of the dominants excluding the other. Some individuals have three and four dominants, and even more, with a like number of tonics.

" The characters with a single dominant are very numerous, and are considered in harmony as the *passional populace,* amounting to about 576 out of 810. Those with two dominants, under the name of *digynes*, are far less abundant; those of three, styled *trigynes,* are still less numerous; and so on. The higher the degree, the fewer the characters. Their numerical proportion is 288, 48, 12, 4, 1. Thus against a mass of 288 monogynes nature only gives 48 digynes, 12 trigynes, 4 *tetragynes*, and 1 *pentagyne*; this last has five dominants.

" Whatever be the influence of the dominant, it does not exclude that of the eleven others, which without having a full swing, generally obtain some empire. You might therefore, in every *monogyne* character, distinguish, after the dominant, four other sub-dominant passions, that exert in gradation the principal influence, and you would distinguish them, according to their dose of influence, into sub-dominants of the first, second, third, fourth degrees—the vice-dominant, counter-dominant, the pro-dominant, and the sub-dominant ; but in order to avoid all complication, we shall name them the four co-efficients, and when only the principal one shall be cited, it shall be called the sub-dominant. Thus we shall say that the monogyne Apicius is endowed with the dominant of taste, with the sub-dominant of ambition ; that is to say, that next to gourmandism, Apicius is principally inclined to ambition, which nevertheless is too weak in his case to be weighed against gourmandism, and becomes a co-dominant. If both had an equal influence over him, he would be a digyne, or character with a double dominant of taste and of ambition. None such exist ; it will be seen that the five sensual passions only reign as sub-dominants in the digynes and other polygynes." [1]

What are the Radical Passions ? The twelve radical passions which Fourier refers to as forming the basis of the 810 graduated characters in the phalanx, which is the unit of the industrial hive or vortex, are divided into three groups.

The first consists of the sensory functions, smell, hearing, sight, touch and taste, all making for *luxism* or the pursuit of luxury. It must be remembered that greater significance is attached to these senses in Fourier's system than is wont. He talks for instance of melomaniacs and gourmands, as if some people's lives were dominated by the *penchant* for music or the craving for victuals. The sex impulse is referred to under the tactile sense (passion) and sometimes termed " tactism " and, at other times, " lubricity " (vol. ii, p. 345).

Illustration of a Taste Monogyne. An example of Fourier's concretization to bring home his ideas is afforded here by the anecdote below, quoted especially because it gives

[1] C. Fourier : *The Passions of the Human Soul*, vol. ii, pp. 297–9 (English transl.).

evidence of his power of observation and faculty for assembling a number of seemingly unimportant events under a significant purview : " It was a tippler, a monogyne with the dominant of taste, the tonic of drinking.   I saw him in a public *diligence* or stage coach ;· he was not a sottish drunkard, but a man gifted with a marvellous instinct for referring all the circumstances of life to wine.   Similar to those mystical personages who see everything in God, this fellow saw everything in wine ; instead of reckoning time by hours and half-hours, he reckoned it by the number of bottles drunk.   Supposing you asked him, ' Will it take long to reach such a place ? ' ' Well ! about the time of drinking four bottles.'   When the horses stopped for a moment, I said to him, ' Do we stop long here ? ' ' About long enough to toss off a bottle standing.'   Now I knew that in his arithmetic a bottle drunk while standing was equal to five minutes, and a bottle drunk while seated was ten minutes.   One of the two coaches on the road, which had bad horses, passed us going down a hill, but he called out to it in a bantering tone, ' Bah, bah, we shall drink before you ' (that is to say, we shall arrive before you, for why do you arrive at all if not to drink ?) One of the passengers made us wait at the station where he had got down ; the passengers complained, and asked, ' What is he after ? he delays us.'   The monogyne replied, ' Perhaps he has not yet drunk his gill ' ; (for why do people delay you except it be to drink ?)   A lady experienced sickness from the movement of the coach ; one person proposed elixir, another eau-de-cologne ; the monogyne cut short the whole by saying, ' You had better drink a little wine, Ma'am ! ' (for what is the remedy for every ·sickness, if it be not wine ?) and he gallantly measured out the dose according to the delicacy of the subject.   Some one ventured to complain of the weather, which was cold and foggy ; our friend took him up severely, and explained that the weather was exceedingly good, because it kept back the vines that would have been exposed to frost by too precocious a vegetation. I listened to him during the moments he conversed familiarly with one of his companions, and nothing was heard but dozens of wine, casks being tapped, beginning to drink the wine, etc. In short, wine was to this man a focus, or a common centre, to which he referred all nature ; a dish was only worth something because it was a help to drinking ; a horse was not worth so much money, but such a quantity of Macon wine in small casks ; whatever subject happened to be discussed in his presence, he knew how to adapt it to wine, with a *finesse* of tact and a pertinateness that men of wit would not have had. He was not on that account a drunkard, but a well-defined monogyne, well characterized by the tonic of drinking. Let us call him Silenus in allusion to mythology ; I shall have occasion to cite him more than once in discussing the monogynes." (*Ibid.* pp. 316–17.)

It may be added by way of digression that Fourier would have this Silenus in his harmonic society as a keeper of a community wine cellar, whence he would supposedly hold a respected place. In that far-off era " the cellar is an immense warehouse, that in like manner discloses all the nectars of all countries ; assistance and advances are lavished in order to facilitate the administration, which delights a troop of sectaries impassioned in its favor." (*Ibid.* p. 343.)

In the second category which he labels " groupism ", we have the " affectuous " passions : friendship, ambition, parentism (or familism) and love.

Fourier's Concepts in Modern Terminology. The distributive passions relate to the economy of the pleasures and labors, their regulation and distribution, for let it be noted that Fourier is a hedonist *par excellence,* and furthermore he assumes pleasure to accompany labor under the proper conditions. These three passions are then the *cabalist,* which " creates piquant intrigues about the merest trifles ", the *papillon* or butterfly passion, which adds zest by affording novelty through variety, and the *composite* passion, the function of which is to dovetail or set in accord the various dispositions. In more modern terminology we should say that the cabalist tendency is one of dissociation, disintegration, catabolism, the papillon is simple alternation while the composite is the associative or integrative function.

The wretchedness and misery which abounds in society is due to the fact that each of the 810 characters in the single phalanx, or 1620 in the double phalanx, cannot play the part for which he or she is destined. The laws and conventions are hidebound and apply to every individual. " Our eternal debates on vice and virtue are void of sense, whilst we are ignorant of the harmonic employments of certain qualities deemed vices, like avarice and inconstancy. Our moralists who would like to run all the characters into one single mould, make all men brothers, all republicans, all friends of commerce, resemble the man who wished all coats to be cut on the same pattern. Before enacting anything concerning good or evil, we ought to know the uses that God assigns in harmony to those inclinations we call vicious, and which are for the most part the finest properties of the human race, like the omnigyne whose infinitesimal gamut, entirely composed of inclinations and excesses ridiculed at present, becomes in harmony the passional diamond and the focus of all social perfection." (*Ibid.* p. 381.)

Superiority of Polygynes over Monogynes. In the state of harmonism, which is the ninth evolutionary stage in society, Nero and Robespierre would develop as superb characters because of their polygyne constitution, which means that they were governed by a set (" dominative ") of several passions. " The polygynes are in the passional vortex what the staff of officers is in a regiment. They form the classes superior to the simple order, inasmuch as they cumulate two opposite developments and unfold them in contrasts in the same individual like the treble and bass of a piano-forte." (*Ibid*. p. 358.) Sometimes he likens the monogynes to instruments of a simple order like the violin or flute and the polygynes (digynes, trigynes up to omnigynes) to instruments of a composite order like the pianoforte or organ on which different parts may be executed simultaneously.

Fourier speaks of the monogynes, *i.e.*, those who are dominated by one passion only, with noticeable contempt. The 576 monogynes of the phalanx of 810 characters constitute the laborers. They are important, in the conduct of the industrial vortex, because of their number, but they must be controlled by the polygynes.

Tolerance Explained. There is a striking passage in Fourier with regard to the difference of reaction to moral exhortation on the part of the monogynes and the polygynes respectively. To the former " Nature has given . . . only one passion as a compass ; they stick to it with desperation ; every other save the sub-dominant having but a feeble influence on happiness . . . They will never listen to fine discourses that advise them to deprive themselves of their chief delights ". . . " It is much more easy to induce the polygynes to listen to (I do not say relish) morality. These, having several dominants, are little moved when one of them is wounded ; they have others for a refuge. Declaim a fine sermon against ambition before Caesar, he will appear to approve you, though no morality can curb his measureless ambition. Though showing some respect for your advice, he will not be disposed to follow it. Here is the secret of his apparent docility.

" Caesar has six passions for his dominants, namely, the four affectuous and two distributives—the alternating and the cabalist. He is only deficient in one of the seven primaries —the composite—as a dominant ; accordingly he has little enthusiasm. He shines on all occasions by his *sang froid ;* he has for super-tonic the thirst for grandeur, for supreme

()

power, one of the shades of the gamut of ambition. He is not on that account insensible to the other noble shades of the passion, such as self-respect ; and if you retail to him a sermon against his *super-tonic,* he listens to it from partiality to oratory ; the moralist can obtain in his case a moment of triumph as an orator, but by no means as a reformer, and perhaps on leaving the place, Caesar will order the passage of the Rubicon. Thus those alone give a fair hearing to morality who are not willing to follow it ; it is only attended to by the 130 polygynes, who lend an ear to it without results ; it also succeeds with a few of the ' mixts '. These chameleons are of all opinions, or contradict them all, for certain mixts of the ascending shades, are contradictory spirits, or pretend to be so ; but in the mass of the passional populace, in the 576 monogynes, who seem to belong to the class that needs correction, since they suit themselves exclusively with one passion, morality finds no disciple for its principles of repression." (*Ibid.* pp. 341–2.)

Contradictory People as Middlemen for Extremes. Students of psychoanalysis will be interested in Fourier's explanation of apparent contradictoriness in an individual's behavior, and still more in his accounting for the transformation of a character into its opposite extreme. Both instances are of course to be found only with the polygynes. " We are very much astonished in civilization at the contradictory manias we frequently observe in the same individual. Such a one appears to us eccentric because he saves his farthings and squanders pounds. Such beings seem to us discordant with themselves. No such thing : they are characters of a composite order ; they are the most brilliant in harmony, but have no office in civilization. They are intended to conciliate in co-operative association two antipathetic monogynes, such as Harpagon and Mondor, characters of extreme avarice and extreme prodigality. In the relations of harmony it is necessary to put these two men in relation with a third, who possesses the two passions in the same degree, to form an alliance of reason between the polygyne Lucullus on the one hand, and the two monogynes on the other. Civilization offers no chances for such an association. Harmony is able to effect it, and thence arises the accord of intervention. . . If, therefore, we find the means of conciliating in a passional league Harpagon with Lucullus, and Mondor with Lucullus, we shall have conciliated indirectly Harpagon and Mondor, although these two persons, as to immediate relationship, would be incompatible in the highest degree." (*Ibid.* pp. 358–9.) Thus they act as middlemen between the two extreme types of monogynes who otherwise would not have been able to understand each other. It is the dual polygyne who is able to effect a *rapprochement*. But civilization is opposed to such polarity in the same individual, who is therefore regarded as eccentric, if not actually pathological. Hence he is compelled by society to make shift as best he may, with the result that he becomes stunted.

Fourier to the Defence of the Neurotic. " As the civilizees [Fourier uses this form opprobriously] of the polygyne class have no means of developing abreast the two opposite propensities of being at the same time avaricious and extravagant, we often see them modulate in alternation, and after having acted a long time in one character, pass suddenly to the opposite extreme, and become new men. I have stated above, that this effect is no more than an eruption of one or other of the two gamuts that had been compressed by education and by circumstances. As this property is frequently manifested, and people are everywhere found who have passed from extreme dissipation to the most regular habits, and *vice versa*, I insist on this well-known effect, to draw from it an indication of the contrasted nature of the composite character bestowed on the 130 polygynes. We must admit it conditionally, and when

we shall have analysed the effort and the influence
of civilization to suppress in each polygyne one
of the two gamuts of his character, we shall the more
easily be convinced of their existence, the more easily
we learn for what uses this twofold nature is reserved
in harmony.

" As for the present the polygynes, limited to one development, may be compared to a man who could only play on
the harp or piano with one hand, and could only perform
a simple part of treble without bass, or of bass without treble.
This passional castration transforms the civilizee polygynes
into social eunuchs, and has prevented any attention being
paid to their property of contrasted development and double
gamut.   The contradictions we see in them cause them to be
regarded as originals, persons more or less inconsistent,
according to their degree, and who require the lectures of
philosophy to be restored to the equilibrium of reason."
(*Ibid.* pp. 360–1.)

Adversary of Philistinism.   Fourier, the omnigyne, has no
great respect for the monogynes of family affection who
" are loaded with excessive praise ; they are the good fathers,
good sons, good cousins, good republicans, persons who
faint with tenderness in their opulent homes whilst their
neighbors are starving.   An omnigyne shines but very
little in these exclusive paternal affections that moralists
and newspapers extol.   He will love his children sufficiently,
but you will see him love and appreciate those of other
people. . . . He will be a father, but little infatuated and
very different from those who are deified every day in
biographical notes under the title of good fathers, good sons,
good republicans ; pure egoists who have no other merit
than that of being good towards themselves and their own
family."   With another happy illustration, this brilliant
Frenchman demolishes the average man.   " Monogynes
believe themselves superior to polygynes as the first fiddle

deems himself superior to the conductor of the orchestra because he excels in solo."

Fourier's outline of character types does not stop with the omnigynes. There are super-omnigynes of various degrees or powers until the seventeenth, only one of which makes his appearance among from two and a-half to three billions of inhabitants. Such a one is the " passional sovereign of the globe ", and Fourier tells us calmly that he is such, for only these possess the " singular property of discovering almost by inspiration the laws of harmony, and I must necessarily be of this degree, since I have arrived at it [this discovery] without any help, without any anterior theory that could put me in the way of it."

I offer no apology for devoting so many pages to this original Frenchman. His far-reaching doctrine could ill be omitted from our treatment ; and unless it is made intelligible, it might just as well be ruled out of the survey. His denunciation of society is of course to be taken with a grain of salt and his utopian plans are vulnerable on the face of them, but no one before him has so incisively shown the relation of the instincts to society, and the effect of conventional morality upon the development or stunting of the innate tendencies of man. His delusion about himself need not blind us to the fact that he is the *unique pioneer of differential or individual psychology*, as may be seen from the present exposition. If his assumptions are unwarranted, his reasoning is clear ; and I believe the application of Fourier's method to a sound theory of instinct, like McDougall's, and employed in the light of present-day knowledge regarding the biological and social sciences, would yield results of inestimable value.

DISCIPLES OF FOURIER

Fourier's stupendous system, though it failed to leave its impress upon psychology, has not been without its adherents who have humanized or personified not only animals and flowers but even stellar bodies and mathematical relations. The physician, M. Edgeworth Lazarus, who, I believe, was the first to use the term " comparative psychology " (1851) exhibits much of the spirit of Fourier's thought, and even his tempestuous style, in his fantastic *Vegetable Portraits of Character*, which is the first volume of a compendium of *Comparative Psychology and Universal Analogy*. This book, published in 1851, was followed by *Love versus Marriage* (1859), another dynamic exposition of Fourierism, at least one phase of it, in which I found the words " introversion " and " extroversion " used in a sense similar to Jung's.[1] The same author has written a *Passional Hygiene*, a *Passional Arithmetic* and a *Passional Geometry* and has translated *Toussenel's Passional Zoology*,[2] which goes to show that more than one scientific worker has taken seriously the *bizarrerie* of Fourier. Of Lazarus not a trace is to be found in the various American encyclopedias and biographical dictionaries.

COMPARISON WITH AZAÏS

In order to realize the tremendous sweep of Fourier's system of characterology we need but contrast with his system the poverty-stricken classification of his contemporary Azaïs, who was renowned in his day as a philosophical writer, and who also dealt with cosmic destinies in his all-embracing works.

Azaïs divides people according as their predominant faculty is (*a*) memory, (*b*) understanding or reason, and (*c*) imagination. Characters of the lowest level are those whose behavior is determined by the mere association of ideas.

---

[1] Since my reading this book, it disappeared from the Harvard College Library, and not being able to find it elsewhere, I cannot verify the reference.

[2] M. E. Lazarus : *Vegetable Portraits of Character* (1851), p. 205.

These individuals are gifted only for the routine in life, are actuated mainly by habit. Characters with judgment and reason in the foreground are known for their sagacity, pursuit of economy, and practical bent of mind, although they lack warmth. As to the characters of the third class, viz., imagination, Azaïs thinks they may be subdivided into two groups, those which are only temporary and intermittent expansions of the judgment type or characterial mean, and the comparatively few that are true imaginative specimens—the creative artists, among whom Azaïs includes the great writers.[1]

[1] H. Azaïs: *Cours de Philosophie Générale*, chap. 25 (vol. viii), 1824.

CHAPTER XI

THE BRITISH WRITERS

The British—and particularly the Scotch—mind does not over-indulge in classification. For this reason we need not look for long lists of types or comprehensive tables of character complexes. There is a good deal of examining the ground-work of the subject, considerable burrowing along side-paths with no effort at reaching finality, *cathedra* fashion.

While, it may be said, the French and, to a less extent, the German writers make classification their goal, the British seem to fall into it as a concession. To be sure, classes are at least implied, but the classificatory tendency is somewhat hampered by an atomistic analysis, a sample of which may be had in Bain's classification that has enjoyed some vogue in the second part of the last century. Bain separated the characters according to the standard division of intellectual, emotional and volitional constituents. With him, however, there is no strict attempt made to distinguish between character and temperament, and on the whole his position is too much that of the phrenologists in that he includes under character the most miscellaneous things, such as virtues, abilities, emotions, and general tendencies—all mixed promiscuously in one grand *potpourri*.

Single Merit of Bain's Essay. One service of Bain's *The Study of Character* has been to emphasize the need of finding a physiological basis for the various differences in character and temperament. The physical seat of spontaneous energy is, according to Bain, to be sought in the conformation of the muscular system.[1] Again some of that power is also due to

[1] A. Bain: *The Study of Character, Including an Estimate of Phrenology*, p. 192.

cerebral currents flowing toward the muscles.[1] " If there be any one point of physical conformation," says Bain in another place, " that regularly accompanies a copious natural activity, it is size of head taken altogether," and still further, " If we were to venture, after the manner of phrenology, to specify more precisely the locality of the centres of general energy, I should say the posterior part of the crown of the head, and the lateral part adjoining— that is, the region of the organs of Self Esteem, Love of Approbation, Cautiousness, Firmness and Conscientiousness —must be full and ample, if we would expect a conspicuous display of this feature of character." [2]

This passage betrays the weakness of that whole school in trying to localize faculties rather than describing and explaining processes. That the influence of Bain is still felt in Great Britain can be seen from the atomistic account of character and temperament given in Shand's book, which, now in its second edition, is an elaborate and painstaking expansion of an article published in *Mind* in 1896.

Jordan's Delineations. Before, however, proceeding to the examination of Shand's views, we must turn our attention to a little book by Jordan,[3] to which Jung devotes a whole chapter in his *Psychological Types*, concluding it with this tribute : " To Jordan, however, the credit belongs of being the first, so far as I know, to give a relatively appropriate character sketch of the emotional types." In this brilliantly written book which Jung admits to have partially anticipated his own divisions, the author sets forth that there are two temperaments, the active and more or less passionless on the one hand, and the reflective and impassioned on the other. The intermediate type is also not to be lost sight of. " There are numberless varieties of character," writes the

---

[1] *Ibid*, p. 193.   [2] *Ibid*, p. 195.
[3] F. Jordan : *Character as Seen in Body and Parentage*. London, 1890 2nd edition).

author in his preface, ". . . many divisions, conspicuous types, intervening gradations, equal or unequal developments, varying combinations. In domestic and social life, intermediate characters produce perhaps the most useful and the happiest results, but the progress of the world at large is mainly due to the combined efforts of the supremely impassioned and reflective, and the supremely active and unimpassioned temperaments."

Jung regrets the fact that Jordan has brought in the element of activity, thus cutting across what might have been a clear antithesis of introversion and extraversion.[1] We are not concerned here with Jung's contentions and criticisms of Jordan, nor do the latter's categories appear adequate. His strength lies in the four rich delineations of the active unimpassioned and the reflective and impassioned man and woman. Jordan wrote before the inauguration of the psychoanalytic movement, but his sketches display a remarkable keenness of insight, and are replete with a psychological analysis which sets off, with a good deal of artistry, seemingly unimportant yet at bottom significant bits of behavior in the various types. Jordan abstractly appeals to physiology for the differences in character. " The physiological actions of the nervous system go to make up character : can these be in any degree gathered from the skin, and hair and bones, and skeleton or figure?" the author asks, and proceeds to show wherein the unimpassioned person differs in appearance and in structure from the impassioned— a procedure which is similar to that of the contemporary schools of endocrinology and clinical morphology, the thesis being that " certain anatomical and physiological peculiarities accompany a certain kind of nerve organization, and denote a certain kind of character ".[2]

A Literary Voice. Courtney,[3] in a popular article called

---

[1] See further, chapter xv.   [2] Loc. cit., p. 61.
[3] W. L. Courtney : *The National Review*, 1890, vol. xv.

"Can there be a Science of Character?" after rejecting
the literary method of La Bruyère and pointing out the
fallacies of the phrenologists, attaches himself, though not
without reserve, to Bain's system and recognizes three types
of characters in accordance with the three-fold division of
mind into volition, emotion, and intellect. First there is
the *energetic* character or temperament (which Courtney
uses interchangeably with the former) marked by strength
but wanting in breadth and far-sightedness. "Such temperaments make admirable assistant masters in a school but not
good head masters." On the *emotional* temperament, this
writer has some interesting remarks, mentioning the part
played by glandular secretions and organic processes in its
formation. True the secretion spoken of deals with the
lachrymal glands, but the observation showed evidence of
a proper orientation. When he tackles the third type, viz.,
the *intellectual* temperament, Courtney is off at a tangent;
for in speaking of retentiveness, discrimination and reproduction as its "three great powers or faculties", he not only
espouses a cause now relegated to a dubious sphere, but is
discussing the subject of intelligence, intellect, talent, genius,
or what-not—certainly he is not in the domain of character
study. And the cause of his going astray is that threefold
division of mind which has played havoc also with the highly
trained French psychologists.

Interest in the study of character had meanwhile been
lagging behind in spite of the impetus which had been lent
it by Mill and Bain. The last decade of the nineteenth
century, which was the most active period for the French
characterologists was unproductive of anything but an
occasional literary article on character. The fascination
which the whole subject of human nature had for the British
apparently was confined to the plots and characterizations
in novels.

Shand Revives Interest in Character. It was Shand who

restored the British tradition in following up the inductive method laid down by his predecessors, and in this sense he may be regarded as Bain's successor, although some of his results are not unlike the findings of the French school represented by Paulhan. Shand's task is to try to build up types of character out of the various instincts, sentiments and emotions. A character for him is only the development of one affective element above the rest. Intelligence and will are totally neglected. He decidedly exaggerates the rôle of the sensibilities of man, and attempts to prove his thesis by showing how one over-developed tendency will have a marked effect on the whole moral and mental constitution of man by giving rise to new tendencies or at least giving them larger scope, and on the other hand by checking other more normal tendencies which interfere with the dominant one. " Every sentiment tends to form a type of character of its own," [1] is one of the numerous so-called laws that Shand formulates in his book.

By way of illustration the following paragraph may be quoted from the same work : " Thus," says the author, " the miser's tyranny over those subjected to him seconds his parsimony, his industry, his vigilance, his prudence, his secrecy, his cunning, and unsociableness, which are the essential means of his avarice. He is secret because he is suspicious, he is suspicious because he pursues ends to which other men would be opposed, and because he has no counteracting trust or affection. He is cunning, because he both suspects and tries to outwit others. He makes a pretence of poverty that no claims may be made on him and that he may justify his economies. He is unsociable because he is secret and suspicious, being engaged in pursuing an object of which others do not approve and which alienates them from him.

---

[1] A. F. Shand : *The Foundations of Character*, p. 123 (first edition).

" The qualities to which we have referred appear to belong to avarice in the sense that its thought, will, and conduct tend to acquire them because they are indispensable to the achievement of its ends." [1]

An Important Issue. Now, the only fault about this treatment is that the fiction of our poets is erected into the ideal or standard type. Shand goes to literature for his illustrations, but, no matter how realistic the character of the miser in *L'Avare*, it is still the creation of Molière, and most miserly people are not nearly so morbid as Molière's character, so that all the other effects which extreme avarice brings on in its train might not be true of them at all. Now, shall we say then, that the true types of character are to be found only among neurotics?

Shall we, furthermore, deny the possession of any character to Kant, Spinoza and Fichte, simply because they did not have this or that sentiment abnormally developed? Unless we settle first of all the difference between the complex characters in literature and the real characters in life about which we are concerned, we should be involved in a hopeless mess. The study of abnormal characters portrayed by dramatists and novelists should be relegated, as Lévy has suggested, to psychopathology. We must begin with the normal characters first, though the abnormal types throw, of course, much light on the subject.

When we say that Raskolnikov in Dostoëvsky's *Crime and Punishment*, or Mishkin in the same author's *The Idiot* is a remarkable character, and that Carlyle had a remarkable character, we are certainly not using the term in the same sense. But in spite of scrupulous attempts at exact definition of the word, this confusion goes on unchecked. Definition, like the law, always admits of some loophole. It is not rigid definition which is indispensable, but rather distinguishing

---

[1] *Ibid.* p. 124.

the various usages of the term, so that we can be put on our guard against misunderstanding. In this respect Shand is by no means the only writer to be taken to task. Throughout the literature on the subject there are several contradictory trends. Particularly is this true about the word *will*, which some use as though it were only equivalent to energy, while others make out of it some entity, some faculty, which is innate and yet can be modified. Still others treat it as a source of good and evil. Such promiscuous use of the term has led to further confusion in the conception of character. We can only get our bearings by first consulting ordinary language, and here we find that energy and will are not synonymous, for we often have occasion to refer to a man who, though strong-willed, determined and resolute, is not possessed of a high degree of energy.

In dealing with the subject, which is still in its initial stages, common usage should play a more prominent rôle than it has been doing in our psychological literature. Even Aristotle condescended to start his investigations with the popular notions of the subject matter under examination.

Analysis of Groundwork by McDougall. McDougall's *Introduction to Social Psychology*, which has exercised a remarkable influence in psychological circles since its appearance in 1908, may be regarded perhaps as the first systematic attempt to study the groundwork of character by examining its constituents and relationships. The merit of this work, which has much in common with Shand's, is the emphasis laid on content, and on the avoidance of formalism, so prevalent among the French characterologists. What McDougall has achieved in this direction is to lay stress " upon the systematic organization of the conative dispositions in the moral and self-regarding sentiments . . . and to exhibit the continuity of the development of the highest types of human will and character from the primary instinctive dispositions that we have in common with the animals ".

McDougall is not interested in the classification of *characters*, but in the *consolidation of character*, which he believes to be dependent on the "organization of the sentiments in some harmonious system of hierarchy ". Like Shand he holds that the predominance of some one sentiment is crucial to the whole development of character. But, though character in the full sense of the word is not the result of a dominant motive or ruling passion alone, such as the love of home, the one master-sentiment "which can generate strong character in the fullest sense . . . is the self-regarding sentiment ".[1] But this needs further to be supplemented in that the "strong self-regarding sentiment must be combined with one for some ideal of conduct, and it must have risen above dependence on the regards of the mass of men ; and the motives supplied by this master sentiment in the service of the ideal must attain an habitual predominance." [2]

Since my own view bears a general resemblance to the foregoing, I might take occasion to indicate at this point that the chief difference lies in the method as also in the emphasis which in McDougall's treatment is laid on the moral side rather than on the intellectual.

Basis of Differences in Temper. If McDougall has not attempted to classify the characters, he has at least drawn up a list of tempers, which word he defines as the expression of the way in which the conative impulses work within man. Since these impulses differ with respect to their (*a*) strength, urgency, or intensity, (*b*) persistency, and (*c*) affectability, there will be eight possible combinations of these qualities, and therefore eight tempers. These may be best presented in the form of a table :—

[1] Wm. McDougall : *Introduction to Social Psychology*, p. 267 (sixteenth edition).
[2] *Ibid.* p. 261.

RELATIONS OF CONATIVE QUALITIES

1. High intensity and persistency, low affectability—steadfast and confident.

2. Low intensity and persistency, high affectability—fickle and shallow.

3. High intensity, low persistency, high affectability—violent and unstable.

4. High intensity, low persistency, low affectability—despondent.

5. Low intensity, high persistency, high affectability—anxious.

6. High intensity, high persistency, high affectability—hopeful .

7. Low intensity, high persistency, low affectability—placid.

8. Low intensity, low persistency, low affectability—sluggish.[1]

I am not sure that these conative attributes can be admitted as the only basic ones (one may conceive, for example, of the rapidity with which the impulses develop and the ease or difficulty with which they hang together as equally basic qualities) and one may doubt whether it can be shown that a given combination of these qualities will in each case yield the particular temper designated by McDougall, but it is interesting to note that there is a resemblance in essential respects between Heymans and Wiersma's three fundamental attributes of character and those of McDougall.[2]   That these

---

[1] Wm. McDougall : *Social Psychology*, pp. 448–9 (sixteenth edition).

[2] As De Froe points out in his *Laurence Sterne* (pp. 97–8) " strength " and " intensity " might corespond with the " activity " attribute of the Dutch investigators ; " persistency " certainly has the same implication as the " secondary functioning " of Heymans and Wiersma, while McDougall's " affectability " evidently is covered by their " emotionality ", but even here, de Froe does not fully realize that McDougall's " affectivity " is " susceptibility to influences of pleasure

investigators should coincide in the number of types and overlap in the categories need not surprise us, inasmuch as the mathematical formula for permutations and combinations would bring about these results. But it requires some stretch of the imagination to identify, as De Froe has endeavored to do, the sanguine character in the Dutch classification with McDougall's despondent temper, or the " sentimental " character of Heymans and Wiersma with McDougall's " anxious " temper. Again the " passionate " or " impassioned " of the former may or may not be " hopeful", and the " apathetic " need not be " sluggish ". This doubtful identification only goes to show how careful we must be in our attempts to reconcile authors or to discover parallels where none exist. (See Chapter XIV for the Dutch account.)

British Counterpart of Spranger's Life-Forms. Mercier's little book on character types [1] is a happy combination of the literary and the scientific, but it is especially interesting that more than half of his eleven temperaments, as he chooses to call the types, correspond to the fundamental forms of Spranger (see Chapter XX). Mercier's portrayals are redolent of British and French characterology of the seventeenth century. There is precision in his demarcations, so that we are not likely to mistake the one division for another, but he does not show anywhere in his discussion how he came to select out of innumerable varieties the eleven which he describes. We feel that each link in the chain is skilfully, even artistically wrought, and yet we are far from certain that the links are in their proper places or that the dimensions are suitable. The artistic temperament, which should really be called something else (neurotic, amoral

and pain ", which is not quite the same as emotionality. Similarly strength of tendency may correlate with activity or is its immediate cause, but we are not justified in identifying the two.

[1] C. Mercier: *Human Temperaments, Studies in Character*, 2n d rev. ed. (1917 ?), p. 18.

and emotional), is contrasted with the temperament of the artist.

" For the keynote of the artistic temperament is selfishness, the dominant is self-indulgence, and the sub-dominant sensitiveness to sensuous impressions. If men are divided into those who feel, those who think, and those who act, then the men of this temperament belong to the first class. They are, indeed, actors, but they are not men of action."

The artistic temperament, on the other hand, depends on the depth or elevation or volume of the emotion expressed, the skill with which it is expressed, and the ability to construct an harmonious and consistent plan.

The religious temperament is rooted in sacrifice, motivated by the desire to propitiate the higher powers, and is displayed in two ways, in self-sacrifice, as in martyrdom, and in vicarious sacrifice, as evinced by the savage, the inquisitor and the Puritan " who deprives his children of innocent pleasures ".

The faddist, again, is " a person who fixes upon some minor phase of conduct and exalts the cult of this mode of conduct into a religion ". The philosopher is recognized by his absorption in theoretical matters, in principles, rules, generalization. Isolated facts, actions, details concern him but little. The practical man. on the other hand, cherishes an aversion for what he dubs theories. He aims at results, regardless of the fundamental principles by which they might be arrived at.

The business temperament which is contrasted with the artistic (amoral) temperament can be distinguished by the capacity for discerning the main issue and sticking to it. Perseverance and promptitude are his chief qualities in action. But neither the business man nor the practical man is to be identified with the man of action who " abounds in energy which is well under control ". Out of this class are recruited the explorers, adventurers, conquerors, pioneers, etc.,

" insensible to fear and contemptuous of danger " because of a consciousness of their own power.

The envious, the jealous and the suspicious temperament complete Mercier's list and require no exposition on my part; their characteristics are too well-known, although we ordinarily speak of them as dispositions rather than temperaments.

Criticism. Mercier's treatment of the subject exemplifies the shortcomings of the merely descriptive schools. We miss in it the *fundamentum divisionis.* Whatever fault might be found with Spranger's life-forms, they are at least *deduced.* There is one principle running thoughout, viz. that of value. Mercier, with his characteristic impatience of the traditional, seems to exclude the classic temperaments deliberately. Description is his forte, but when we ask why he jumps about from affective or emotional qualities like jealousy, envy, and suspicion to intellectual and volitional characteristics as distinguishing marks of his types, we are at a loss for an answer. Why does he not include the irritable, the vain, the fickle, etc., as categories in his character scheme ?

Moreover, if the business man is one who seeks out the important issue and sticks to it, is not the true philosopher a business man ? And has he not made room for superstition in his rather crude envisagement of religion ? The mystic element in religion does not seem to occur to him. Negation is perhaps one of the chief features of religion, but is its purpose always propitiation ?

The compass of the various temperaments is strikingly unequal in Mercier's presentation. The " artistic " temperament really covers the whole personality of an individual, but the envious or jealous person may be like the philosopher, the practical man, the artist, etc. in all respects but one. It is as if countries and counties were grouped together for the purpose of classification according to boundaries. What vitiates Mercier's attempt is his leaning toward the practical, as he himself describes the trait, without delving into motives, purposes, cultural tendencies.

A Psychoanalytic Flavor. Belonging to the British school, but without taking into consideration the much-needed information which other writers can supply, is Hugh Elliot's *Human Character*—a collection of essays rather than a unitary treatment. The psychoanalytic element in the book may readily be detected in such a sentence as this: " To understand character, we have continually to be shredding off the externals and going beneath them. The true significance of a motive might almost be said to be inversely proportional to the ease of discerning it."

The following passage which, if not wholly acceptable, is at least thought-provoking reveals the direction of the current more strikingly.

" The direction of a person's interests and attention is thus a far more important point in his character than the opinions which he holds on the subjects in question. A tyrant and a slave for instance are much more alike than either of them to a free citizen. For both a tyrant and a slave have prominently in their minds the conception of subordination " . . . " The teetotaler is a potential drunkard, just as the prude is a potential rake, and the slave a potential tyrant " . . . " In all spheres, the views entertained by any person are less significant for a diagnosis of his character than the subject on which his attention is focussed. . . . The fact is deeply rooted in the physiology of the nervous system. The electrical manifestations which accompany a feeling of pleasure are more similar to those which accompany a feeling of pain than to those which characterize indifference ; and in all human life, pleasure far more easily converts to pain than to indifference."

Causes of Character Differences. Among the causes to account for differences in character, the author believes the following to be the most important :

(1). The variations in the volume of the normal current of disposable mental energy, i.e., in some people, mental life is strong, in others it is weak.

(2). The fact that some people are governed more by the permanent deeper feelings than others who are guided by the feelings of the moment.

(3). Differences in suggestibility.

(4). The ratio of the strength of the mental current to its compass, i.e., " the stream may run torrentially through a narrow gorge, as in the fanatic, or it may flow placidly over wide meadows." [1]

(5). The composition of the feelings making up the mental current. " Some men are intellectual, others emotional, others again abound in active energy." [2]

Throughout the book, Elliot repeats almost *ad nauseam* the central idea of Le Bon, Freud, and other champions of the unconscious, viz., that intellect plays no part in shaping our motives, that " the bulk of human activities are blind and unreasoning " and that " deep and obscure emotion " is the driving force, not the intellect, which is only a tool in the service of the former.

---

[1] Compare here Otto Gross's concentrated and narrow *versus* the shallow and broad types, in the chapter " Suggestions from Psychiatry ".

[2] H. Elliot : *Human Character*. 1922.

CHAPTER XII

I

THE ALIENISTS

The subject of character seems to have had a peculiar fascination for the French, since, beginning with Fourier, they have maintained an unflagging interest in this field, culminating in the active period of the nineties when half a dozen important works on character appeared. That the study in France should have been begun by a social philosopher and passed through the hands of psychiatrists before being taken up by psychologists is noteworthy, as compared with the fact that in Germany characterology was the monopoly for a time of philosophy and pedagogy, and only lately has psychiatry taken an active part in the shaping of its destiny.

Another item of distinction which may be mentioned is the detachment of character from the moral sphere. In Germany, and to some extent in Great Britain, character discussions usually begin and end in ethics. France, to be sure, has not wholly neglected this application of character ; for education and conduct are represented by men like Payot and Queyrat, but certainly the bulk of the literature is devoted to the psychological phase, and even where the two are treated in the same work, they are sufficiently separated to avoid confusion.

Bourdet. An early treatment of character, much after the fashion of McDougall's in his *Social Psychology*, though of course more fragmentary and sketchy, is to be found in Bourdet's *Des maladies du caractère*, the first edition of which appeared exactly 50 years before its British successor, in 1858.[1]

Bourdet's work, colored by Comte's philosophy, would be considered to-day a sort of handbook on mental hygiene. Starting out with the various functions of the brain, he classifies them into instincts, affections, sentiments and impulses—that aside from the " faculties ", such as the spirit of synthesis, the spirit of analysis, generalization, co-ordination and communication. As to the instincts, he recognizes egoistic and altruistic classes and includes among the latter : attachment, veneration and kindness (or sympathy). The military instinct and the industrial instinct are regarded respectively as destructive and constructive.

With this groundwork, the author proceeds to discuss the various ailments of character according as the individual deviates from the normal with respect to this or that function. Unlike the later French characterologists, he does not classify characters as such, but through the affective ingredients which go to make them up. The instinct of property, for instance, gives rise to three objectionable deviations, viz., cupidity, avarice and theft, and several tendencies just the reverse, such as prodigious generosities, great financial ideas, and noble tastes for artistic expenditure.

Bourdet writes from a social point of view, and he seeks to employ all the tools at his command in order to produce a serviceable guide toward preserving one's moral and mental equilibrium. But his eclectic method, in which philosophy, physiology and (of a dubious nature in some instances) psychiatry are introduced as grist to the mill, would even to-day be fraught with serious disadvantages.

Azam's Method. More direct and suggestive is Azam's *Le caractère dans la santé et dans la maladie*, but if anything less scientific, in spite of the renown of its author and the commendatory foreword of Ribot. Azam's method is, as

---

[1] The second edition, which is before me, appeared in 1878.

Ribot tells us, comparative, tracing character in animals, in the human individual, in states of health and disease, and even in groups such as nations. The plan is excellent, but he falls far short of executing it. The bulk of the book is devoted to the description of various traits, after the simple classification of good and bad characters and those which are good or bad according to the circumstances. There is much information and entertainment in these short sketches of the curious, the hypocritical, the vain, the tender-hearted, etc. There is only this thing lacking in it which characterizes Fourier's work—system. Mental elements are not sufficiently analyzed, hence all traits, qualities, propensities and tendencies are put on an equal footing. We need not be surprised then if Azam, wishing to prove that character changes in ill-health, only convinces us that the invalid's *disposition* takes a turn for the worse.[1] For this reason, it might be proper, were it not for the instructive references and stimulating side-issues which the author introduces, to place Azam's account under the head of literary characterology. In the last part of the book, however, a number of important questions are raised, one of which, that of the localization of character, we shall have to revert to in Chapter XXXVII.

II

THE PSYCHOLOGISTS

We leave the alienists and turn to the psychological writers, the first of whom to have brought out a systematic work on character is the genetic psychologist, Bernard Pérez, for whom character and personality, as for practically all of the French characterologists, are synonyms. Pérez discloses a behavioristic streak, for the basic principle with him is

---

[1] E. Azam : *Le caractère dans la santé et dans la maladie* (1887), pp. 190 ff.

movement or *action*. As a movement may be quick, slow or vehement, we obtain, through a series of combinations, six different classes of character. They are the active, the slow, the vehement or passionate, the actively intense (*vifs-ardents*), the slowly intense (*lents-ardents*), and, finally, the balanced characters.[1]

Pérez's Classification Behavioristic. Now, whatever of value there may be in such a simple classification, it is clear that we cannot adopt it, if for the reason alone that movement cannot be the pivotal point of personality and *a fortiori* of character. It was evidently the *reaction* that Pérez was emphasizing as a mark of character. That it is easier to discern different kinds, or rather different rates, of movements than anything else in the way of people's reactions, is a fact which probably nobody will care to dispute, but the crux of the question lies in this: whether it is a safeguard, whether movement is not after all merely an indication, and not the most essential indication, of one's inner make-up.

Are we not frequently baffled at seeming inconsistencies which we cannot clear up ? Do we not see people who are constantly in a bustle, rushing about from morning till night, and yet accomplishing very little ; while others who walk with a great deal of poise, speak with marked deliberation, and give the impression as if they were extremely slow and indolent, yet achieve wonders in comparatively brief periods ? In other words, appearances deceive ; and a quick external reaction may not be coincident with a quick internal reaction. We all know that quick apperception does not always go hand in hand with fluent expression. The rapid thinker is not always the glib talker, and to resort to the resultant as our last appeal is neither psychological nor philosophical.

---

[1] B. Pérez : " Le Caractère et les mouvements," *Rev. Philos.*, 1891, vol. xxxi, and *Le caractère de l'enfant à l'homme*, 1891. The first " e " in Pérez variously appears with and without an accent even in his own works.

We might as well classify character according to noses and jaws, for we may assume on general principles that a certain type of nose and jaw goes with a certain kind of character.

In the study of character, more than anywhere else in psychology, our aim should be not merely to discover correlations, but to find out *the causes of the correlations*. If we see a man walking very quickly, it may be that he is naturally brisk, but there is also the possibility that, being slow and dilatory, he has neglected something important which he is now trying to make up—hence his bustle. We can never be too sure as to which group a particular person fits into, for we do not know how much allowance to make for circumstances, and in that respect, therefore, we should never be able to compare any two individuals.

Ribot—Founder of New School. The next few years saw several serious attempts on the part of French psychologists to grapple with the problem of character. Ribot in 1892 laid the foundation for what might be called the *facultative division of character types*, which characterizes nearly all the French schools and which has its source probably in Bain's account. The article [1] in which he first developed his views is marked by a directness of treatment that makes up for the comparative brevity with which the subject was treated. First of all, what constitutes character ? Ribot asks. The earmarks are noted as unity and stability. This already commits him to an *innate* conception of character. " A true character is innate." For the purpose of simplification, Ribot rules out forthwith two large classes of personalities which lack either unity or stability or both. These are (*a*) the amorphous, the products of chance and circumstance who " once caught in the machinery of life . . . act like everyone else " and (*b*) the unstable, " changing from instant to instant, by turns inert

---

[1] Th. Ribot : " Les diverses formes du caractère," *Rev. Philos.*, 1892. This article appeared later somewhat revised as a chapter in his *Psychologie des sentiments*.

and explosive . . . Acting in the same manner under different circumstances, and varying their actions in the same circumstances, they are indefiniteness itself."

A Hierarchy Proposed. Excluding these two categories, Ribot aims to establish a classification analogous to the botanical. The genera of character are the merest framework, practically nondescript. The species embrace the pure types—forms it is true, yet real. The third general order in the hierarchy comprises the mixed or composite forms (varieties of character) and lastly there are the substitutes which he calls *partial characters* (*cf.* the concept of displacement in present-day psychoanalysis, yet without the suggestion of abnormality, as Ribot takes up abnormal or morbid characters in a separate chapter.)

Ribot in his treatment of character leaves out of consideration the factor of intelligence entirely. The two functions that are fundamental for him are feeling and action. In this way he derives his two large divisions of character : the sensitive and the active, according as feeling or energy predominates in the individual. The apathetic class, possessing a low degree of both elements, is added by way of supplement. Out of the more comprehensive classes he builds a hierarchy of character types. Among the sensitive may be enumerated (*a*) the humble, marked by excessive sensibility, shallow or mediocre intelligence, and no energy, (*b*) the contemplative, characterized by a keen sensibility, acute and penetrating intellect, and no activity, (*c*) the emotional type, combining the extreme impressionability of the contemplative with intellectual subtlety and activity. Two sub-classes belong to the active characters, comprising the mediocre minds and the powerful intellects, technically called the mediocre active type and the extremely active. The apathetic class is composed of the purely apathetic with little sensibility, little activity and little intelligence ; and the calculative type is endowed with little sensibility and activity but with a practical intellect.

More combinations yield us the sensitive-active kind, the apathetic-active, the apathetic-sensitive, and the temperate.

It will be seen that, after relegating the intellect in the first place, Ribot smuggles it in to make room for new groups and varieties that could not have been introduced on the basis of feeling and action alone.

Ribot's scheme is no more psychological nor less logical than those of his predecessors, but the notion of a hierarchy that he suggests seems to be a valuable innovation which may be used in the future, after we reach some more satisfactory classification.

Paulhan more British than French in his Classification. Paulhan in a more specialized work, *Les Caractères*, approaches the subject from a different angle. He attempts to go to the root of the matter so as to discover the *modus operandi* of the apparatus which is responsible for differences in character —with the result that he lands in atomism.

Deriving his principle from the English associationist school, Paulhan regards the organization of character as the result of a systematic association process among the constituent elements of one's mind. These images, ideas, desires, and what not are welded together with reference to a certain end that characterises the individual. All that makes towards this end is reinforced, all that is antagonistic to the general purpose of the individual is inhibited. In this way we obtain a sort of metabolism which gives rise to various grades of character organization in accordance with the strength with which certain tendencies are welded together and others driven apart. In the final analysis, character depends on just how well or how poorly the various elements can harmonise in the individual under the guidance of one main tendency. Thus Paulhan would have it that there are balanced characters and unbalanced characters, coherent and unified characters, and characters that are incoherent and not unified.

Fouillée's Objections. Fouillée in his *Tempérament et Caractère* devotes a good deal of space to criticizing Paulhan's doctrine ; and the objections may be summarized as follows : (1) Paulhan's classification is uninforming, though it is not difficult to accept it. (2) He puts the cart before the horse when he tries to derive difference in character from his law of systematic association. It is in virtue of the possession of a certain character that such a law would operate in an individual in one way and not in another, but to describe the reinforcement or inhibition of ideas, images and desires, by merely saying that such processes do take place, does not in the least explain why the law should operate differently in different minds.[1]

Ribot's Criticism. Paulhan has had to bear the brunt of other attacks as well. Ribot, for instance, reminds him that characters are governed by feelings, not by associations, that contrary or contradictory characters like de Musset's are not moved by ideas but by unconscious impulses. Furthermore, he points out that if the alteration or oscillation of such characters is to be explained by contrasted associations, it would be necessary to invoke the principle of physiological contrast (such as in color contrast) rather than the psychological opposition of ideas. The alternation would then be due to fatigue, partial exhaustion. Above all, it ought to be considered that unstable characters do not go from one thing to its opposite, but rather from difference to difference. Thus association by contrast is ruled out as an explanatory principle.

In Defence of Atomism. Paulhan, in his *atomistic* presentation, seems to be closely allied to the British schools, and his position among the French writers is more vulnerable on that account. There is something foreign in his mention of relations among the numerous tendencies which criss-cross one another in so many ways ; and his attaching importance

[1] A. Fouillée : *Tempérament et Caractère*, pp. 122 ff.

as regards character development to the fact that one is of a visual type and another an audile, calls forth surprise in the French camp ; above all, the vast number of combinations which may result from the consolidation of the various tendencies, associative and qualitative, such as social, vital, and organic traits, seems to bewilder them. Lévy [1] rejects Paulhan's classification as impractical and abstract and as not dealing with realities.

In the second edition of his work (1902), Paulhan defends himself with great aplomb, maintaining that the method which he pursues is *analytic*, as contrasted with the *concrete* approach of his critics whose classifications are purely formal, deriving their authority from the faculty psychology. To say that one is an active or sensitive type tells nothing worth while about the person. The concrete types will find a place in his scheme too after the proper analysis, but the simple cataloguing according to three great orders of psychology is inadequate.

As to Ribot's objection that characters are not governed as a rule by conscious processes, Paulhan agrees and explains that his principle of association by contrast is intended to operate on a physiological basis (" reaction to passions too long arrested or to the exhaustion of tendencies which have been too long dominant ").[2]

We need not of course go further into the controversy, which will be summarized toward the end of the chapter. The chief merit of Paulhan's book, to my mind, lies in the wealth of biographical material which the author employs to good purpose. In one passage he adduces a number of illustrations that might be used in corroboration of the *compensation theory* in the case of organic or acquired inferiority. Byron's and Lemercier's precipitate tendencies are attributed to their infirmities as an effort to triumph over the injustice of nature.

---

[1] A. Lévy : *Psychologie du caractère*, 1896, pp. 196 ff.
[2] Fr. Paulhan : *Les caractères*, 1902 (2nd edition), p. 38.

Idées-Forces. In an extremely suggestive book,[1] Fouillée, one of Paulhan's chief critics, develops a theory of character which seems to be based on his pet doctrine of *idées-forces*. The elements of character to him are ideas and will-power with feeling as a mediator. Not unlike Bain, he has his three main divisions of intellectual, sensitive and voluntary (used as a synonym of "volitional" in this chapter) characters, which again he divides into sub-classes: the intellectual types into the speculative and imaginative varieties, and again, from the standpoint of their method of procedure, into the intuitive and inductive minds; the sensitive[2] class into (a) those who possess little intelligence and little will-power, (b) those who are endowed with an energetic will but with little intelligence, and, finally, (c) those who have little will-power but have a great deal of intelligence. The adjectives "emotive", "impulsive" and "reflective" respectively may describe the three sensitive types. The same method of permutation and combination Fouillée follows in discussing the main voluntary divisions. Here we have: (a) those who have little sensibility and little intelligence, that is to say, the obstinate and perverted; (b) those who have considerable sensibility and little intelligence, such as the headstrong and violent—a class from which criminals are recruited—and, finally, (c) the "voluntaries," who possess a great deal of intellectual power but little sensibility. They are the cold and energetic calculators.

All through the book Fouillée emphasises the part played by the intellect in shaping and determining a man's character as

[1] A. Fouillée: *Tempérament et Caractère*, pp. 122 ff.

[2] "Sensitive" perhaps is not so good a rendering as "sentimental" or "emotional". "The *sensitifs*, from the physiological point of view," says Fouillée (loc. cit., p. 136), "are those whose nervous system, and especially the cerebral part of it, is originally constituted in such a way as to 'play' practically alone with an intensity which is often out of proportion to the external excitations."

against the views of Schopenhauer and Ribot that intelligence is a negligible factor in its relation to character, and that the very concept of character presupposes an innate disposition that is fixed and immutable. Illustration after illustration is adduced in confirmation of his thesis that intelligence has actually changed the behavior of many notable men; and there can be no doubt but that Fouillée's contention is sound, except that it suggests that originally there must have been some disposition in these men to want to change. Intelligence acts only as a means, but the will takes the initiative. It involves really the hoary issue whether or not determinism in the ultimate analysis implies fatalism.

In the Interest of Pedagogy. If Queyrat's little volume,[1] of which the fourth edition (revised) appeared in 1911, was first published in 1896,[2] the same year in which Lévy's *Psychologie du Caractère* was brought out, there is a striking coincidence that the Belgian Jew and the Frenchman should have arrived independently at the same conclusions.

In his introduction, the author takes occasion to excuse his endeavor to add another classification to the number already put forth, on the ground that we must have a classification as simple as possible, if pedagogy is to profit by it. This simple scheme is actually built on the faculty view initiated in France by Ribot to whom, incidentally, the book is dedicated, and proceeds in the direction of Lévy's observation that it is the predominance of the one faculty, two faculties or equilibration of the three which counts. As a matter of fact, there can be no closer agreement between the two writers.

Queyrat recognizes nine normal characters, three semi-morbid and three diseased characters. In the first division,

---

[1] F. Queyrat: *Les caractères et l'éducation morale* (4th edition). 1911.

[2] This is implied in a footnote on p. 23, where the words "Note de janvier 1896" in parenthesis would signify that the subsequent references did not appear in this original footnote.

governed by the marked predominance of only one " faculty " or tendency, we have (a) the emotional, (b) the active, and (c) the meditative or intellectual. The second division, in which two faculties are simultaneously predominant, yields us (a) the active-emotional or passionate, (b) the active-meditative or voluntary, and (c) the meditative-emotional or sentimental. The third division, based on the balancing on different levels of the three different faculties contains (a) the equilibrated character, (b) the amorphous, and (c) the apathetic. Since one or more of the three faculties may function irregularly or intermittently, we might add (a) the unstable, (b) the irresolute and (c) the contradictory characters. Lastly the diseases of character embrace (a) hypochondria, (b) melancholia and (c) hysteria.

We may designate these five main classes as (a) the pure, (b) the mixed, (c) the balanced, (d) the irregular or abnormal and (e) the psychopathic, to use a more recent terminology.

Queyrat achieves his end if simplicity is his aim, but the perfect symmetry of his table raises a suspicion in our minds as to how much of the scheme is psychological and how much of it—logical. The descriptions of the various types follow Ribot pretty closely, and the copious illustrations from historical persons, which lend the work its chief value, are in the vein of French characterology as a whole, which displays such a wide knowledge of biography and history.

Queyrat's Samplings not Satisfactory. Of course there is no reason why many of the celebrities who are mentioned among the pure types could not at the same time be contrary or undecided; in fact contemporary psychography and pathography would establish the untenability of Queyrat's arrangement of his material in many respects. What he and others of his countrymen have accomplished is simply to take out incidents and mental habits from the lives of well-known individuals and label them; but granted that Spinoza or Newton or Leibniz was a meditative type, that

Q

Caesar belonged to the active group, it is still possible that Spinoza was a balanced character, while Caesar might have been the contrary. Socrates is cited as an example of the balanced type, yet he might easily be regarded as a pure intellectual. One feels that Queyrat might have improved his simple table, if the fourth and fifth divisions were subordinated to the others.

The anecdotes which are given, too, do not in many instances prove the point. They may illustrate *moments, incidents* of one's life, but not necessarily traits, let alone full characterizations. At best these samplings are indications, not complete evidence, and it is to be feared that in the light of even a modicum of psychoanalysis, the incidents would receive at times different interpretations.

Lévy. In a work of unusual breadth and steeped in the humanities, by Lévy,[1] we find another basis for classification. He recognizes that all attempts at classification of character must necessarily remain artificial, but, since that is the case, he says, we ought to fit our scheme into the three great manifestations of mental life, viz., intelligence, feeling and will. The resulting classification would then hinge on the amount of blend there is in the individual. To Lévy it does not matter so much whether it is intelligence or feeling that is predominant so long as we recognize the fact that some one faculty is more marked than the rest.

Thus he obtains three classes : (1) the exclusive or unilateral types, characterized by the predominance of one of the three so-called faculties or functions ; (2) the mixed type where two of these faculties are highly developed at the expense of the third, and where there is possibly a conflict between the two elements, the one having the upper hand at one time, the other at another time, with intermittence of vigor and apathy at intervals ; (3) the perfectly balanced characters which may be the result of great deficiency of

---

[1] A. Lévy : *Psychologie du caractère*, 1896.

all the three elements or else may indicate a beautifully harmonious organization.

Lévy would add under another rubric the morbid characters, for, says he, there are diseases of character, such as hypochondria, melancholia, hysteria, etc. But these, he concludes, come under the head of psychiatry rather than ethology.

So far as I can see, Lévy differs with Ribot only (a) in assigning a legitimate place to instability under the mixed types and to the amorphous characters under the equilibrated rubric, and (b) in recognizing intelligence as a prime category, like affection and will, in the indexing of character.

Clinical Neurology. Regnault's project of a classificatory scheme ought to be mentioned here, not only because it varies widely from the other French classifications, but also for the reason that its conclusions are based on considerations similar to those which have been put forth recently by Kretschmer and Ewald. What has united these investigators in different countries is apparently the *psychiatric bond*.

The mental phenomenon, observes Regnault,[1] passes through three stages: first, the level of sensation, then the stage of association and colligation, assimilation with other processes (none of these terms is actually used by Regnault, who merely speaks of the sensations stirring up the brain), and finally, there is the expression phase of the circuit.

People will differ widely as to each of these three different departments; for instance, on the sensory level, one may get stronger or more intense impressions than another, one may make greater use of the higher senses (vision and audition) than his fellow-being, etc. On the elaborative side, we can conceive a number of things happening.

" The sensation (*sic*) may cross the brain without provoking either sentiments or ideas, in other words, leading directly to a suggested act."

---

[1] F. Regnault: " Sur une classification naturelle des caractères," *Rev. de l'Hypnot.* 1898, vol. xii.

The sensation sets into action a group of cells, rouses a sentiment, or it may excite many groups of cells or many ideas, whence the most important one will bring on the act, in this case deliberative.

When these possibilities are applied to character, the situation offers greater complexity. The sensation may cause an act of imitation or suggest an opposite course of action (both obstinacy and caprice, which differ from each other only as regards duration, come under this head). Furthermore the suggestion may not only be accepted but even magnified.

The sensation may excite a certain group of cells which are easily thrown into vibration—the basis of the feelings. The affective qualities and their relationship present a variety of characters, according to the intensity, constancy, rapidity, translatability into action, etc. We may thus have the emotive (intensity), the constant natures (singleness of feeling), fickle characters, incoherent, passionate, impulsive, impressionable, the cold-blooded—all involving the relationship of the feelings.

The ideational characters are grounded in the sensation exciting a number of groups of cells. Here we have those who associate few ideas (the simple minds), those who connect their ideas poorly (the false), those who associate well (the intelligent) ; and these latter may be ranged into literary people, i.e., those who possess many ideas feebly connected, the scientists whose ideational fund is comparatively meagre, but well articulated, and the true philosophers who are expected to concatenate solidly a wealth of ideas. Or the individual may have some ideas along a special line, whence reasoning with him could be done satisfactorily only in that field. ·

As regards the mutual influence of the feelings and intelligence, restraint or performance of an act may be exercised by the one or the other, i.e., the feelings or reason.

With respect to the motor end of the impressional circuit, we may, following the nature of the act, distinguish the slow or phlegmatic, the rapid or the violent, and the moderate. .

Regnault's crude physiology does not satisfy us, but his endeavor to free himself from the faculty view, so rampant in France, and to consider the *elements of character* merits our attention.

Historically it has a place as representing the movement in French psychotherapy, the termini of which were the Salpêtrière and the Nancy schools.

Types on a Scale of Social Achievement. In order to follow the original plan of including as many different points of view as possible in this inquiry, let us tarry a while to consider the classification of a Roman Catholic representative. Bulliot, in a paper read before the International Congress of Psychology in Paris [1] showing the influence of the anatomical and physiognomic doctrines, attributes two phases to character : the psychological and the physiological. Temperament is classed with the physiological constituent. Psychologically, character is marked by the predominance of one faculty or function of the individual over all the others. Physiologically, character is constituted by a certain individual make-up (temperament, cranial structure, general constitution of the organism) which effects the subordination of the other functions to the main one. Thus every simple character is a synthetic whole composed of two elements, the physiological and the psychological, or derived from a physiological factor which governs the psychological character. Complex characters are fashioned out of the simple characters.

In consonance with the study of Ledos,[2] Bulliot recognizes five classes of temperaments "which supply the material to character", but in examining types of character, Bulliot

---

[1] P. Bulliot : " De la classification des caractères et de la physiologie humaine," IVe *Congrès Internat. de Psychol.*, Paris, 1901.

[2] E. Ledos : *Traité de la physionomie humaine*, 1894.

finds more than five psychological faculties or functions dominating individuals. Their number in fact is at least seven, if not eight, and they might be envisaged as a scale perhaps according to their social value.

First of all there is the primitive man, characterized by the predominance of the instinct of self-preservation—the ordinary laborer. The imaginative type comes next, and then the affective type whose function is to be charming, to express beauty, love, joy. The active or combative type, to be recognized by the sharp and energetic features, receding forehead and muscular frame, is the fourth type.

The intuitive type possesses a nervous temperament, an oval face, slender form and often angular contour. Curiosity is the *motif* of the intuitive type. Such an individual is keen to learn, to see new things, is dominated by an incessant search of new ideas but he is easily fatigued, and is incapable of protracted exertion. His instability goes hand in hand with the unwillingness to be governed by habit.

The characteristics of the reflective type—the reasoner, the theoretician, the systematizer, the man of great will power—are as follows : on the physiological side—a melancholic temperament, the features marked by perpendicular lines, to the exclusion of curves, and the eyes deep set ; on the psychological side—sensibility underdeveloped, attention highly concentrated inwardly, imagination cold and constructive, inclinations serious and positive, intelligence of a calculative sort, plans well thought out and slow to mature, conscience highly developed. This type is inclined to be misanthropic, exacting, severe, inflexible, with a will-power much above the average.

The seventh type corresponds to the man of practical sense, the balanced and socially attractive individual. He is the typical head of a family, candidate for office, public spirited citizen, pastor, and community worker. His chief qualities are practical reason, judgment, authority and sociability.

The supreme type is the *radiator*, the great leader of men, who not only represents a harmonious combination of functions but possesses his faculties in a striking degree. Sometimes he is the unrecognized genius burning with excessive pride. This synthetic character corresponds with the synthetic temperament, which in spite of a nervous make-up, is endowed with inexhaustible energy, capable of making the greatest sustained efforts. Psychologically, Bulliot invests these characters with all sorts of excellences, a piercing eye, the vision·of an eagle, a prodigious memory, an indomitable will and lofty conceptions, but he imputes to them inordinate haughtiness and superhuman ambitions which, as in the case of Napoleon and Alexander, precipitate their fall. The article is accompanied with illustrations for each type.

Bulliot's classification suffers from the same defect as many others, viz., basing his descriptions on *ex hypothesi* formulations, the description suiting the particular dominant faculty, as he calls it. Nevertheless the curious thing about these eight divisions is the resemblance which they bear to Jung's revised eight types (*q.v.*) ; and it is for this reason that so much space was devoted here to the explanation of Bulliot's types.

Malapert. The classification of Malapert [1] is along the same line as that of Fouillée. For him there are primarily four classes of characters : (*a*) the intellectual, (*b*) the affective, (*c*) the active and (*d*) the voluntary. The supplementary classes are the apathetic, whose sensibility is very small, and the perfectly modulated type in whom there is no predominance of this or that character element.

In the four main divisions, there are the following subdivisions. The sensitive may be fickle and vivacious, emotional or passionate. The intellectual may be analytic, reflective

---

[1] P. Malapert : *Le caractère*, 1902, and *Les éléments du caractère et leur lois de combinaison*, 1906 (2nd edn.).

in a practical sense or speculative and engaged in constructive work. As regards activity, there are the inactive, active and reactive types. Lastly, among the purely voluntary types, we find the men without will power, i.e., those who carry on a routine life; and the amorphous and unstably impulsive. Again, we have the incomplete "voluntaries", comprising the weak-willed, the wavering and capricious, and, finally, the men with great will-power who are complete masters of themselves.

Ribéry. Lastly we may mention, among the French character studies, the doctoral thesis of Ribéry,[1] who follows pretty closely in the footsteps of his teacher Ribot, carrying out the idea of a hierarchy of characters more consistently perhaps than the latter. At the top of the table may be set down the amorphous, i.e., those without any definite characteristics. Then come the sensitive, divided into two groups : (*a*) the affective, (*b*) the apathetic. The passionate may be either stable or unstable, and the apathetic may be of the slight or the deeper sort. A combination of the active and the sensitive yields us a new class—the sensitive-active with its sub-classes ; the affective-passionate, the emotional-passionate and, lastly, the perfectly balanced or modulated character.

Ribéry admits that these are only empty forms which the innumerable individualities may fill out in a general way only. The number of conceivable combinations and permutations is legion, but what Ribéry endeavors to do is to provide us with a formula that we can use to our heart's content. His general classification follows the botanical or zoological scheme with its classes and sub-classes, orders and sub-orders, its species and varieties. The method is deductive, the combinations being derived, according to the author, from general psychological principles.

---

[1] Ch. Ribéry : *Essai sur la classification naturelle des caractères*, 1902.

SUMMARY OF THE FRENCH SCHOOLS

What is apparent about the French writers on character is the general adherence to the tri-partite division of the mind in their classification. The issue between Paulhan and his opponents is something which occurs again and again in psychology. It is the difference between the *genetic or empiristic* view and the *nativistic*. Paulhan, and to some extent this is true of Bourdet, was influenced by Comte, and that possibly explains the kinship with the British Associationist school whose representatives were, as is well-known, in sympathy with the French positivist.

Ribot and his associates might be considered nativists in that they believed that primarily we are born in such and such a mould, and the elaboration of the various tendencies and their interrelations will depend on this original cast. Character is there to begin with, according to them, and its formation is directed in a definite way. Paulhan builds character up out of a multitude of elements which, though in themselves probably inborn, may enter into numerous relationships thus resulting in different character types.

Paulhan's doctrine on the whole would find favor with the majority of the American investigators, especially those who have a leaning in the direction of a mechanistic or behavioristic psychology. Its chief defect is that it takes up so many factors that it is impossible to state anything definitely with regard to their interrelations. We are lost in a veritable maze of laws, tendencies, and types which are hypothetical and rarely applicable. It must be said, however, that Paulhan has gone farther than any of his contemporaries in France to account for oddities in character.

CHAPTER XIII

THE TEUTONIC SCHOOLS

Passing on to the German characterologists, we notice that they have not been so prolific in this field as the French psychologists; and the little that has been done by them has not been taken account of in the French works. Their writings, too, exhibit less homogeneity than do the French, nearly all of which are grouped around one central idea in classification. We may properly speak of a French *school* of characterology, but it would not be correct to apply the word in the singular, when referring to the German writers on character. The Germans laid more stress on temperament, perhaps because it affords a more definite scope for physiological explanation. Hence we find Julius Bahnsen in an elaborate work on Hegelian principles (though his guiding *motif* came from Schopenhauer) attempting to deduce the various types of character from the temperaments—a procedure at which Meumann shakes his head in disapproval.

Wundt has not much to say on the subject of character, except in its relation to temperament and other qualities.[1]

Emphasis on Polarity. The gist of a brochure by Sternberg [2] is this: we must not try to summate qualities if our aim is to arrive at a scientific characterology. It is above all necessary to trace contrasts in a given character. A positive element never makes its appearance without the negative being in some way touched off. Sternberg is probably thinking of compensation in his stress of polarity, but he nowhere mentions this term. Illustrating his thesis, he

---

[1] W. Wundt : *Physiologische Psychologie*, vol. iii, p. 637 (5th edn.).
[2] Th. Sternberg : *Charakterologie als Wissenschaft*, Lausanne, 1907.

cites the relationship between sadism and masochism, which as Apfelbach later expounded, are inherent in normal man. Even the pathological sadist, the writer claims, has his masochistic moments, and the masochist at least in phantasy turns sadist.

Principle of Organic Causality. Likewise with other traits, every character stimulus releases two opposing tendencies in different degrees, thus producing a tension. The normal trait is that which is statistically predominant, but the " contrary " trait is never completely crushed. Sternberg, who seems to have been influenced by Fichte, sets up the doctrine of contrasts as a heuristic principle in characterology, and is inclined to the belief that through various circumstances, such as exhaustion or other nervous conditions, a change may take place from one trait to another as in the well-known oscillation between excitation and depression. In fact, we are to understand as a *fundamental principle of organic causality that the more an excitation or depression exceeds the normal, the greater tendency is there for the hyperstimulated process to turn to its opposite*, just as in the sensory sphere of vision and affection.

Character Parallels. Since we are dealing with contrasts and restrictions, our character curves will of necessity take the shape of a zig-zag, allowing for plus and minus relations in the most complicated ramification ; and yet these relations are not really quantifiable. When we compare two individuals with regard to certain traits, it is not enough to say about them that A has so many traits of a positive kind, and B has so many of a negative kind. They are entirely different *wholes*, just as red and blue, or C and D are respectively two different colors and two different tones. But just as the vibration length and vibration frequency afford us a scale of comparison, so two individuals are comparable as a result of the analysis and collation of traits, and the synthesis of character is best brought about by setting up a hierarchy of trait parallels, especially when comparing two contrasted individuals after Plutarch's fashion. Sternberg's little book contains, at least in its negative aspect, the germ of the modern " Struktur " movement, so prevalent in German psychology to-day.

Many Stimulating Thoughts. There is much suggestive material in Sternberg's little book, unsystematically arranged and dashed down in outline. We are impelled to reflect on such statements as that morality is not fundamental in the concept of character ; that there is a relation between the logic of character and its ethic, so that a defect seen through the one is carried over to the other standpoint ; that aesthetics plays a central part in characterology in that it is the medium through which the perceiver grasps the perceived, especially when the logical phase of character is viewed through a moral perspective, or *vice versa*, the moral phase through a logical perspective; and finally that characterology is both a science and an art, an art-science, if adequately described. The feature, however, which stands out most in the pamphlet is the emphasis laid on polarity and the intimation that a metabolic principle may obtain in the sphere of character similar to the process in nerve excitation.

KANTIAN ECHOES

Heteronomous and Autonomous Characters. The Kantian tradition is represented in the inaugural address on character and world-outlook by Adickes, and in the compact little book by Elsenhans, referred to earlier in Chapter VI. Adickes, undertaking on a miniature scale what Jaspers has later done in larger proportions, namely, to analyze philosophical tendencies in the light of personality, harks back to Kant's famous division in the *Critique of Practical Reason* of the autonomous and the heteronomous will. Elaborating on this dichotomy, Adickes recognizes in the heteronomous—the character type of the masses—those who are moved *not by inner necessity, but by authority,* by the sentiment of the public, by what Mrs. Grundy will say. Of this character type there are three varieties : those people who are governed wholly by material considerations (utility, the " mess of pottage "), those who are the slaves of custom and habit, and lastly the individuals who evince a craving for novelty. ˙Eliminating the first class from our consideration as beneath notice, we have the two contrasted species of the heteronomous genus to deal with—the man who is steeped in the routine of tradition, and the one who is constantly changing his views with the advent of every new idea, as if by throwing aside the old, he is rearing himself above the crowd. Imagining himself to be a leader, an innovator, he is in reality only an echo, a reflection of every bright light. His *Weltanschauung* is not experienced within, but is merely mimicry, reflex.[1]

Inner Compulsion. The second genus, the *autonomous,* comprises several varieties whose common characteristic, however, is the inner necessity of their life attitudes. Whether they belong to the dogmatic type which˙ brooks no opposition and craves security in certainty, in decisiveness—or whether they incline to the agnostic type which is filled with scruples and doubts, their views are rooted in an inner compulsion. Metaphysics and religion are the domain of the dogmatic, whose *not being able to think otherwise* makes them feel that the objective facts *cannot be otherwise.* Theory of knowledge circumscribes the field which attracts the agnostically inclined (sometimes called " positivists ").

A Valuable Distinction. Apart from the application of the original dichotomy to philosophical systems or attitudes, the Kantian distinction of autonomous and heteronomous, from the standpoint of standards and values, is far more important than that of subjective and objective, or introverted and extraverted. I should not hesitate to affirm that character

[1] E. Adickes : *Charakter und Weltanschauung,* Tübingen, 1907.

properly belongs only to the autonomous, and the vast majority of people, making up the heteronomous class, though not wholly characterless, lack that element of inner regulation which marks the man of worth.

Formal and Material Aspects. The Kantian, and perhaps also Germanic earmarks of Elsenhans's treatment of character, are to be seen at once in the separation of formal and material phases, as well as in the direct appeal to the will. The formal qualities of character, and therefore of the will, are recognized as consistency [1] (*Konsequenz*), force, including persistence, and lastly independence. The material phase refers to the direction of the will, whether it is " good or bad ", and the standard of the " good " or " moral " character is, according to Elsenhans, Kant's categorical imperative.

In the chapter on terms, I have already had occasion to intimate that most of the discussions of character are cluttered up with too many distinctions which are not fundamental to the subject. I should be the last person to deny that " force " is not something different from " persistency " or from " independence ". Of course they are all personality traits, but the question is whether they strictly belong to character. If Elsenhans had looked deeper into the matter, he probably would have realized that a *consistent character cannot be anything but independent*. Why duplicate qualities then ? Again " good " and " bad " have an honored place in ethics, but are not in order when the *psychology* of character is on the table. In sum, the characteristic of consistency, if understood not merely as a *rule or uniformity governing one's own acts*, but as a *standard governing the relation between*

---

[1] Th. Elsenhans : *Charakterbildung* (1908), pp. 11 ff. The word *consistency*, as used in this sense, differs greatly from my own use of the word later on ; and it should therefore be pointed out that the German word *Konsequenz* aptly describes uniformity of acts, but does not necessarily refer to the *objective* standardization of conduct which would demand the same rights for others as for oneself. Individual uniformity is secondary to inter-individual consistency.

oneself and others, is the only one of the qualities which should be accepted, according to the point of view developed in this book.

Meumann's Physiological Theory. More promising, however, is the account of Meumann in his *Intelligenz und Wille*, where he expounds a physiological theory of character. Meumann, like Wundt, defines character as a disposition of the will, and thinks character quite independent of the feelings.[1]

After discarding the attempt to derive character from any form of affective life, he says, " We should come much nearer the truth if we traced back the intensity or energy of the will to an elementary strength of the will dispositions themselves. It must then be a physical basis that lends its force to the will act. In the last instance it is to be sought in the nervous energy of men. He who is endowed with great energy for motor innervation and movement, and in addition possesses an intensive and easily evocable association between the sensory parallel processes of his goal ideas and between the external movements, has in these qualities the foundation for energetic physical activity. And the man whose central nervous system, especially whose cortex is the seat of numerous sensory cells with a large stock of physical energy and whose functional sensory dispositions are possessed of great energy, will have thus the foundation for mental energy."[2] The corollary to be drawn from this suggests that men with weak nervous constitutions have little will energy ; and the flagrant negative instance of Kant is explained away by Meumann in assuming that Kant's physical weakness stopped at the brain, and that the philosopher's central nervous system, and especially the brain and those parts of it in which the parallel processes leading to mental activity took place, were endowed with an enormous amount of energy.

[1] E. Meumann : *Intelligenz und Wille*, Part II, chapt. iii.

[2] *Ibid.* p. 237.

In the above we have, according to Meumann, the first of the fundamental properties of the will, which gives rise to pure volitional types of character.

A second property is the time relation. The " will " activity may be transient or lasting. He who can manage to expend a relatively equal amount of energy and develop for all tasks a lasting intensity possesses an enduring will. Here, too, Meumann, profiting by the results of Mosso, Kraepelin. and Stern, traces this property back to the way in which the stock of nervous energy operates in different people, and their aptness to be easily fatigued or not, also to the various stages of the work at which fatigue is likely to set in.[1]

A third property is to be found in the degrees of development that the will attains in various individuals. The will that is guided by one principle or a system of principles to which all other things are subordinated will form the consistent character. Sporadic outbursts of activity will form the inconsistent character.

The disposition to act instinctively and impulsively on immediate ends and its opposite tendency, viz., acting with reference to more ultimate purposes, yield us a fourth property of the will. Aligned with that is the attentive type of the will, the root of which is a concentrated attention and the perseveration of goal ideas (static, as opposed to dynamic, activity).[2]

Another type of pure will form is derived from the manner in which people will approve or disapprove of a certain course of action. Some will be led to behave in a certain way through the co-operation of their feelings directly, while others will not act until they have considered and turned over in their mind all the reasons by which their course might be ratified. In this way we obtain the wavering type, and the one who quickly makes up his mind.

[1] *Ibid*, p. 243 ff.   [2] Loc. cit., pp. 238-9.

Finally, among the pure will forms, may be mentioned the habitual or mechanical or routine characters, that is to say, the individuals who have a tendency to get into certain grooves of conduct. So far we have dealt with *pure* will forms.

The second large division of will forms is the affective order, and it is here that Meumann finds eight fundamental properties in the feelings. (1) With reference to quality, they may be either pleasant or unpleasant. (2) As to intensity, they may be of various degrees. (3) In respect of time, they can persist in consciousness for a longer or shorter period. (4) The feelings may be excited with greater or less ease. (5) Their effect may be transitory or more lasting and reverberate in consciousness. (6) They may be classed as to the manner in which they develop, some feelings having a more objective basis than others. Again, the content of the idea may influence us, or the particular form in which we experience it may excite the feeling. (7) Connection with other contents of consciousness or the degree of fusion forms another category. (8) Their relations to us may be different. We can objectify our feelings ; for instance, when we say a " cheerful day ", or " a pleasant neighbourhood ", we read our own feelings into those objects, or else we can subjectify the feelings by ascribing them to our own inner condition.

Through such an analysis, Meumann is able to construct an elaborate scheme of the temperaments according to the combination of the different attributes of feeling a man possesses.

The third large class of will forms is called " intelligence forms of the will ", by which Meumann means forms of the will that have their origin in the effect of certain fundamental intelligence forms on the will ; for, says Meumann, properly speaking, intelligence forms of the will are only forms of intelligence that are translated into action, just as the affective forms also are to serve the purpose of the will or activity.

In this third class there are three categories : (a) that which

R

is responsible for differences in mental productivity, reproductivity and unproductive thinking in man, (*b*) comprising differences in intellectual independence and dependence, (*c*) embracing differences between analytic and synthetic thinking and between intuitive and discursive thinking.

It will easily be seen what an immense stock of character types can be had out of the manipulation of so many forms in different combinations.

Meumann has perhaps overstepped the limit in the drawing up of numerous classes and forms, but he, more than anyone else in Germany, has given us a solid foothold for our problem and has pointed out the direction in which we are to attain our object.

A learned Layman in Contrast with Meumann. Lucka's scheme [1] is somewhat interesting, not only because he takes the point of view of the worldly man on the subject, but because he has recently been recognized as one of the most prominent fiction writers in Germany. Character to him is not so much what differentiates one man from another as the attitude a man takes toward the external world. He sponsors the philosophical aspect of the subject. It must be on the ground of worldly experience that he divides men into four, or rather two wider classes and two narrower sub-classes. We begin with the naïve who make no distinction between reality and value, who are always on the spot to act because they, as a rule, do not realize the import of their acts. They make the soldiers, the speculators, and the adventurers. Then there is, secondly, the mediate class, the reflective people, who not only have experiences, but ponder over them. They often waver and hesitate, because they see so many relations of which the naïve man has no idea.[2] The man of the moment is our third type. For

---

[1] E. Lucka : " Das Problem einer Charakterologie," *Archiv. für die gesamte Psychologie*, 1908, vol. xi.

[2] We immediately perceive in these Jung's introverts.

him there are only incoherent experiences. He lacks the continuity of the subject. He is perfectly passive without being able to create anything new out of his impressions. He is reproductive but not productive. His life is made up of impressions alone. (4) The productive type, represented by men like Goethe, whose very memory function necessitates a recasting of experiences, constitutes just the opposite. His life is directed outward, beginning with his own personality whereas the reproductive type brings the outward world into his own. Spontaneity marks the productive individual who never merely learns, but is continually experiencing.

Lucka, though he is abreast of the literature on the subject, disregards the *psychology* of character entirely, and trusts solely to his insight into things. His view of character belongs to the class of observational accounts, approaching in content, though not in form, to the scattered brilliant *aperçus* contained in La Bruyère, La Rochefoucauld, Jean Paul and Schopenhauer. The newer schools to which Lucka's views seem most closely aligned are to be found in what now constitutes the *Struktur* movement; and in some measure there is an overlapping between Lucka's types and those of Spranger, who will be considered in another chapter. To Lucka " character " is " the disposition of an individual psychic organization to receive impressions from the world about (in the widest sense) in a definite way, and to react to them in a definite manner." Character, in Lucka's vocabulary, is to be translated as a " characteristic attitude toward the world ".

Klages' Pigeon-holing of Qualities. Though Klages' *Prinzipien der Charakterologie* might properly be brought into relation with the other German treatments of character, it would take too much space even to give the merest outline of Klages' classification which is marked by a complex architectonic. The capacities of men, he believes, form the stuff or texture of character, while the strivings or conations constitute its quality. Furthermore, the structure of character is determined by the organization of the material, and is indicated by the ratio of all the driving forces of the individual and his resisting or inhibitive tendencies. The *personal reactivity* quotient then would be the result of the formula $\frac{R}{D}$, where D stands for the driving forces and R for the resistance.

When we begin to look into Klages' tables, we are confronted with a rather perplexing list of differences which are pigeon-holed into various categories, such as differences of quantity (full and empty) ; differences of distinctness (warm and cold) ; differences of mobility (heavy and light) ; differences of quality (deep and shallow). Klages is very careful to find a place for every quality and trait, but his mode of procedure smacks of Hegelian dialectic, and the presentation lacks clarity, so that, with all his discerning observations and eagerness to save us from general fallacies, he is apt to be confusing. The confidence with which he makes certain statements, such as that, though we say " *Es* reizt mich ", we never use the same quasi-passive construction in the case of willing, would be shaken if he took cognizance of other languages.[1] Similarly his tabulation and schemes do not carry conviction. Under deficient self-preservation, he lists in the ethical category—injustice, unreliability, " characterlessness " and unscrupulousness. It would seem that the very people who possess these negative traits were born with an exaggerated instinct of self-preservation.

---

[1] It is well to examine a concept from the point of view of its popular usage or etymology, but Klages places too much emphasis on linguistic forms. As a matter of fact, the untutored person scarcely uses the verb *to will* ; and *willing* is most frequently employed by the man in the street in the sense of *desiring*. In Yiddish the quasi-passive construction with the verb " to will " is often used, but in the sense of desiring " Es vilt zich mir " is the equivalent of " I should like ", with the implication of the desire being due to organic sources.

Of all the recent writers on character in Germany, Klages has been the only one actually to create a school, which however is confined to the literary people. It cannot be denied that he has specialized in this branch of knowledge, and his researches on handwriting in connection with character,[1] which to him is bound up with the reactivity of the individual, have widened the scope of his possibilities, but it is partially because Klages has occupied himself with a mass of details that he is exposed to the danger of not seeing the forest because of the trees. The *minutiae* on which he dwells may be important in *special* connections, but if each individual is to be measured in every particular as proposed by Klages, then the classification of characters becomes a practical impossibility. In the mode of approach to the problem and the results, there is a great deal of resemblance between Klages and Paulhan.

Character and Work. For a number of years Kraepelin has laid great stress on individual differences in the working curve. It was at his instance that many investigations were conducted, principally in Munich, with the purpose in view of discovering fundamental personality traits. The word *Arbeit* seems to have loomed large with Kraepelin, for not only was his periodical named *Psychologische Arbeiten*, but the term appears very frequently in his articles. Kraepelin has been instrumental in furthering our knowledge about the working curve, as a result of the painstaking experiments on practice effects, habituation, fatigability, recovery, etc., but to regard differences in fatigability and adaptation to work among the underlying bases of personality is certainly taking a great deal for granted ; and it is only after about *twenty* years of hopeful endeavors that Kraepelin reluctantly admits the complications involved in such experiments as his pupil

---

[1] L. Klages : *Die Probleme der Graphologie*, 1910. *Handschrift und Charakter*, 1920.

Lange [1] has been conducting, and rather ungraciously attributes the difficulties to flaws in the method, which he supposes might be obviated in the future.[2] Lange, it must be said, accomplished his task most conscientiously, and if he was not able to establish any correlations, even in the narrow field with which he was concerned, he at least posed a number of serious questions, such as whether there is a *single* capacity for practice gain, or *any one* type of *fatigability*. Thus it seems as if unwittingly Lange queries the very presuppositions of his master's ambitious project.

DIMENSIONAL VIEW OF CHARACTER

Sex Types. There is perhaps no more intriguing treatment of character than Apfelbach's [3] who might well be considered a disciple of the youthful Weininger, mentioned in Chapter V. Apfelbach, of course, does not go so far as to say that the " lowest man is infinitely higher than the most worthy woman ". Nor does he believe with his master that woman is non-moral. But the fact that this writer shares the opinion that fundamental in the synthesis of character are the ingredients of sexuality, i.e., masculinity or femininity, as well as what he calls by the generic name of psychomodality which embraces the qualities of sadism and masochism, at once makes it clear that the thread runs back to the author of *Sex and Character*.

Like him, Apfelbach thinks that all persons partake of male and female elements in different ratios, but whereas Weininger was satisfied that all else could be inferred from this quantitative relationship in a given individual, his follower prefers to regard this polarity simply as one dimension which must be combined with other dimensions to provide us with a true profile. The typical woman, e.g., is certainly not the

[1] J. Lange : " Zur Messung der persönlichen Grundeigenschaften," *Psychol. Arbeiten*, 1923, vol. viii.

[2] E. Kraepelin : "Bemerkungen zu der vorstehenden Arbeit," *ibid*.

[3] H. Apfelbach : *Der Aufbau des Charakters* (1924).

logical thinker, nevertheless, a woman may be endowed with a masculine form of thought and *vice versa*.

Apfelbach will probably meet with little resistance in setting up the distinction between the male and female elements in both man and woman. *Einfühlung* (Empathy) is claimed as a special mark of femininity, so that every good actor must *ex hypothesi* be of a feminine cast of mind, unless he plays only parts which correspond to his own character. A formula is given even to determine the masculinity or the femininity of the children. Thus if the father's and the mother's masculinity are greater than unity the offspring will be endowed with masculinity ; if they total less than unity, the offspring will have a tendency to appear feminine in their make-up.

Psychomodality. But the dimension of psychomodality requires more attention. This dimension comprises the two contrasted traits : sadism and masochism, not to be taken in the sense of perversions but rather in that of ascendance and submissiveness.[1] (The terms positive and negative algolagny, literally " pain lust ", have been coming into vogue more recently to supplant the more commonly known words formed from proper names.) The sadist, according to Apfelbach, is energetic, courageous, enterprising, aggressive, full of vitality. The masochistic type is marked by lack of will-power, shyness, reserve, submissiveness and a sweet disposition. Pure psycho-modal types are as rare as pure sex types. There are all sorts of imperceptible gradations.

All conquerors, warriors, leaders in action are set down as sadists. Among the masochistic persons are the poets and composers, Schubert for instance. The masochistic man is somewhat at a disadvantage, but the sadistic woman is often a misfortune. She makes a shrewish, ambitious, pleasure-seeking wife, apt to ruin her husband and family by her unmotivated and unreasonable demands. She will brook no

[1] Much as in F. Allport's *Social Psychology*, 1924, p. 119.

opposition and gives vent to the feeling of hatred in an extreme measure.

The author devotes a good deal of space to sketching the sadist's and the masochist's tendencies in various situations : in sport, in science, in religion, and so on. The sadist, for instance, is *descriptive* ; the masochist *explanatory*. The former has a flair for details, especially in botany, anatomy, morphology and histology, also in analytic chemistry (quantitative rather than qualitative), while the masochist is the generalizer, the philosopher who is seeking ultimate solutions to problems. The sadist is an experimentalist in science and after persistent endeavors might come upon a discovery. The masochist, then, brings this discovery into line with other discoveries and formulates a general principle. As a scientist, the former is hasty in his utterances and is inclined to radical negations. In polemic, he is not objective and therefore useless. Jealousy and hatred move him to annihilate his opponent. The masochist, on the other hand, is moderate in his criticism ; more conscientious and tender in his dealings with adversaries.

Psychomodal Types of Thought. It is time, however, to summarize the characteristics of the four types of thought, viz., (*a*) masculine, (*b*) feminine, (*c*) sadistic, and (*d*) masochistic.

(1) *Masculine type of thought* : highly developed logicality in the formation of judgments ; grasping of the essential, and objectivity.

(2) *Feminine type of thought* : looseness of logical connections, deviation from the essential, inclination to use metaphor, lack of objectivity, muddled judgment and predominance of subjective coloring.

(3) *Sadistic type of thought*. Keen interest in details and the accidental, little sense for the general and causal ; preference for the concrete and descriptive.

(4) *Masochistic type of thought.* Hankering for problems, striving after deep-rooted explanations, and interest in the general and causal.

It is evident that four combinations are possible; and vector formulae are introduced to illustrate the exact relations of the types in different individuals.

Much as I should like to continue the glittering analysis of the sadistic and masochistic types in all branches of endeavor developed most ingeniously and supported by many illustrations of a specific nature,[1] we must not forget that there are other dimensions of character to be considered.

The Affective Dimension. Emotionality constitutes a third dimension of character. Here we have the division of (*a*) hypo-emotional, and (*b*) hyper-emotional. Emotionality, which is likened to the pedal of a piano determining the intensity of the tones, or in the case of man, the events of his life, is made the basis of temperament by this author as we have seen in a previous chapter.

Idealism draws upon emotionality with a masochistic background, so that there might be more room for inhibition of elementary forms of satisfaction, thus facilitating sublimation which is the stamp of all idealism. The realistic bent is brought about by a slighter degree of emotionality combined with a sadistic disposition and a lower moral level.

Morality. The fourth dimension of character is that of morality with the bi-furcated division of (*a*) morally adequate and, (*b*) morally defective. The unscrupulousness and unreliability of the latter in various spheres is well pictured, but space limitations will not permit of further citation except to point to the four classes of delinquency in accord with the

---

[1] Even musical instruments, poems, and musical compositions are classified according as they are sadistic in appeal or masochistic. Thus Grieg's *Solveig's Song* is masochistic, while Paganini's *Witches' Dance* is sadistic. The 'cello is a masochistic instrument; the piano, intended for the sadist.

dimensional table. Of the four classes, two belong to the
erethic (sthenic, active, energetic) and two belong to the
apathetic (asthenic) type. The highwayman and the swindler
are of the erethic sort, yet the first is *masculine*, sadistic, and
hyper-emotional in his make-up, the second is on the other
hand, *feminine*, sadistic and hyper-emotional. In the apathetic
group, there are the hypo-emotional types of delinquents—
the suggestible accessory who is feminine and masochistic,
and the vagabond who is also masochistic but masculine.
Thus Apfelbach's dovetailing seems to proceed without a
hitch.

Intellectuality. In the dimension of intellectuality, there
is a distinction made between special intellectuality which
validates and gives direction to the special functions called
specific intellect, including memory, judgment, etc., and
combinative capacity. Both parts together, the special and
the specific, go to make up the total intellectuality of a person.
The different functions operate differently with persons
of different psychomodality ratios. Thus the memory type
comes into its own with the feminine sadistic constitution,
where the logical causal relation of the material learnt is
negligible. With the masculine masochistic constitution,
however, the judgment type reaches its fullest development
and the emphasis is then laid on the logical and abstract
rather than on the concrete. It need hardly be said, in comment on Apfelbach's distinction, that experimental psychology offers no ground for such a sharp opposition between
judgment and memory. Men of great philosophical insight
are often better at remembering nonsense syllables than those
who are good rote memorizers of meaningful material. Our
author is given to making dichotomies, hence his occasional
aberrations. In general, however, despite his brilliancy, true
Geistreichkeit, he follows a sound course in his presentation,
and his conclusions are bound to arrest our attention whether
we accept them or not.

There is still a sixth optional dimension which must be mentioned—the accessory elements, consisting of the altruistic and egoistic impulses, which should not, according to Apfelbach, be confused with the morality dimension. Many "morally insane individuals" as he calls those who are unreliable in conduct, are anything but selfish, and a number of those who are normally adequate, he maintains, are egoistic.

Combinations of Character Types. Representing each of the six dimensions enumerated by the symbols A B C D J F and designating the positive pole by a capital letter and the negative by a small letter, Apfelbach obtains a table of 64 character types. Some of these combinations he analyzes by way of illustration from historical examples or personal knowledge. To select at random : combination 4 is represented symbolically as a b C D J F which signifies a feminine, masochistic, hyper-emotional, morally and intellectually adequate, and frank nature. In this case, the man would be a gentle, contemplative, sentimental type, a lyric poet, or as an actor a youthful lover ; with a little more masculinity, he might be a novelist or even an essayist. As a scientist, he would choose the non-rigid branches such as archæology, history of art, literary criticism, philology, etc. The woman of this type would develop into the true ideal motherly wife, possibly with an erotic sentimentality. Combination A B C d J F, i.e., the masculine, sadistic, hyper-emotional, highly unmoral, intellectually adequate and open nature, would yield the ingenious, violent criminal who deliberately plans and executes a major crime in broad daylight. If F is negative, brutality marks the crime and if J is negative, the ingenuity is missing entirely, and only the brutality remains.

Certainly if we grant Apfelbach's premise that his dimensions are the only ones or the most important in the characterial constitution, the many interesting conclusions which he has drawn therefrom stand uncontroverted, but even if we do not go with him all the way, his side of the story sounds plausible.

German Idealism in Switzerland. Returning to Germany we note that sufficient interest has been aroused there to warrant the publication of three periodicals devoted to problems of character. The most solid of these is the *Jahrbuch der Charakterologie* which began to appear in 1924. The *Zeitschrift für Menschenkunde*, with an applied and psychoanalytic slant, followed in 1925, while *Der Charakter*, which in on a popular level, stressing the inspirational and betraying a streak of the occult, made its *début* in the same year.

Some of the essays in the *Jahrbuch der Charakterologie* will be taken up in later chapters where they fit in better with the subject matter. The majority of the articles in these periodicals, coming under the purview of characterology, are listed in the bibliography.

Meanwhile we must not neglect to mention a German work which has recently appeared in Switzerland, although it too may well be considered under the rubric of the philosophy of character. The fundamental concepts of person, personality and character are here defined rather scholastically in such a way as to cover generalities but not the differentiated body of observations on personality that have been made lately in several neighbouring fields of knowledge. Personality is regarded as an essentiality of a particular kind, something spontaneous and subjectified. More precisely personality is defined as the psychically understood structurally and genetically complex individuality as we encounter it in typically human conduct.[1] "Character is the unitary totality of reactive possibilities, and therefore qualities, of a person." It is thus a particular phase of personality. Finally the study of personality in its individual manifestative possibilities would be equivalent to characterology.

[1] P. Häberlin : *Der Charakter*, 1925, p. 37.

The trouble with such definitions is that they contain terms which are far obscurer and certainly more complex than those defined. If we should be called upon to place Häberlin in a characterological chart, there could hardly be any question but that he would come under the more idealistic wing of the interpretative psychologists, with a religious note underlying his conception. Häberlin approaches the question of individuation with awe and is content to dispose of it as a mystery. In Chapter XXVII we shall see how this author's view of character does not rest on psychological principles but on philosophical presuppositions.

Dynamic Synthesis. Some of the leading German schools and movements are reflected in the most recent work on character, the comprehensive volume [1] by the aesthetician Utitz, who has also brought out the *Jahrbuch der Charakterologie*, now in its fourth year.

It would be impossible to do justice to this book, which covers partly the same ground as the present treatment, in brief compass. Utitz, in spite of his fondness for repetition and metaphor, and use of a feuilletonistic style *ad libitum* to the extent of underscoring the obvious, has assembled a large number of problems growing out of the recent studies on character, as approached from the various fields of human endeavor. The theme which this author harps on again and again with slight variation of instance and phraseology is that character must comprehend all phases of one's behavior, that we ought not to ask after the fundamental only. The interesting concept of " Stratification " (*Schichtenstruktur*) which crops up also in other German works, refers to the layers of characteristics. Courtesy or friendliness, for example, may be shown by an otherwise morose person for business reasons, but it may also be, and usually is, the expression of a spontaneous quality. In the friendly person, the trait then is

---

[1] E. Utitz : *Charakterologie*, 1925.

" deeper " ; in the grouchy fellow who makes an effort to smile, the trait is more on the surface.

Levels of Character. It is the same with other forms of behavior.   The lie as an event and the lie as a charactero-logical datum are two different things. Many different motives can be adduced in seeking the antecedents of the deliberate deception.   Naturally he who lies in order to alleviate suffering does not tap the lying trait to the same depth as one who wishes to escape punishment or who wants to make a particu-larly good impression in some regard, or the pathological liar. The lie emerges from different levels. Yet we need not, on that account, make the mistake of disregarding the more superficial levels, and reach our conclusion on the basis of the fundamental layer only. Quoting Georg Simmel, whose philosophy has apparently, together with Stern's psychology, formed the foundation for his characterological development, Utitz identifies himself sufficiently with the *Struktur* movement in Germany to insist that a part or single phase of a character has no significance except with reference to the whole. Even the single trait must be envisaged as a theme with variations. Utitz might have also brought the analogy of the ordinary tone which is constituted not only by the funda-mental but by its overtones as well.

A character then consists of a synthesis of levels. Even the most apparently contradictory character has its laws governing this contradictoriness, and every one of our actions may be grounded in several different levels of motivation at the same time. In conduct there is seldom an excluded middle. We may be philanthropic both because it affords us pleasure to help others, and also for the reason that it titillates our *amour-propre*, or because we are likely to be honored for it or perhaps receive commercial advantages in return.

In another passage [1] the author talks of fundamentals and necessities in character, or characteristics of a primary,

---

[1] Loc. cit., pp. 255 ff.

secondary, tertiary, etc., degree. Stern, as we shall see in Chapter XXVIII, asked: What is genuine, and what is spurious in a character ? Utitz poses the same question, merely using the words " necessary " and " contingent " instead. But he is at the same time anxious to explain that the contingent or accessory is of value in estimating the necessary or primary and is to some extent affected thereby.

The keynote of the whole book is that the variations, deviations, or seeming inconsistencies in character must be taken account of, and the illustrations from everyday life are supplemented with analogies in art. Utitz has well expatiated on the dynamics of personality, the relationship between an act and its mainspring, but really psychoanalysis has pre-empted nearly all these issues in its own technical way. Perhaps it has gone too far in its advance, but then much of the exposition in Utitz's *Charakterologie* appears common-place to any one with a smattering of Freud's teachings.

In this work is to be found the fault that might be ascribed to much of contemporary German philosophical writing : categories are added unnecessarily and distinctions are made which, though perhaps logically valid, are psychologically without significance. Utitz, as is not unlikely, must have come under the influence of the phenomenological school of Husserl, although Simmel and Stern have contributed considerably to his outlook. When one begins to speak of characterological dynamics, characterological rhythmics, weight, intensity, direction, dimensionality, etc., it is time to ask where the catalogue will end, and whether some of the cases treated under several rubrics may not be envisaged under one purview. It is easy to draw distinctions. Any act or trait can be seen somewhat differently when associated with a different field of knowledge. Is it, however, incumbent on us to take this difference seriously ? As literature—yes, but as science—no ; for we shall only be impeding our own course by putting obstacles in the way.

Serial Classification.   Utitz rightly urges that we need not be deterred by the magnitude of the task, but this salutary exhortation loses its force when the task is needlessly complicated.   In his classification, for instance, he arranges the characters in series: vocational characters, *weltan-schauliche* (according to world outlook) characters, psychopathic characters, ethical characters, criminal characters, one-dimensional and multi-dimensional characters, material and purposive characters, national characters, period characters, culture or civilization characters, endogenous and circumstantial characters and finally accomplished and empty characters.   This programme is enough to paralyze our whole inquiry.   Not that we should question the soundness of most of the distinctions.   Surely all might admit that the age in which one lives, one's race, and one's general view of life (*Weltanschauung*) would in some degree affect one's endogenous character, that even the vicissitudes of life will color one's personality.   Unless, however, we restrict our exploratory expedition, we shall be scurrying about aimlessly.

This constitutes perhaps the chief reason for Utitz's failure to reach specific conclusions, in spite of all the vast material at his command, so that his treatise remains a *methodological* discussion, by no means sterile, and yet not likely to lead the way for the perplexed.   It is further to be remembered that the more categories, the more room for dichotomies in those very categories.   Thus the *anschauliche* character may actually *live* his *Anschauung*, or merely *profess* it.   He may be an agnostic or materialist and yet lead a spiritual life or he may be an idealist in his philosophy and live on a low plane.

Reconciliation of Standpoints.   Utitz has endeavored to steer clear of extremes, but he has not shown how to reconcile them.   In general he is inclined to ground the science of character in individual characters, not in formal types (Ideal-bildungen).   Yet the class character may serve as a pattern for an inductive or empirical treatment (Kasuistik).

Neither the empirical phase of character which concerns itself with individuals only, unmindful of any type which the individuals might fit into, nor the formal aspect which is exemplified by phrases like " the artist ", " the scientist," " the rigid character," is useful in and by itself. Both halves must function if we are to have a real characterology, where actual facts in life are subject to method.

For that matter, Utitz might have drawn for support on the Kantian conciliation of the *a priori* and the empirical. Certainly individuals could not be recognized as characters, unless there was a ready category to embrace the particular cases, whether this category is suggested in books or generalized and abstracted out of numerous personal experiences, which at first must have registered but vaguely, and in terms only of likes and dislikes but not as objective discernment. To illustrate, as children we judge people according as their individual acts give us pleasure or discomfort. We say A is good if he entertains us, gives us presents; B is bad or naughty if he teases or scolds us. We gradually then build up the type " a good man ", " a just person," etc.; but it is only in mature adult life that we grasp the meaning of characteristics that are not based on dealings with ourselves, and above all, that are complex and subject to alternation. For this reason the concept " sanguine " or " manic-depressive " is an instrument the value of which we too seldom stop to consider. Without such formal categories at hand, we should have been groping in the dark, as indeed we do, before we derive the necessary information.

On the question of the interpretative *versus* the descriptive, Utitz again is disposed to make concessions to either side, but he rightly points out that we are not at all clear as to the essence of an interpretative or understanding psychology. All that we know of it is that it is bound up with the senses and their interplay—meanings in subjective form. The

s

explanatory psychology is a little better off in that all are agreed that to explain is to indicate causal connections. But the value school, which is identified with the interpretative movement in psychology, has this advantage : it makes allowance for a striving or purpose, a drive which is the core of character and which is not out of accord with a causal inquiry into the relationships of the character elements. In this point Utitz seems to have fallen in with Stern's personalistic view (cf. chapter XXVII).

CONCLUDING NOTE ON GERMAN CHARACTEROLOGY

Since another chapter will take up the more typically Germanic movement represented by the *Geisteswissen-schaften* and the *Struktur* schools, the remarks here will be confined to a few critical observations. In the first place, the German writers tend to introduce a fair dose of philosophy in their discussions. This is true especially of the more recent characterologists. Whether they align themselves with any particular system or not, they are invariably certain to refer to philosophical works. The alliance between philosophy and psychiatry is stronger in Germany than anywhere else ; and the influence of the newer tendencies in German philosophy and psychology manifest themselves in psychiatric circles by the use made of the concepts of value and purpose.

Many of the German articles and books on character display a wide knowledge of the work done in Germany, but take little cognizance, if any, of investigations undertaken else-where. In justice, it must be admitted that comparatively few studies are being carried on in this field outside of Germany, but there is no effort made to become conversant with these foreign angles, so that the numerous discussions are eminently Teutonic in character, with the result that there is an over-emphasis of certain problems at the expense of others. Words like " endogene ", " Schicksalcharaktere ", " Kasuistik ",

" Lebensverfassung ", and others have become stereotypes in the various presentations.

There is a great lack of systematic historical *exposition* of views on character. Either a man will present his own theories adequately (Kretschmer) or else he will cover a vast territory *alluding* to scores of characterologists without revealing the burden of their claims (Kronfeld, Birnbaum). The survey then becomes a huge *feuilleton* ; and not even Utitz's comprehensive work is free from this criticism.

On the other hand, there is no denying that in Germany (and Austria) issues have been picked out and demarcated with singular clarity in spite of frequent digressions to dwell on some side-plot, or occasional enthusiastic lapses into platitudes decked out in a slightly new terminology. If the German characterologists were only to assimilate and incorporate into their studies proportionally as much of the foreign material as they do their own findings and in addition make an endeavor to expound the results rather than to accumulate allusions in edition after edition of the same book, the task of students in this whole field would be half accomplished.[1]

[1] It is encouraging to learn that W. Rink is now working on a comprehensive history of characterology. At least so we are told by Th. Lessing in his monograph "Prinzipien der Charakterologie", *Deutsche Psychologie*, 1926, vol. iv, No. 2, p. 50.

CHAPTER XIV

I. A DUTCH ACCOUNT

The laborious comparative study of Heymans and Wiersma in which the character traits of thousands of persons were treated statistically on the basis of both biographical and questionnaire material resulted in, or rather began with, the selection of three fundamental criteria for the rating of character, viz., activity, emotionality and the preponderance of either the primary or the secondary function, and the statistical tabulation of numerous traits or responses relative to the above criteria. The criteria of activity and emotionality need no explanation, but the curious designation of " primary functioning " refers to such qualities as " easily comforted ", " changeable sympathies ", " ever interested in new impressions and friends ", " easily reconciled ", " apt to change occupation or course of study ", " often takes up with great plans which never are realized ", etc. The preponderance of the " secondary function ", on the other hand, yielded such data as tenacity, " clinging to old memories," " hard to reconcile," conservatism, " influenced by future prospects rather than by immediate gain," and so on.

On the basis of the three divisions according to the fundamental criteria, Heymans and Wiersma have set up eight types of characters after this fashion.

(1) *Amorphous*—the non-emotional non-active with predominant primary function.[1]

---

[1] G. Heymans and E. Wiersma : " Beiträge zur speziellen Psychologie auf Grund einer Massenuntersuchung," *Ztft. für Psychologie,* 1906–9, vols. xlii–xlvi, xlix, and li.

(2) *Apathetic*—the non-emotional non-active with predominant secondary function.

(3) *Nervous*—the emotional non-active with predominant primary function.

(4) *Sentimental*—the emotional non-active with predominant secondary function.

(5) *Sanguine*—the non-emotional active with predominant primary function.

(6) *Phlegmatic*—the non-emotional active with predominant secondary function.

(7) *Choleric*—the emotional active with predominant primary function.

(8) *Impassioned*—the emotional active with predominant secondary function.

The chief value of this extensive investigation lies in the detailed delineation of a given type by affixing numerous qualities to the individual in varying degrees. The application of the results of the questionnaire to the miser is in itself a very interesting study which appears to approach the truth more nearly than a similar study by de Fursac.

What the Dutch authors have done is to supply us with a ready chart, which brings to light correlations among the hundreds of traits catalogued, and at the same time affords a grouping scheme according to the basic criteria and correlations. The eight separate classes which they obtained fit in well with the results of the French school, except that a much more empirical method has been employed by the former.

In other respects, however, we miss a theoretical basis both for the concept of character and its categories. We must proceed on an arbitrary plan in the first place, and in the last analysis the correlations are of statistical value more than of practical application in individual cases. The spendthrift, for instance, is domineering in 31% of cases, mercenary in

20% of cases, unselfish in 48% of cases, but how about *this particular* spendthrift under examination ?

Biographical Material. In another German periodical,[1] Heymans develops the same ideas on the basis of results obtained through the biographical method. Taking his data from the sketches of both famous and notorious persons in different walks of life, he has no difficulty in assigning to nearly all of them a place in his classificatory scheme. Perhaps the most important part of this study, however, is the brief analysis of the hundreds of traits which the author enumerates as preliminary to relating them to both the traditional four temperaments and the three fundamental qualities mentioned above. Thus, to take several instances of his results, a domineering tendency is found among the impassioned three times as often as among the other types. Ambition and vanity are coupled with those in whom the " primary function " is predominant, and are favoured by low activity. Their maximum is reached in the nervous type and their minimum in the phlegmatic. Interest in conventional distinctions such as nobility, orders, etc., is greatly developed among the nervous, and to a large extent, among the sanguine. The nervous are given to literary or scientific jealousy. Happy marriages which, Heymans takes care to point out, though in no way signifying a trait of character, yet are not without a certain symptomatic value, form the rule among the easy-going sanguine people and the exception among the nervous. (Apparently he does not attach sufficient weight to the element of *choosing* in which the extraverted sanguine person, tinctured with conceit and not over-burdened with scruples, often has an advantage over others. The facts still remain the same, but the inference that the sanguine person is best to get along with is much less obvious when all things are considered.) The choleric and the phlegmatic make better friends than

[1] G. Heymans : " Über einige psychische Korrelationen," *Zt. für angewandte Psychol.*, 1908, vol. i.

the sanguine and especially the nervous. Conscientiousness is to be found among the types with predominant secondary function. The sanguine and the nervous are least scrupulous, while the choleric are just about average. The nervous are inclined to pose, and are relatively unreliable with regard to communications and promises. Shyness is a trait of the sentimental while forwardness characterizes the sanguine and the choleric, who are also less prone to be formal than the other types.

Heymans compares his main types with those of the French-writing characterologists (Letourneau, Lévy, and particularly Malapert) and furnishes us a number of curves based on the Bayes formula to show the probability that a certain trait will appear with a given type.

But what is the primary function to which Heymans refers so often, and how does it differ from the secondary function, which, all in all, seems to be the more desirable property?

Primary and Secondary Functions. It is easy to see—at least that is my interpretation of the difference—that what characterizes the former concept is *change*, lightness, lack of endurance and ready susceptibility to objective stimulation, while the latter concept entails the qualities of seriousness, solidity, endurance, and great susceptibility to ideational stimulation. The one class should correspond within certain limits to Jung's extraverts, while the other would answer to the introverts.

From a letter the author wrote in answer to my inquiry, the following quotation will make the matter clearer :—

" The terms *Sekundärfunktion* and *Primärfunktion* have indeed been borrowed by me from Otto Gross, who first introduced them in his very suggestive little book *Die cerebrale Sekundärfunktion* (Leipzig, 1902). As this title indicates, he took the matter physiologically from the beginning, but the facts alleged by him are psychological ones, and I have found his distinction very useful for psychological purposes. So for me the *primary function* of ideas or other mental contents signifies nothing else but their mental efficiency as long as they are conscious, and their *secondary function* nothing else but their efficiency when thay have sunk below the threshold of consciousness."

Gross's Original Theory. The term secondary function, then, has originated with a psychiatrist and has been employed in a rather different sense, yet the division of types on this basis corresponds to Heymans'. For this reason, especially as the phrase has been mentioned in several books, besides the articles of the Dutch psychologists (Webb's *Character and Intelligence*, Jung's *Psychological Types*, De Froe's *Laurence Sterne* and Otto Gross's monographs) it would be well to state the physiological theory with regard to the secondary function as propounded by the Austrian psychiatrist Otto Gross.[1]

The latter believes that every *nervous process arousing an idea in the mind perseveres*, after its proper function has been fulfilled in bringing about a mental content, *for some time as an after-function* which, however, no longer has anything in consciousness to correspond with it; and yet this after-function determines the course of the subsequent associative activity in the mind. The original process which is attended by consciousness Gross calls the primary function. The after-effect which perseveres he styles the secondary function.

Much is made to depend on the duration and intensity of this secondary function which, if heightened in both respects, goes with a *narrowing* of consciousness, while if lowered or diminished it bespeaks the *broadened* consciousness. In this distinction we have the principle of the two abnormal types, the one exhibiting an inferiority with a contracted consciousness; the other an inferiority with a shallow consciousness. Whatever the physiological explanations of the two types, they answer Heymans' dichotomy both in name and

[1] Otto Gross: *Die Cerebrale Sekundärfunktion*, Leipzig, 1902, pp. 10 ff.

description, while Jung in an extended exposition of Gross's theory identifies the shallow-minded individual, whose secondary function is of brief duration, with the extravert, and the concentrated individual, whose prolonged secondary function allows of the incubation of ideas, with the introvert.[1] But we shall have to revert to Gross's division in the chapter " Suggestions from Psychiatry ". Meanwhile the digression was necessary in order to avoid confusion because of these somewhat different usages of the same term.

The curious thing about Jung's usage is that after practically adopting Gross's terminology in the technical acceptation, he proceeds in a later chapter to employ the phrases in the ordinary sense, " primary function " signifying " leading function ", and " secondary function " meaning the less important, complementary or auxiliary function.

Secondary Function as a Psychological Constant. Heymans has more to say on the meaning of the terms " primary function " and " secondary function " in his book on the psychology of women. A certain development of the secondary function is presupposed in the following of an argument, or even the understanding of a somewhat complicated sentence, inasmuch as the several parts of the argument or of the sentence cannot all be present in consciousness at once, and yet in spite of their absence they must all contribute to the comprehension of the material. This influence of the total past on the present is significant in that it constitutes a " relatively constant complex of factors which brings unity and coherence into life, and in the case of inevitable changes is able, through its restraining power, to effect a gradual veering about in the place of the sudden impulse. The secondary function, when highly exaggerated, leads to melancholia, and paranoia. It is often the cause of sterile brooding, a reduced sense of reality and lack of presence of mind, as well as slight adaptability. The preponderant primary

[1] C. G. Jung : *Psychological Types*, pp. 514–5.

functioning, on the other hand, is to be associated with super-ficiality and incoherence ".[1]

Heymans' inductive method and conclusions have been embodied in other researches, chiefly in Holland. De Graaf,[2] for instance, in his doctoral dissertation attempts to apply his master's findings to well-known historical characters, with special reference to the part played by morality in the expression of the primary or secondary function. With him, character seems to be inseparably bound up with morality ; and one might detect a theological atmosphere in this study.

De Froe[3] makes occasional use of the concepts " primary function " and " secondary function " in his psychological, in a sense virtually psychoanalytic, biography of Laurence Sterne, the humorist ; and .Briedé has employed the same method in her characterological study of physicians.[4]

II. RUSSIAN DISCUSSIONS OF CHARACTER

Objective Psychology and Personal Reflexes. The omission of references to Russian investigators is apt to give the impression that characterology has made no advance in Russia. The truth is that studies on character have been undertaken there as well as in Poland for some time, but unfortunately the works and reports are for obvious reasons inaccessible. This is true particularly of Lazursky's *Outline of a Science of Characters*, the second edition of which appeared in Russian in 1908, and which, as Bekhterev would imply in his *Objective Psychology*, is concerned with the classification of characters in various manners.[5]

---

[1] G. Heymans : *Die Psychologie der Frauen*, pp. 54–5, 1910 (1st ed.).

[2] H. T. De Graaf : *Temperament en Karakter*, Groningen, 1914.

[3] A. De Froe : *Laurence Sterne*, Groningen, 1925.

[4] F. Briedé: "Die Psychologie der Mediziner." *Zt. f. angew. Psychol.*, 1926, vol. xxvii.

[5] In his monograph on individuality about to be abstracted, Lazursky mentions several Russian characterologists, among them Lesshaft, Lossky, and Virenius.

Bekhterev himself, who is not primarily a psychologist, has nevertheless been very influential in directing psychological thought into objective channels. Extending the methods of Pavlov, famous for his conditioned reflex experiments, he attempted to create a science of reflexes in which character naturally would become a highly complex set of reflexes. Purposive strivings are for him merely " *personal reflexes* " in which past traces in the nerve substance are revivified so that they serve as determinants in a given act. If one rests after becoming fatigued, the reaction is an instinctive reflex; but if the same person goes on working in order to complete an urgent task, the past has influenced the act and we are dealing therefore with a personal reflex. It is these internal factors, former traces, which lend to the act the appearance of spontaneity. The personal reflex is different from other reflexes only in being actuated more by elements in the organism than by external stimuli.

In vain do we look for an explanation of just how a mere trace becomes revived in order to effect a certain result, how, in other words, you can build up a purpose out of associations only. That does not enter into the present topic. Bekhterev speaks of a " psychic individual " but to him this individuality is constituted by a nexus of nervous reactions.

Some personal reflexes govern the physical individual, i.e., the sum of physico-chemical properties which are connected with the welfare of the individual. Others again are bound up with the psychical individual, and may run counter to the well-being of the organism. Herein we have the basis for *egoism* and *altruism*, according as the personal reflexes rise into the one sphere or the other. The more independent the personal reflexes are of organic considerations, the more social they are in their scope, the more articulate does the character of the individual at issue become. In fine, then, character is merely a word to designate the functioning of the personal reflexes without regard to organic well-being.

Objective types. With this as a starting point, it is easy to throw off the yoke of introspective psychology and to cease speaking about subjective traits such as goodness, senti- mentality, etc.   We should rather take into account the relation of the cerebral mechanism of the individual to the external world. In so doing we should obtain such types as the *speculative, artistic, active* and so on. The first is characterized by the wealth of associations, the second by the development of aesthetic reactions, and the third by the facility of carrying out external (overt) reactions. "Each of these terms signifies a modality of functioning which predisposes the psycho- neural mechanism to certain reactions in preference to others, and enhances the determination of the personal reflexes." [1]

The linking of character types with the various qualities of the associative process as basis is in familiar vein. It runs extensively in the French literature, but Bekhterev's enumera- tion of types is *mirabile dictu* just as much related to his exact apogee, Eduard Spranger and his value-characters, as to the French characterologists. Thus we see how divergent paths will yet lead to the same destination. Reflexology and the *Geisteswissenschaften* meet at the same point as regards classification, however much they differ in their premises and methods.

Inductive Programme. If Lazursky's chief work on character is not translated, we at least can get a glimpse of his views through the German translation of a shorter study on individuality,[2] where the author discloses himself as belonging to the same school as Heymans. True, Lazursky's interest seems to have been primarily pedagogical, and his endeavors in this monograph are most closely connected with the subject of differential psychology.   His method, however,

[1] V. Bekhterev: *La psychologie objective* (French trans., 1913), p. 450.

[2] A. Lazursky: " Über das Studium der Individualität" (trans.) *Pädag. Monogr.*, 1912, No. 14.

of categorizing characters consists in following up individual characteristics, both subjective or endogenous, such as stability, sensitivity, etc., and objective or exogenous, dealing with acquired qualities (education, social status). In the course of the procedure, the material collected should indicate with regard to each individual not only the presence or absence of a given quality or tendency, but its intensity, its specific forms and peculiarities, its developmental stage and finally its scope or reach.

Static Method. It is clear that this author has not dealt with the *dynamic* aspects of personality. *Every quantitative account, whether statistical or not, must of necessity remain static,* for as soon as one begins examining the relationship of traits *analytically*, not merely correlations of traits, the statistical value of the data becomes impaired.

To say that Lazursky does not realize that there is also a dynamic phase of personality in addition to the static would be doing him an injustice. He does speak of supplementing the static method of observing the changes in reactions, the fluctuations, and the calling forth of one tendency through another which is closely related or co-ordinated with it under a central regime. Furthermore he notes that the *tension* of a certain tendency may be changed, when its expression in one direction facilitates its course in other allied outlets, although the *potential* of the disposition remains the same.

For all that, Lazursky, writing under the sway of the experimental movement, and with the possibilities of differential psychology fresh in his mind, does not conceive the dynamic problems as we know them to-day. Compensation does not occur to him, nor does he attempt to compare the data from normal persons with those gathered in the clinic. His position is made clear in the first chapter of his compact monograph, where he outlines the advantages of the quantitative method as against the qualitative ; and elsewhere he shows himself to be wholly in disagreement with those who claim that the individual must be understood in an intuitive way (Einfühlung). He insists on a systematic record of all the facts relative to a given individual, and these to be gained (a) experimentally, (b) by means of a questionnaire, and (c) through objective observation. The third method he recommends for the purpose of a psycho-social analysis, embracing the observation of all the individual's relationships to his environment.

The weakness of a purely inductive method becomes perceptible as we glance at the elaborate programme drawn up by Franck and Lazursky (in the appendix) for the study of individuals. The questionnaire material in all its details is of no slight value to the investigator of individual differences, but unless he goes into the reasons for such and such an attitude or relationship on the part of the subject, there will be a significant gap in the results. Even if the reasons discovered for a given type of behavior are not trustworthy they are yet better than no reasons at all. Nevertheless the programme for the systematic investigation of individuality proposed by Franck and Lazursky contains the most methodical approach by way of the questionnaire; and whatever fault is to be found with it really marks every questionnaire.

Classification According to Niveau. Lazursky, taking issue with his predecessors who attempted to draw up classifications of characters, contends that all the stress had hitherto been laid on the psychical content of traits, and not on the *psychical niveau* of the character, i.e., the stage of development which a character might reach. The elements that enter into this psychical *niveau* are : the amount of activity, together with the degree of complexity, co-ordination, and consciousness (*Bewusstheit*) of the individual expressions. The higher the organization, the higher the *niveau*, and the greater the degree of these qualities. On the basis of this organization, we have three types of individuals : (a) those who play a negative rôle in society, who are scarcely adapted to their environment, (*b*) those who are simply moulded by the environment, and finally (*c*) those who are masters of their fate. The pure types will be found only where the exogenous (environmental) factors correspond with the endogenous make-up of the individual. Where, however, the circumstances of life, as often happens, are not co-ordinated with the inner make-up of the individual (for instance when a man of talent is forced to engage in menial work) the character-type is no longer pure, but of the mixed order. There are also transition types. At the bottom of Lazursky's classification is the unification of the subjective and objective factors of personality in the interest of society. The *motif* here is therefore socio-pedagogical.

III. A HUNGARIAN VIEW OF CHARACTER

An appealing theory is set forth in a work called *Charakter und Nervosität* by the Hungarian psychiatrist, Jenö Kollarits. Evidently influenced by Ostwald, who regarded chemical properties as specific, inasmuch as any change in them would alter all the other properties in the substance ; while the physical properties such as color, temperature, electrical condition, etc., because of their readier variability, he considered arbitrary arrangements, Kollarits proceeds to establish a physico-chemical view of character which he traces from inorganic matter to organic beings. In raw substance, character resides or subsists in the molecular motion of the chemical reaction. In man, character inheres in or is grounded in the chemical reaction of the nerve substance. There is only this difference : while inorganic substance changes when the chemical reaction is varied, the nervous system of man maintains a permanent set of reactions which are only enforced with repetition ; and for this reason character cannot be said to change except in so far as the brain has undergone a complete transformation in its structure.

Character as a Physico-Chemical Property. The type of chemical reaction, however, does not altogether determine this character of substances. The rate of the reaction enters in as a secondary factor. Two kinds of conditions account for inorganic characteristics: (1) hereditary (if that is at all applicable here), specific, structural, endogenous, (2) exogenous, extraneous. In man these conditions are paralleled in (1) the specificity of the nervous system and (2) the stimulus which releases or varies the reaction. Character *then is a physico-chemical property of the nervous system* which represents, in its material phase, the specific type of reaction and, in its formal phase, the rate of the reaction. The latter is often associated with the concept of temperament.

Feeling-Tone in Relief. The particular type of reaction is the result of both feeling and intelligence (cognition), with emphasis on the former since it serves as a guide to intelligence ; and accordingly characters must be further classified with reference to feeling-tone. A character may be marked by general feeling-tone or specific feeling-tone. Exaltation and depression are the ingredients of the general kind. Elements of specific feeling-tone are particular qualities, like courage and cowardice, which in themselves may be only special manifestations of euphoria or depression.

Turning again to our affective categories, we can appreciate that a character may be (*a*) inclined to pleasantness, (*b*) indifferent, (*c*) inclined to unpleasantness. Kollarits, in common with all the mechanistic and hedonistic writers, exerts himself greatly to prove that all our moral dichotomies, such as " good " and " bad ", are at bottom derivatives of feeling tone, either in connection with one's own experience or in sympathy with those of other people, or through education, suggestion, etc.

Kollarits is anxious to treat his subject in a *naturwissen-*

schaftliche sense, and therefore analyzes a number of qualities with a view to examining their claim to inbornness. The touchstone which he applies in every case is that of pleasantness and unpleasantness. Laziness and industry, cowardice and bravery are all special character traits only in so far as they reveal the affective tone of the person in relation to the acts which usually are considered (say) " brave " or " cowardly ". In themselves the reactions are devoid of significance.

As regards the type of reaction, based on the feeling tone, we have seen that three classes are possible, viz., (1) pleasantly toned and corresponding to euphoric, (2) indifferent, and (3) unpleasantly toned corresponding to the depressive type; but the majority of people oscillate between the first and the third categories, in accordance with the nature of the stimuli. Now, if we only consider that a feeling may be strong, in which case it is given the name of affect, or weak, our scheme will finally contain the following divisions :

(1) Pleasantly toned euphoric character.
    (*a*) calm euphoric.
    (*b*) excitable exalted euphoric.
(2) Indifferent.
(3) Unpleasantly toned, depressive character.
    (*a*) calm depressive.
    (*b*) excitable despondent depressive.

A possible addition to this scheme is the euphoric-depressive character, oscillating between the first and third classes.

Formal Phase. So much for the material phase of character. But there is also the question of temporal attributes of the reaction which constitute the formal aspect. An act may be premature or delayed, quick or slow, strong or weak. Such attributes (and Kollarits does not tell us that the latter are qualitative rather than temporal) depend on the strength of the feeling as well as of the stimulus. Excitable, euphoric and depressive characters react quickly only because of the strength of their affect; calm euphorics react perhaps a little more quickly than the calm depressives, while the indifferent characters react most slowly of all.

What part does intelligence play in the act? Kollarits answers that by referring it to the feeling-tone. The excitable euphoric, for instance, will be more inclined to tackle a social or a scientific problem in the interest of mankind. All his associations will thus be directed toward this end. The calm depressive or indifferent character will pursue such questions with less zest, and consequently with no success. As a rule, the high euphoric holds out great expectations to himself; the depressive regards every. task as purposeless. Here Kollarits cites Ostwald's classification of great men into classic and romantic types, corresponding, as he supposes, to the two divisions under discussion. At this point an important observation is made by the author. He professes to have noticed that on many occasions, in cases of doubtful diagnosis, the deciding factor will be the character of the physician. If a euphoric, he is apt to consider the disturbance a curable neurasthenia or hysteria, since his mind is bent on curing, while the apathetic or indifferent practitioner is likely to pronounce it an incurable organic ailment.

The relation of Kollarits's character types to the time-honored table of temperaments is too close not to be perceived. In fact the correspondence is almost perfect. The sanguine temperament stands in apposition to the euphoric type, the melancholic to the calm depressive.; the phlegmatic to the indifferent character, and lastly the choleric answers to the excitable euphoric. Kollarits, like many psychiatrists of to-day, as if by way of compensation for the exploitation of the doctrine of the temperaments on the part of their colleagues for many centuries, seems to have a predilection for the term " character ", assigning his reason for the preference to the fact that " temperament " is not a clear concept, and at most can apply to the *formal* attribute of character, viz., the speed of reaction.

Connection between Character and Autonomic System. There is yet another point of interest to consider in Kollarits's theory. Character is according to him connected with visceral phenomena, and he argues thus : since one and the same nervous system has been uniformly built up in its various parts, it is not reasonable to suppose that the one part would function above the norm, while another would react at a speed less than the norm. The conclusion is, therefore, arrived at that the autonomic system and the cerebro-spinal system must function on a parallel basis, as, for the rest, commonly observed in such cases as heightened tendon reflexes going hand in hand with heightened vaso-motor reflexes. Furthermore even the popular mind has sanctioned a certain correspondence between character traits and visceral reactions, since sudden peristalsis has become an abusive metaphor for the " fly-off-the-handle " type of behavior.

Kollarits may be one-sided in his naturalistic conception of character, omitting what I should regard as its core, but he has presented at least a consistent theory and, as already intimated, one which would appeal to many people of a mechanistic bias. Yet it would be unjust to call Kollarits a mechanist in the extreme sense given to the word to-day in behavioristic quarters. If he represents the physico-chemical view of mind, he also, however, makes heredity the chief source of character.

IV. CHARACTEROLOGY IN ITALY

The Italian writers on character mainly confine themselves either to its socio-pedogogical and ethical phases or else envisage it under some psychopathological aspect. Latterly, as has already been brought out in Chapter V, the interest in clinical morphology (physical constitution) as related to the endocrines has been aroused largely through extensive researches that have originated in Italy. It is hardly to be expected that such a relatively inaccessible literature would receive more than a passing notice at the hands of foreign authors, and in mentioning the abstract of a paper on character by Fr. Del Greco[1] read at the International Congress of Psychology at Geneva in 1909, my intention is merely, as a preparatory step, to bring into relation one or two of his remarks with my own views.

The central plot of a general ethology according to Del Greco is the psychology of personality, which falls under two different purviews: (1) the physio-biological, embracing the studies of temperament and constitution, (2) the psycho-social, comprising the problems of intelligence and character. But since character stands for a superior intellectual and to a certain extent instinctive and psycho-organic activity, the fundamental task of the science is to discover the manner in which our self-conscious and rational expression is integrated (*s'integrano*) with the subsconscious and instinctive part of us. In other words, Del Greco's problem, which he seeks to solve through the suggestion of the unification of an ideal, is tantamount to asking how the biological or physiological can be merged into the social. The ideal, which is to reconcile the two and bring about the profound change, is formed through images of those personalities who affect our imagination and who cause us to wish that they assimilate with us. These then are the psychological stimuli of our ideal whose function, in its turn, is to transfer our psycho-biological capacity (*virtualità*) into a unitary conscious manifestation which is fixed, typical, and active (*vissuto*).

V. A SOUTH AMERICAN VIEW

The Argentinian Areco, perhaps in order to overcome the great difficulty of classifying the various temperaments and

---

[1] Fr. Del Greco: " Il Problema Fondamentale della Etologia," *VIème Congrès International de Psychologie à Genève*, 1909, pp. 638–40.

characters, has conceived a simple scheme.[1] One might judge that character to him is to be measured by the deviation from the mediocre or average. Since he considers the thinking function the chief characteristic of man, he practically disregards the normal man as mediocre, nondescript, drab. The abnormal are then ranged into two classes, (a) the *evolutive*, which constitutes the talented people and the geniuses, (b) the *atavistic*, which comprises the delinquent and the feebleminded. The first are designated as positive ; the second main division is regarded as negative.

The chart illustrating the article is interesting. Here we have a nucleus and nucleolus of grey mediocrity in the centre of a rectangle, intersected by a horizontal line and two diagonals, making really six lines. The right half of the rectangle is reserved for the positive qualities and their possessors ; the left for the negative. On the right, then, we shall have the ascending diagonal of originality emerging out of the zone of mediocrity and culminating in genius ; while on the left there will be its continuation, the descending diagonal of imbecility ending in idiocy. On the left, again, the diagonal of delinquency in the upper section has its continuation, after intersecting at the nucleus of mediocrity, in the lower right diagonal of immorality, while the horizontal line on each side of the nucleus represents, on the right, all degrees of talent—and on the left just undifferentiated crassness and crudity, both, however, still falling under the head of normality.

From the chart it is evident that the author does not subscribe to Lombroso's theory of genius as a species of degeneration. The genius may be immoral, but immorality is still in the positive half of the rectangle, though in the lower section. Only the combination of delinquency and immorality indicates moral degeneration.

[1] H. P. Areco : " Los Temperamentos Humanos," *Archivos de Psiquiatria y Criminol.*, 1913, vol. xii.

PART III
MOVEMENTS AND METHODS

CHAPTER XV

If the difference between the abnormal and the normal is only one of degree rather than of kind we may well hope to obtain valuable data from the field of psychiatry to elucidate the more obscure regions of psychology ; and it is only recently that the seemingly regressive method has been adopted. Again, I shall not attempt to catalogue all the references showing what psychiatrists have to offer to the student of character but will content myself with the more direct treatments.

For many years the *rapprochement* between psychiatry and character came through the endeavors of the French alienists (Bourdet, Azam)[1] largely because it was natural for the French, who led the world in studies of the abnormal, to broaden their territory and discover points of contact with other fields of research

Toward the end of the last century, however, the Germans have been taking over the hegemony in linking up psychiatry with psychological problems and particularly with the study of personality and character, until at present, it would seem, characterology has become a sort of *Nebenfach* with German psychiatrists.

Koch's Pioneer Work. But before the two branches of science could become neighbors, it was necessary to delimit the nearer end of psychiatry, and, for the purpose, segregate it from the mainland. This was effected by Koch, first in a handbook of general psychiatry,[2] but especially in

---

[1] *Vide* Chapter X.

[2] J. L. A. Koch : *Leitfaden der Psychiatrie* (1888). In this work a whole chapter is devoted to the description of psychopathic inferiorities which term dates from that year.

In this early book Koch divides mental inferiorities into two general

Die psychopathischen Minderwertigkeiten (Psychopathic Inferiorities), a work which is referred to by both Kraepelin and Ziehen in their respective textbooks of psychiatry, and which probably contains the germ of the subsequent inferiority complex doctrine, though Adler nowhere mentions Koch in his writings. By his systematic and clear presentation of the numerous psychopathic types which had come under his observation, as the director of an insane hospital, Koch was perhaps unwittingly drawing attention to the fact that the distance was but short between the institutional cases and the character defects of the normal person. In his *Nervenleben*, etc., and a monograph called *Die abnormen Charaktere*, he further explored the boundary lines between normality and abnormality, with the result that he became almost an apologist for the psychopath, whose inferiority was nevertheless understood to be caused by a diseased condition of the brain.

In the former book,[1] he plainly states that " by far the majority of those who suffer from psychopathic inferiority are not less adequate (*schwächer*) than the average person. Many of those psychopathically inferior tower above other people, exhibit great talent, fine feelings and are energetic in action, possess noble characters and are scholars, prominent men ". In his *Psychopathische Minderwertigkeiten*, he even goes so far as to relieve himself of the paradox that " many inferior persons (*Minderwertige*) are *mehr wert* (i.e., of greater

classes, viz., innate and acquired. Each of the two groups consists of inferiorities in different stages. (*a*) the dispositional stage, (*b*) the stigmatic stage, and (*c*) the degenerative stage, but furthermore even the psychopathic disposition may be either *latent*, where the condition often regulates itself before arousing any suspicion, or *manifest*, when it expresses itself in a psychic tenderness. The psychopathic disposition falls within the normal compass, while the degeneration may well come under the rubric of psychiatry, the true borderline being the psychopathic stage with its well-defined symptoms.

[1] J. L. A. Koch : *Das Nervenleben des Menschen in guten und bösen Tagen* (1895), pp. 62–3.

value) in their psychic life than many others who are perfectly sound ".

Koch's book of " inferiorities ", which is now undeservedly forgotten, has bridged the gulf between the abnormal and the normal by actually disregarding the more serious mental disturbances, psychoses, etc. In his *description* of the innumerable symptoms of the neurotic,[1] he nowise falls behind the skill of the Freudian schools of to-day, and moreover, his balanced standpoint is stamped on all his writings, as when he remarks that it would be a " great folly and a fatal mistake to seek psychopathic inferiorities *everywhere*. They are most unusually prevalent, more so than is supposed, but they do not exist everywhere ". Orthodox psychoanalysts might well ponder Koch's warning against taking every bit of unusual behavior as an indication of psychopathic inferiority, as if anything short of the ideal normal behavior were a sign of impaired mental health. With characteristic discernment. Koch insists on the distinction between a *physiological* condition, perhaps only temporarily induced, and a *pathological* state of hereditary origin, or if acquired, at any rate of long standing. Haughtiness or irritability may in its merely physiological but normal stage resemble the same traits on a pathological level, yet they have on either side their own peculiar earmarks.[2]

Janet's Psychological Conception of Neurosis. The *Dissociation* school formed primarily by Janet (*La désagrégation psychologique*),[3] and more definitely established by Prince in a number of studies, has further advanced our knowledge

[1] See especially pp. 19–41 of his *Die psychopathischen Minderwertigkeiten*.

[2] J. L. A. Koch : " Abnorme Charaktere " in *Grenzfragen des nerven- und Seelenlebens*, 1900, vol. i, p. 193.

[3] Pierre Janet : *L'automatisme psychologique*, part ii (1889). The term " psychisme inférieur " employed by Grasset and Janet and signifying a type of subconscious activity should not be confused with Koch's term " psychopathic inferiority ".

about the relationship between the normal and the abnormal in their diversified forms.   Here we were given not only descriptions but tentative explanations which were bound to figure in ascertaining the causes of character formation.   Nor should one under-estimate the significance of Kraepelin's endeavors to furnish a psychological key to the psychoses, even if he afterwards abandoned his own enterprise and let others continue his labors.

Wernicke's Sejunction.   Concepts introduced later by psychiatrists, who approached the subject with an eye to the groundwork of psychology, were invaluable in that they could be applied with appropriateness to personality forms.   One of these concepts is *Sejunction* (much like *dissociation*) used by Wernicke to explain the origin of delusions, which so contradict reality.[1]   *Sejunction* is a term favored by Otto Gross in his *Über psychopathische Minderwertigkeiten* and compared by Jung in his *Psychological Types* with the concept of *introversion.*

Advance of Freud.   The greatest impetus, however, given to the progress of our borderline study came through Freud and his disciples.   The concepts of repression, displacement and compensation, particularly the latter, were of the greatest significance in understanding the continual give and take between general and abnormal psychology.   To be sure, the phenomenon of conflict, as shown in another chapter, was nothing new and even the mechanism of compensation was more than hinted at by previous writers.   Yet there has been an enormous advance in our insight of the subject, as may be gathered by comparing the problems handled, let us say, twenty-five years ago with those of to-day.

At the beginning of this period, Tesdorpf has adumbrated much of what is worked on at present.   It is interesting that he should, unlike the practitioners of to-day, resort to the

---

[1] C. Wernicke: *Grundriss der Psychiatrie,* 1906 (2nd edition), pp. 109 ff.

theoretical and thereon base his definition of a pathological character. His analysis of the subject leads him to recognize the unconscious motive in many actions.

Tesdorpf's Analysis of Character. In quest of a definition of character applicable in judgment on the insane, Tesdorpf [1] comes to the conclusion that the classification of character must proceed along the lines indicated by J. S. Mill, when discussing the attributes of the mind in his *System of Logic*. These three attributes are *quantity*, *quality* and *relation*. It is the qualities of character which determine the kind of character one has. The number of qualities varies in different individuals, thus resulting in the division of *simple* and *composite* characters.

As to the relation of the character qualities to consciousness, we can readily see that while some act unconsciously, others appear to have conscious motives. Hence we may talk of *conscious* and *unconscious* characters. But this relationship is only a special case of a more general relationship which has a triple approach. In the first place, we may consider the qualities (*a*) as related amongst themselves, (*b*) as related to internal or external influences, (*c*) as related to inner psychic states. The last is the most important of the three, and corresponds to the above division of conscious and unconscious characters. Now with regard to the first of these relations, i.e., the relation of qualities among themselves, we may distinguish beween harmonious or consistent characters and inharmonious or contradictory characters, according as the qualities are in consonance with one another or not.

A third set of characters, viz., the impressionable and comparatively unimpressionable, issues from the consideration of the relation between the qualities of character and the internal or external influences on the individual.

---

[1] P. Tesdorpf : " Sur l'importance d'une définition exacte de ce qu'on nomme caractère pour notre jugement sur les aliénés," IVᵉ *Congrès Internat. de Psychol.*, Paris, 1901.

So far only *relation* has been dwelt on as one of the attributes of the mind, which form the basis of a classification of characters. With our attribute of quality, we cut across the three large psychic domains, obtaining the division of (*a*) characters of sentiment (from the affective domain), (*b*) characters of understanding (sphere of intelligence), and (*c*) characters of the will (volition). *Uniform* characters are those which may be referred to only one of the three great departments of the mind, while a *multiform* character partakes of two or all three of the mental provinces.

The attribute of *quantity*, as applied to character, makes room for still another division according as the character qualities are pronounced or slight.

An Important Conclusion. A pathological character is accordingly one in which a pathological alteration manifests itself in deviation of the customary behavior and is due to illness. This alteration may affect any one of the relations and phases of character. Thus the pathological influence which certain types of insanity will exert on character, may be studied together with the complementary question, that of diagnosing mental diseases through the avenue of character.

It appears that only of late has this latter suggestion of Tesdorpf been followed up by his profession. And within the last few years, both sides of the revolving question have been studied by Boven in Switzerland, Rosanoff in the United States, and Kretschmer and Ewald in Germany.

Psychosis and Personality. Boven[1] proceeds from the facts of character to diagnose psychoses on the supposition that the diversity of psychoses corresponds with the diversity of characters; allowing, of course, for combinations of traits and temporal factors, one might, according to this writer, say that the particular type of character an individual possesses will be responsible for the psychosis he develops.

---

[1] W. Boven : " Caractère individuel et aliénation mentale," *Jour. de Psychol.*, 1921, vol. xviii.

As Jastrow[1] expresses it, "A temperament becomes a more or less marked liability to a specific type of abnormal complex."

The same general principle, operating however in the reverse direction, leads Rosanoff[2] to deduce a theory of personality in conformity with the classification of psychopathic types, which, according to him, consists of (a) the antisocial; (b) the cyclothymic behaving like a swinging pendulum; (c) the shut-in or autistic, and (d) the epileptic personalities. In the normal individuals the various personality types are more or less mixed, and it must be remembered that not only is the normal individual safeguarded because of the low index of the peculiarity or the fortunate combination producing a more desirable blend, but also on account of the inhibitory factors and greater stability of the nervous system.

Character and Physique. The psychiatric treatment of character and temperament is not a sporadic attempt. It has a number of representatives and seems to be spreading. In a carefully worked out monograph which has passed through several editions and which has now appeared in an English translation, Ernst Kretschmer finds a distinct relationship between what he calls character and physique.* Taking a large number of clinical cases for material, and charting the chief physical characteristics of the patients, he establishes the following four types: (a) asthenic, that is, of slight physique, (b) athletic, or muscular, (c) pyknik, or plump, (d) hypoplastic, or regularly undersized for the most part, though, as in infantilism, certain parts are apt to be especially small. The temperaments are divided into *schizothymic*, from which the schizophrenic patients are recruited, and *cyclothymic*, which forms the basis of the circular psychoses. Each of the two classes is sub-divided into several popular

---

[1] J. Jastrow : *Character and Temperament*, p. 320.
[2] A. J. Rosanoff : "A Theory of Personality Based Mainly on Psychiatric Experience," *Psychol. Bulletin*, 1920, vol. xvii.

types, such as the "gushing jolly people", "the quiet humorists", etc.

The author apparently does not think that he is invading psychological territory with psychiatric methods; for, says he, "It must be pointed out clearly from the very start that the designations schizothymic and cyclothymic have nothing to do with the question of sanity, but are terms for large general biotypes . . ."

"The words, then, do not indicate that the majority of all schizothymic persons must be psychically dissociated and that the majority of all cyclothymic people are subject to periodic fluctuations." [1]

Kretschmer's application of his classification to both ordinary individuals and men of genius, though teeming with suggestive characterizations, suffers from the defect of all books on character analysis, viz., the characterizations are made *ex post facto*, and the most solid theoretical observations will be of no avail so long as there are no fundamental principles to guide us in making individual judgments.

Before we leave this account, it would be well to reproduce here his definitions of the concepts *constitution, character* and *temperament*. By constitution he understands the collection of all individual qualities which depend on heredity. Character is to him the mass of affective and volitional reactive possibilities of an individual as they have come about in the course of his life development, and include therefore not only hereditary dispositions but also physical and psychical influences derived from the environment and experience.

Naturally, after broadening the concept of character to include practically all mental traits, Kretschmer is obliged to reduce the term "temperament" to a heuristic concept ("*noch kein geschlossener Begriff*"). In common with other writers he bases temperamental differences on chemical

---

[1] E. Kretschmer : *Körperbau und Charakter* (3rd edition), p. 154.

reactions in the body, and claims the cerebro-glandular apparatus to be the organs of the temperaments.

As to the two main temperamental divisions, Kretschmer's cyclothymic temperament, from his description, would correspond to Jung's extraverted type, while the schizothymic person may easily be recognized as the introvert.

Kretschmer's studies on the relation between the build of man and the disposition to particular psychoses has stimulated a number of other investigators to check up on the measurements. Olivier, Sioli, and Meyer, Jakob and Moser, and more recently Henckel, Wyrsch, von Rohden and Gründler, et al. (see bibliography for titles of their researches) have in general confirmed Kretschmer's results, but the findings nevertheless, do not seem conclusive on methodological grounds, and there are just as many writers who question Kretschmer's interpretations (Bumke, Jaspers, Michel and Weeber, Wilmanns, Möllenhoff, and especially Kolle).

No Character to the Insane. But we should bear in mind that, after all, personality types are not exactly the same as character types, though there is a tendency to identify the two orders of facts in most accounts. It is really here that we have an opportunity for revealing a significant difference between the two. It is this : While much may be inferred from a patient's psychosis as to his original temperament traits, there is little information to be gained as to his character, except through a method of extensive reconstruction. It is precisely for this reason that the insane are considered irresponsible. In a word, the affective pattern of the normal individual has merely been thrown into bolder relief when he becomes insane, but his character complex has been so twisted that it loses its very essence. *There is no character to the insane.*

Application of Heredo-Genetic Method. Kretschmer has been fortunate in gaining a wide hearing and having his conclusions discussed by a number of psychiatrists. One of his

U

followers, Hoffmann, undertook to study the hereditary basis
of character by tracing the striking traits to parents and even
other ascendants ; for it is his contention that there is greater
danger in ignoring certain components or phases of a personality
than in complete error. What he believes to be responsible for
many a discrepancy between two reliable investigators is that
they do not make allowance for complementary data. Taking
up a number of actual cases, he shows how various *fusion*
types have derived their components from different
ascendants. Compensation he thinks of as an hereditary
function,[1] which belief both separates him from the psychoanalytic schools and also sets a stumbling block in his way ;
for compensation is a mechanism which, by hypothesis,
complicates the original conditions. It accordingly becomes
exceedingly difficult to discern which human quality is a
direct inheritance, and which is the result of the general
hereditary function of compensation ; and considering that
every individual has for his or her more immediate
predecessors two parents and four grandparents, the quandary
becomes even more perplexing.

Hoffmann, who combines a genetic method with the programme of his master, is thereby able to fit the data obtained
in the examination of a Swedish community tree not only into the
framework of Kretschmer's two main types, the cyclothymic
and the schizothymic, by
mentioned before, and also to connect these character forms
with the physical constitutions which are thought to run
parallel with them. The study seems to be utterly uninfluenced
by psychoanalysis, and accounts for sexual anomalies, like
inversion of normal sex activity, on the principles of
genetics and endocrinology. The endeavor to trace qualities

---

[1] H. Hoffmann : " Über Temperamentsvererbung," *Gr. des Nerv.-
und Seelenlebens*, 1923, No. 122, p. 46.

" The individual does not seem to compensate as it suits him, but
just as his germplasm prescribes."

that are sometimes contrasts in the make-up of an individual to different lines in the family tree is certainly not to be disregarded in spite of the conjectural state in which most of the results must rest for the time being, in the absence of more accurate knowledge regarding the laws of heredity.

Components of Character according to Kretschmer and Ewald. The more recent monograph[1] of Ewald likewise is grounded in Kretschmer's foundations of character. The four components of character, viz., impressionability, retentivity, intrapsychic exploitation, and the readiness with which a given experience is worked off through the muscles or glands, are combined variously so as to form two general classes of " emotionals " and "intellectuals", the first subdivided into active (sthenic) " emotionals " and passive (asthenic) " emotionals ", and the second into the unimpassioned active intellectuals and unimpassioned phlegmatic natures. Each of the subdivided classes consists of four groups, so that in all there are sixteen types, as in Bahnsen's system of which Kretschmer's and Ewald's scheme is so reminiscent.

But since Kretschmer's work is the inspirational source of Ewald's, it behoves us to turn to the former for the systematic exposition of the components of character. Kretschmer's approach[2] is through the *temporal development* of the experience from its entry until its exit. What determines the course or fate of this experience ? First of all it is the *impressionability* of the individual ; his *retentivity* preserves the experience, not only by preventing its issuing forth into action, but by retaining it as an active factor in mental life. The degree to which this is carried on will depend on the *intrapsychic activity* whose function is that of moulding and elaborating new affective, ideational and volitional forms out of the original impression.

[1] G. Ewald: "Temperament und Charakter," *Monog. aus. d. gesamtgebiete der Neurol. und Psychiat.*, 1924, No. 41.

[2] E. Kretschmer: " Der sensitive Beziehungswahn," in *Monog. aus d. Gesamtgebiet der Neurol. u. Psychiat.*, No. 16 (1918).

But the process must come to an end after its various vicissitudes, of rising and sinking, assimilating and being assimilated, until it finds its egress either intra-psychically through a free all-around association in the reservoir of ideas, or else centrifugally in vocal, affective or will reactions (*Abreactivity* seems to be the nearest equivalent to the German term *Ableitungsfähighkeit*, but it should not be confused with the psychoanalytic " abreaction ", or catharsis).

We see then that Kretschmer casts aside static views of character for the dynamic. The experience is not the atomized laboratory experience but the complex experience of everyday life ; and the adoption of Lipps' expression " psychic force " leads him to re-introduce the terms " sthenic " and " asthenic " long known in character treatises. Even these, however, receive a dynamic twist and a more definite connotation in this presentation. The sthenic or forceful quality of character is determined (*a*) by the affective level, the intensity with which something can be experienced ; and therefore connects with the impressionability phase of character, (*b*) by the affective duration, which brings in (*c*) the factors of retentivity, and (*d*) affective dischargeability. A compulsion neurotic may be sthenic as regards (*a*) and (*b*), but lamentably deficient as to (*d*) and consequently is to be set down as asthenic in comparison with the chronic grumbler. The *driving force* of ethical conduct is attributed to the sthenic elements of the constitution, while the delicacy of ethical feelings is ascribed to the asthenic components, so that Nietzsche's derivation of altruistic ethics from the asthenic instincts in man is given support by Kretschmer's conclusions.

Five types of Psychopathic Reactions. The psychopathic character, which the author defines as one likely to call forth abnormal disturbances, in response to experiences, more readily than the average character, is subject to five types of reactions : (*a*) primitive, (*b*) avoidances, (*c*) expansive reactions and developments, (*d*) sensitive reactions and developments, and (*e*) purely asthenic reactions.

The *primitive reaction*, which in its typical form occurs in childhood as a grasping of a bright object, or as a cry in pain, has been called a " cortical reflex ", and in the psychopath manifests itself in immediate responses, reckless and uncontrolled. It is the reaction of the morally insane, the born criminal, the impetuous, etc.

Avoidances are those reaction-forms which occur in hysteria, and whose characteristic is the derailment of the experience into the unconscious where it continues to run its course instead of being exploited by the conscious. As in the primitive reaction the avoidance is an escape from the elaboration process which every experience normally undergoes before being discharged into action. Thus the hysteric's repression or relegation leads to a steady conflict, the outcome of which manifests itself in primitive reactions of the explosive type.

The *expansive reaction-form* belongs to the sthenic character and as a rule is a mark of health. With an egocentric leaning, pronounced retentivity and good intrapsychic activity, the expansive sthenic type proceeds energetically along the most direct lines, resisting obstacles, but avoiding them when they are not to be removed. The expansive psychopath, however, is handicapped by having an asthenic drawback in his sthenic make-up, whether it be supersensitivity or irritability or something else of this sort. Paranoia would be the aggravated state of this reaction-form.

The *sensitive* type of reaction, on the other hand, points to a defect on the side of the dischargeability of the experience. Compulsion ideas are the result of the stalling of this process. Anxiety and scrupulosity are the attending states. When the condition has reached a climax, *inversion* takes place, that is to say, the primary experience is inwardly directed and assimilated into a group of ideas which had been overelaborated into a secondary thought mechanism that is only associatively related to the primary experience but has not been developed out of it. This secondary accretion is like a foreign body which receives undue attention at the expense of the primary experience. A repressed love experience, leading to conflicts and self-accusation of sin and sensuality, was symbolically inverted into a compulsion phantasy of a snake (symbol of seduction) choking the patient. This secondary thought mechanism or foreign body came into being after a conversation with a friend who spoke of the temptation of the serpent in Genesis as signifying seduction. The normal intrapsychic activity, after the love experience, was repressed ; and the inversion into the unconscious, with the consequent compulsion phantasy bordering on hallucination, was the only outlet.

Finally there is the *asthenic* reaction, which is a simple depression without even the energy of the sensitive compulsion neurotic, whose impressionability and retentivity at least are not wanting. The asthenic psychopath is sad and weary without being able to gather sufficient force to worry. Thus Kretschmer presents his five types of psychopathic reaction-forms and four main groups of character types, the hysteric not being included as a character type.

Ewald's Formular Elaboration.—We can now turn back to see how Kretschmer's character scheme fared at the hands of Ewald. The most important feature of Ewald's method,[1] apart from its painstaking elaboration of the combinations further illustrated with case histories, is that a formula is attached to each of the sixteen types which are subsequently considered according as they are endowed with a greater or less drive, and also as they belong to a higher or a lower level. In reality then we have sixty-four possible sub-types.

The formula for the ideal character is :—

$$\frac{E_{10} - R_{10}}{Tr_{10} - R_{10}} > I.A._{10} - L_{10}$$

[1] G. Ewald: Loc. cit.

where E stands for impressionability, the upper R for retentivity of sentiment experiences ; the lower R represents the retentivity of instinctive (Tr.) experiences ; I.A. refers to intrapsychic exploitation (*Verarbeitung*) of the experiences and control and L the reactivity factor or working off of the experiences.

Thus every case may be expressed by a formula which immediately shows the weakness or strength of a given character component in the individual under examination. To take an instance : In group 8, consisting of impressionable natures with defective retentivity, intrapsychic activity and motor reactivity, there are the following four formulae corresponding to that particular type :

	With Less Drive	*With Greater Drive*	
Lower Level	$\dfrac{E_{25} - R_{10}}{Tr_{10} - R_{10}} > I.A._{10} - L_{10}$	$\dfrac{E_{20} - R_{10}}{Tr_{22} - R_{12}} > I.A._{10} - L_{12}$	Lower L
Higher Level	$\dfrac{E_{15} - R_{8}}{Tr_{10} - R_{9}} > I.A._{7} - L_{6}$	$\dfrac{E_{14} - R_{8}}{Tr_{16} - K_{9}} > I.A._{7} - L_{9}$	Higher L

It should be noted that the defect of a certain component is not to be measured absolutely but in relation to another component. For this reason L_{12}, though manifestly indicative of a greater motor reactivity than the average which is 10, is incommensurate with the amount of impressionability E_{25}, with the result that the individual's experiences are not sufficiently exploited psychically or expressed in action. Such persons give vent to their feelings at most in passive weeping. They are receptive, yielding characters, too often taken advantage of and used as tools until, in their weakness of will, they completely collapse and find themselves in a sanatorium.

The differences between the indices of the various components are significant, inasmuch as a divergence greater than 10 indicates an abnormality in the individual, while, on the other hand, all the indices may be reduced to a certain extent, i.e., below the average, without the person coming into this class. That a component with a too low or, again, a too high index is undesirable may be seen from the formula typifying a contentious school teacher with ideas of reference, who took the most insignificant incident as a personal slight and spent precious hours in forming plans to punish the culprit, who usually was never discovered.

Formula for the paranoid type

$$\frac{E_{20} - R_{25}}{Tr_{22} - R_{30}} > I.A._{14} - L_{20}$$

What was especially at fault here appears to be the excessively high retentivity of experiences affecting the ego complex in the instinctive sphere which, as will be seen, is also highly charged.   The working off of the experiences retained (i.e., the irritation which keeps accumulating from day to day) is also expressed by means of a high index.

Physiologically, the relation among the different components is to be sought in the relative predominance of the cortex over the brain stem or *vice versa*. Since, argues Ewald, the affective-volitional and instinctive components have their seat in the brain stem and the retentive and intrapsychic functions are associated with the cortex, then the dislocation of the ratio between cortex and brain stem would signify a redistribution of component indices. In certain post-psychotic cases, Ewald thinks the balance of power is moved in favor of the brain stem, accordingly resulting in a heightened sensitivity and lowered mental control.

DESCRIPTIVE vs. INTERPRETATIVE APPROACH

Psychiatry has taken over in its camp the controversy which had been carried on in the ranks of psychology. On the one hand are ranged those who with Klages and his large following, or better, the majority of the French characterologists, look to descriptive schemes in solution of the problem ;

on the other hand are arrayed the representatives of the various nuances of the *Geisteswissenchaften* school, who claim that characterology is a phase of the *verstehende* (interpretative) *Psychologie*, that the individual must accordingly be studied as a totality.

A clear presentation of the main objection against the descriptive attempts to fathom the depths of character is to be had in Kronfeld's recent work on psychotherapy where he declares " The very nature of individuality is to be unique (*einmalig*) and indivisible. Every sketch can only encompass such traits as could be subsumed under a general concept, in other words, only such traits as one individuality has in common with another. This we call typical because of its recurrence in a number of individuals. It is clear, however, that in such a procedure, we are constantly grasping only one part of the individuality, not the whole. This part we abstract because it seems to us the essence of the personality in question, and at the same time to represent the typical in the sense above. We rely in this matter on our ability to emphasize. And then we substitute the part for the whole ".[1]

Furthermore, Kronfeld calls our attention to the fact that an apparently simple type may be psychologically quite complex, and that the abstractions do not correspond with realities, because they include so many different shades, which, in spite of a descriptive class name, nevertheless possess their own distinctions ; whereas if the abstractions are further analyzed into so many sub-varieties, they dwindle into mere trivialities.

Instead of trifling with raw schemes, this author advises us to examine the foundations of character from a biological and genetic standpoint, but the plan of the structure which Kronfeld proposes is terrifying because of its stupendous magnitude. With all the kaleidoscopic show of possibilities

---

[1] A. Kronfeld : *Psychotherapie, Charakterlehre, Psychoanalyse Psychagogik*, 1924 (1st ed.), p. 12.

in human behavior, it dawns upon us that we must make concessions to the descriptive view, if we are to collate the facts into some system.

IS CHARACTEROLOGY THE SAME AS PSYCHOLOGY OF TYPES ?

Although enthusiastically supporting a leader at whom Kronfeld cavils more than once, Prinzhorn,[1] evidently a reverential disciple of Klages, nevertheless reaches almost the same conclusions, and brings out the further difference between characterology and the psychology of types. Types, he holds, may be set up in innumerable ways, all according to the purpose of the codifier, his particular point of view. In the structure of character, however, the variations allow of so much latitude that scarcely a pair of correlations may be thought of which cannot be found in one and the same individual. Man is not like iron or cotton batting, always in one state, but fluctuates from one pole to the other. Only the dominants of a quality complex can be kept in sight, so that for practical purposes, an individual may be labelled according as the one swing is preponderant or the other. But types must be handled, if we are to deal with characterological problems, statistically. The types must be recognized first, then recorded and ranged in some order or classification.

When we study, however, an individual *qua* individual, it is different. Then it must be realized that our task becomes infinitely complicated, for we are dealing with a complete indivisible concrete totality.

It is only natural that psychiatrists should have sensed these distinctions better than theoretical psychologists, since in their experience, what is ordinarily taken as average, or simple, presents contradictions and conflicts that baffle their understanding. And yet for all the strictures of Kronfeld and

---

[1] H. Prinzhorn : " Psychiatrische Wege zur Charakterologie," *Archiv f. Psychiat. u. Nervenh'ten*, 1925, vol. lxxvi.

the admonitions of Prinzhorn, it is curious to note that both
in orthodox psychiatry and psychoanalysis, recognized leaders
have set up very simple types which are constantly referred
to (Kretschmer, Gross, Jung), although the most recent
tendency is to belittle this method.

Interpretative psychology with its best devices, its appeal
to *Einfühlung* and phenomenological intuition (derived from
Husserl's philosophy) cannot help us without a concrete key
to the significant qualities of man, and their mechanisms.
Klages' tables of qualities is at fault because it is *static*. It
does not take into consideration *traits in operation*, their
origin and transformation. On the other hand, the Freudian
system, which is undoubtedly *dynamic*, is not sufficiently
solid, makes too many moves that are not wholly accounted
for. The ideal approach is to harmonize the static and the
dynamic, that is to say, to begin with tendencies that are least
disputed and study the mechanisms by which these tendencies
change in accordance with the circumstances both external
(stimuli) and internal (governing principles).

SUMMING UP

We must now pause to see whether psychiatry is justified
in claiming a hold on the subject which heretofore was con-

principles. But has it contributed significantly to the problem
of character?

In answer, one might suggest that the chief contribution
has consisted in transferring the study of character from the
confines of the academy to the vast expanse of life with its
myriads of complexities and varieties. Clinical observations
always yielded invaluable data which formerly were disregarded by psychologists as falling beyond their scope.
Latterly the alliance recognized the value of reciprocity with
the result that, as we have seen, the problem of types has

become central in the various phases of psychiatry, etiological, diagnostic, and therapeutic, while the application of the facts in abnormal psychology to the mere forms set up in theoretical psychology has served to substantialize them at least with sound hypothesis and to point the way to further investigation.

A Hopeful Sign in Consolidation.   What above all is cause for rejoicing is the *common nucleus to be found in so many writings which approach the subject from diverse angles.* Intimations of many of our present day conceptions have been foreshadowed in numerous works, but it is the harmonizing of these hints with recent findings and the agreement of the more outstanding psychiatrists amongst themselves which make us feel that we are " warm " in our unceasing search. Different inquirers may employ different names and terms, but on analysis it will be discovered that the burden of their contention converges in the same direction ; and every new convergence serves to consolidate the structure erected by workers who at first, as in early biblical times, did not understand each other's language. The disagreement is often only on the surface.

Quantification of Data.   Another hopeful sign is the application of quantitative methods to test the theories. Kretschmer's views, for instance, regarding the relation between physique and character or psychopathic disposition would lack the weight attached to them at present were they to be grounded in pure generalizations; and if Ewald's formulae of the different components of character could actually be worked out on a standardized plan, we should by that much come nearer the possession of a true picture of the mechanism of personality or character in the broad sense.

It is only by collating the whole array of findings in the psychiatric and psychoanalytic spheres that we can expect to derive common denominators out of the seemingly confused mass of theory. What if the compensation concept in psychoanalysis is of a slightly different tint from that in Anton's view? What if there is a slant on introversion which Wernicke's sejunction does not cover? The essentials are of a kind. Usually the more recent term, as is quite natural, contains an amplification or at least a lead toward a broader system. How well, after all, the " secondary function " in Gross comports with the " secondary function " in Heymans and Wiersma ; how suitably Gross's neurological theory makes provision for such personality types as schizothymic, sejunctive and introverted !

Definite Mechanism Indispensable. What, however, must constantly be kept in mind is that a classification without reference to a definite mechanism, no matter how tentatively explained, will always remain sterile. We may classify people into those who prefer carrots and those who are fond of turnips, and for all we know these tastes may mutually exclude each other and thus furnish us with another vein of inquiry, but since we are still far off from the time when tastes will be *scientifically* accounted for, our dichotomy remains a mere curio.

On the other hand, idle speculations, though industriously and laboriously conceived, are not to be mistaken for exposi- tions of neurological theories. We must remember that the nervous system in its operation as a whole is such a *terra incognita* that thousands of hypotheses are possible as to its working. We should demand first of all, then, of every new exponent that he make himself familiar with the generally accepted, orthodox, or conservative body of facts before plunging ahead afresh, and secondly that the theory advanced be not only possible but at least plausible, which requires as a minimum condition that it does not come into conflict with more or less established evidence.

What we Must Avoid. The danger of individualistic or *autistic* theorizing in a realm which is not amenable to experi- mental control is too great for us to pay attention to the innumerable attempts made, in many cases by means of diagrams, to secure our support of a view which is too loose to be subjected to a rigorous examination, just as a melodrama is too often laden with strange coincidences to even permit of realistic questioning.

The most profitable results will originate from the deliberately restricted lines of investigation initiated, however, in pursuance of a significant objective and only after the whole field serving as a locus for the study of character has been comprehensively surveyed. The mastery of the broader issues in all their ramifications may not be found in the investigator who would be waiting to follow up an isolated problem in all its intricate and irksome aspects. In that case it would be proper for the man of knowledge to direct the course of action in others with a proclivity for detailed research.

Shock Treatments. Whether the various shock treatments that have been administered within the last decades to mental patients has thrown some light on the inner core of personality has not been definitely established, but the advance made through such daring or desperate operations as frontal lobotomy and lobectomy has opened up a new field or rather has caused the *rapprochement* of two otherwise independent disciplines—surgery and psychology. Hence the new hyphenated branch called psychosurgery.

Psychosurgery. To those of a previous generation surgery meant the removal of pathological tissue, perhaps an infected area, or else the grafting of tissue or mending of impaired organs, but to cut away part of what was regarded as the most essential physiological substance would have been thought most fanciful until Egas Moniz electrified the world by reporting his extraordinary measures to treat patients suffering from hopeless depression. Thus, severing the connection between the frontal lobe of each hemisphere and the epithalamus would lighten the mental load of the patient, though at the expense of judgment and discrimination.

Naturally, too, the sense of responsibility would dwindle, since the inhibitory function which, before the operation, had been exaggerated, has now been reduced to a minimum. Inasmuch as inhibition and responsibility are pertinent to the whole constitution of character, it stands to reason that tracing their origin through such therapeutic experimentation should be of service to the understanding of character.

Psychosomatic Medicine. Like many other recent developments, psychosomatic medicine is not really new. Its germ may even be found in antiquity ; for is not the Latin proverb *mens sana in corpore sano* an expression of the close connection between mind and body ?

In a number of couplets and also prose passages, Goethe speaks of the artificial severance of things which were intended by nature to remain inseparable. In a sense, then, he might rate as a pioneer in psychosomatics. It was, however, his *alter ego*, the illustrious poet and dramatist, Friedrich Schiller, who has given us the first compact treatise on psychosomatic medicine, in his dissertation written as a candidate for the medical degree. It is curious that this gem, which first appeared in print in 1780, when Schiller was hardly more than 20 years old, is never referred to in the psychological or medical literature and, in fact, is seldom included in his collected works.

To prove my contention that this noble prodigy was at least one of the early pioneers who recognized the close connection between body and mind, particularly in disease, it would be best to reproduce a few scattered passages of this inspired little work.

A sensation which pervades the whole soul affects in a corresponding degree the whole structure of the body— heart, blood vessels and blood, muscular fibres and nerves ; from the powerful and important impulse of the heart to the insignificant tension of the hairs on the skin . . . Every part of the bodily life becomes more intensely active. . . .

Therefore it is that a condition of the most exalted soul-delight becomes, for the time being, a condition of the highest bodily welfare . . . .

This conclusion is corroborated most evidently by those patients who are cured by joy. Send him whom home-sickness has reduced to a skeleton back to his native country, and he will again be blessed with blooming health . . . Sailors drifting about on the ocean and prostrated by the want of bread and water practically recover their health and strength at the sound of " land " shouted from the mast-head. It would be a great mistake to ascribe this change exclusively to fresh food. . . . Joy will bring about a more intense action in the nervous system than any tonic which the pharmacies can furnish, and may even remove obstructions in the tortuous canals of the intestines which no dissolvents, not even mercury, could reach . . .

The shiverings that seize the one who is about to commit, or has committed a criminal act are the same chill that shakes the fever patient. The nightly startings of those who are tormented by remorse, which is always accompanied by a feverish beating of the pulse, are real fevers . . .

Schiller further dilates on the seeming exceptions, as when a sudden joy might produce a shock or when an onset of rage might " terminate the most obstinate constipation ", or fright relieves " old pains in the limbs and incurable paralysis ", or dysentery " has removed infarctions of the portal system and the itch has cured melancholy and rage ". As Schiller puts it in his somewhat antiquated phraseology, the law reduced to simple terms is " that the universal sensation of physical harmony is the source of psychic delight ; and that animal discomfort is the source of psychic discomfort ". Finally, we have a dictum which sounds the very essence of psychosomatic medicine, viz., " *Man is not soul and body ; he is these two substances inmostly united.*"

More articulate, however, was the effort of Jacobi who especially pleaded the cause of somato-psychic medicine, while Ernst v. Feuchtersleben may very well be spoken of as the founder of the systematic conception underlying which is " the psychophysical totality of man ".

That indigestion is often psychogenic was known for a long time even by the ordinary practitioner. The very phrase " nervous dyspepsia ", in use perhaps half a century, attests to this. W. F. Cannon's experiments, in which emotional conditions were induced, conclusively proved the psychic phase of digestion, but certainly even 25 years ago, it would have been thought extreme to associate asthma or cancer with mental states, whether conscious or unconscious.

It is not easy to single out the chief protagonists of psycho-somatic medicine, such as we know it to-day. Georg Groddeck is assuredly one who has emphasized the etiology of organic disease as lying in the unconscious.[1] S. E. Jelliffe, Franz Alexander, Flanders Dunbar, Therese Benedek and others have assisted in placing the branch, common to both psycho-logy and medicine, on a scientific footing, largely through the contributions published in the *Journal of Psychosomatic Medicine* and its monograph series.

[1] G. Groddeck's *Der gesunde und kranke Mensch* (1913) as well as *Das Buch vom Es* (now available in English), and his " Unconscious Factors in Organic Disease " which appears in *Exploring the Un-conscious* (English translation London, 1933) may be considered the first hard planks of the psychosomatic platform, with the grain running in the direction of the mental.

x

CHAPTER XVI

THE PSYCHOANALYTIC APPROACH

Offhand it might seem that psychoanalysis and psychiatry could go hand in hand in their approach at least, even if their results should turn out to be divergent, but in reality the presuppositions and standpoints are different from the very start. The psychoanalytic camp is inclined to stress the cause of the disturbance as a determinant of the disorder; the orthodox psychiatrist, though in the past seeking the entire cause of the evil in a special incident or series of incidents, has at last come to recognize that the same stimuli would react differently on different individuals. Now, if there are different types of diatheses in organic as well as in mental diseases of a functional nature, it stands to reason that each diathesis is correlated with a certain personality type.

Character and Anal-Eroticism. Since 1908, when Freud published his paper, *Charakter und Analerotik*, a number of his disciples have attempted to show that certain traits of character are connected with the sex impulse and the excretory functions. Freud started out by relating three traits to anal-eroticism, to wit: orderliness, parsimony and stubbornness, but within a few years of the publication of his original article the list had been increased to a score or more. The whole problem of motivation which Freud has raised may, of course, be considered as a vast contribution to the study of character,[1] treating it from a hitherto unknown angle,

---

[1] The extent to which psychoanalysts are prone to employ a definite term in a colourless way can be inferred from the mere title of Van der Hoop's account of the psychology of Freud and Jung; for, though the book is called *Character and the Unconscious*, there is hardly a direct reference to the first term of the title in the whole presentation.

but it is evident that I must confine myself to the more specific references which seem to centre about this peculiarity, so much made of by psychoanalysts.

How Freud has come upon his peculiar theory, he does not tell us. He merely assures us that " no theoretical anticipations . . . played any part in its production ". In later life, the original infantile interest in the excretory act is supposed to be supplemented by the love of money (parsimony). To be sure, Freud is not in a hurry to complete the circle with the three aforementioned traits. He leaves the door open for more traits to be linked with the sexual zones ; and his disciples were not slow to accept the hint.

Toward the end of the original paper which was reprinted in the second series of his *Schriften zur Neurosenlehre*,[1] Freud finds himself under the obligation to add that " One must take into account moreover whether other character complexes might not indicate a connection with the excitement of definite erogenous zones. Thus far I am acquainted only with the inordinate ' burning ' ambition of former enuretic persons. At any rate it is possible to give a formula for the formation of the ultimate character out of the constituent impulses. The permanent character traits are either unchanged continuations of the original impulses and their sublimations or else reaction formations [2] to offset them ".

Freud's Original Scheme Supplemented. No sooner had the master given the signal than his disciples picked up the clue and began to find varieties and sub-varieties of the original triad. Blüher [3] introduces a new division, separating the interest in the *act* from the interest in the *region*, and he

---

[1] An English translation of this essay appears in his *Collected Papers*, vol. ii, 1924.

[2] A reaction formation in the Freudian sense is the building up of a trait which keeps in restraint and hides another trait. The repressed trait is frequently the contrast of the reaction formation.

[3] H. Blüher : " Studien über den perversen Charakter," *Zentralblatt für Psychoanalyse*, 1914, vol. iv.

believes that perverseness of character can be traced to this double infantile habitus. Jones, Sadger, Brill, Federn, von Hattingberg, Glover, Abraham, Ferenczi and Andreas-Salomé all do their bit toward amplifying, elucidating and expatiating on the basic thesis of the pontiff of psychoanalysis. The upshot of this whole speculation, as reported by Jones in the last paragraph of his chapter already referred to, shows us at once that the diagnosis in this particular case is not far from the horoscope readings of astrologers, at least in respect of form. " It will be seen," concludes Jones, " that the total result is an extremely varied one, owing to the complexity of the interrelations of the different anal-erotic components with one another and with other constituents of the whole character. Some of the most valuable qualities are derived from this complex, as well as some of the most disadvantageous. To the former may be reckoned especially the individualism, the determination and persistence, the love of order and power of organization, the competency, reliability and thoroughness, the generosity, the bent toward art and good taste, the capacity for unusual tenderness, and the general ability to deal with concrete objects of the material world. To the latter belong the incapacity for happiness, the irritability and bad temper, the hypochondria, the miserliness, meanness and pettiness, the slow-mindedness and proneness to bore, the bent for dictating and tyrannizing, and the obstinacy, which with the other qualities, may make the person exceedingly unfitted for social relations." [1]

The anal-erotic thread, once passed through the eye of the psychoanalytic needle, became useful in sewing up all sorts of phenomena and incidents, if only the stitches were not so loose. Thus, elaborating on a news item relative to the death of an internationally known capitalist, Coriat [2] points out the

[1] E. Jones : *Papers on Psycho-Analysis*, 1919, p. 688.

[2] I. H. Coriat : " Character Traits of Capitalistic Instinct," *Psychoanal. Rev.*, 1924, vol. xi, pp. 435–7.

special delight the man took in possessiveness and showing off his wealth, and relates this and other traits to anal eroticism. Among the latter are noted the following : hate in regard to the possibility of deprivation, avariciousness, yet with no desire for living well, even to the point of wearing shabby clothes, overtenderness to children, and his own family in particular, perseverance, pedantry, and a childish narcissism, which, Coriat thinks, reveals the reaction formation.

What is a capitalistic instinct ? We know that there might be such things as acquisitive and aggressive instincts, but is there such an inborn mechanism as to make one a capitalist ?

URETHRAL CHARACTER

As might have been expected, the cue given by Freud on the anal character was only the signal for further explorations, and soon many other " characters " were discovered. There is, e.g., the urethral character which correlates with a consuming ambition, harking back to the child's period of competition in the matter of urination. Ernest Jones formulated the theory in 1915, after Freud has observed the connection between urethral activity and a burning ambition.

Sadger was not long in bringing to the fore some case histories of urethral eroticism, producing a number of extraordinary memories dating from early infancy, a doubtful hypermnesic phenomenon, especially when it dates from the first year ! Thus he tells us that one of his patients " remembers quite definitely " that every time his third sister would pick him up, at that age " liess ich es los ".[1]

The sexual connections here may be placed to one side, since our concern is with the character traits, and in this province, we note Sadger's observations on the sublimated varieties of urethral eroticism in the form of sports and voca-

[1] J. Sadger : " Über Urethralerotik " : *Jahrbuch d. Psychoanalyse,* 1910, vol. ii, p. 414.

tions. Thus, he associates such original impulses with all activities that centre around water : swimming, rowing, sailing. Sailors, sea adventurers, and yachtsmen are recruited out of this urethral class. The great interest in marine engineering, watermills, turbines, and hydraulic works is also derived from the same source.

Sadger further sees in the preoccupation with wells, canals, etc., which artists show, a sublimation of the urethral erotic tendency. He mentions particularly a well-known painting of Rembrandt and Hermann Hahn's Brunnenbuberl. We may have expected someone to go a step farther and inform us that the urethral erotic will choose drowning as the favourite form of suicide.

Since Sadger was one of the earliest collaborators of Freud, and as he was not yet bound to the later edicts of the psycho-analytic regime, he could still quote from Adler, and better still, he could, forty years ago, at least attribute the tendencies to hereditary factors, e.g., bladder or prostate trouble in the family, although he naturally did not eliminate the habitual handlings of the child's phallus on the part of the parents.

Sadger has written a useful clinical account, but as has been the case ever since, the interpretations are highly con-jectural and the applications are even more so.

It was left to Ernest Jones to formulate more or less the theory of urethral erotic character along the lines of Freud's system, and no one, I believe, can be counted upon to do this more faithfully than Jones.

Recording a case of compulsion neurosis in which the patient was constantly at pains to single out some special advantage for himself in the lavatory, such as using the first urinal, or else the last (" last but not least ") so that, in his own estimation, he would come out on top, Jones[1] attempts

---

[1] E. Jones : " Urethralerotik und Ehrgeiz ". *Intern. Ztschr. f. Psychoanalyse*, 1913, vol. iii, pp. 156–7. This article was not in-corporated in any of his books.

to account for the association between the traits of ambition and rivalry (which this behaviour would point to) and the sphincter urethrae, rather than the sphincter ani. He assigns three reasons for this circumstance (a) micturation often takes place in the company of others (especially in the case of men) which permits comparison and rivalry ; (b) the variability in the process as compared with defecation (speed, distance, height, volume, etc.) due to the anatomical difference involved ; (c) pride in the matter of directing the flow.

Jones, as may be seen, does not take his lead this time from the phrase " burning ambition "—haphazardly supplied by the master, but in British empirical fashion attempts to find the genetic basis, although with hardly greater success ; for are we to conclude that none but the urethral-erotic individual can be ambitious, or conversely, all who have been ambitious (and that means everyone who has achieved distinction) are cases of urethral eroticism ?

In a shorter communication, E. Hitschmann appears to confirm Sadger and others who have written on the subject ; and particularly is he guided by the words of Freud, the reference to a " burning ambition ", but in general, he does not offer anything new.

" We do not know of the existence of a urethral character as we do of an anal one, but two traits can be empirically deduced in persons who were formerly urethral erotics. They are a ' burning ' ambition and the predilection for playing and working with water. Intellectual ambition particularly is often strongly developed in obsessional neurotics, not without connection perhaps with the ' omnipotence of thought '. Excessive bathing and washing seems to be in close relation with urethral erotism.

"Statistics prove the strong development of urethral eroticism in obsessional patients." [1]

[1] E. Hitschmann : " Urethral Erotism and Obsessional Neurosis," *Intern. J. of Psycho-Analysis*, 1923, vol. iv, p. 119.

Yet Jones tells us that " Freud has confirmed my conclusion that the general association between hate and anal
erotism is important, and that a high development of this
combination is the most specific characteristic of the
obsessional neurosis." [1] But if so, then what becomes of the
statistics which Hitschmann enlists as proving the urethral
origin of obsessionals ?

The ambition which has been linked to urethral eroticism
is supposedly the resultant of the struggle against the shame
involved in the urethral erotic conflicts ; for just as the fear
of being eaten is centred in the oral phase, and the fear of
being robbed of something precious emanating from the body
is the core of the anal phase, so shame represents the urethral
phase. [2] Ambition then develops to live down the shame, to
nullify it with a vengeance.

Writing in 1924, Coriat describes in detail a case of enuresis
in a young woman whom he had been analysing ; and,
although she apparently had some rectal irregularity too,
he treats hers as a typical urethral-erotic case, and lists all
her proclivities and idiosyncrasies as definitely connected
with her pregenital development : Her hate, jealousy, constipation, fear of water and crossing bridges (we have seen
that others have found the opposite, the love of water in
urethral-erotics) neatness, her feelings of being misunderstood,
sensitiveness about her rights and a wish to dominate—all
these are supposedly bound up with her urethral eroticism,
but we have other tendencies as well.

As a child she took pleasure in playing with soap, enjoying
the heavy lather. She would like to play with matches,
watching them burn, and would pass her finger through the
candle flame (as what child would not ?), but this must be

---

[1] E. Jones : *Papers on Psycho-Analysis* (3rd ed.) p. 560.

[2] O. Fenichel : *The Psychoanalytic Theory of Neurosis*, 1945 (Norton),
pp. 69, 139.

introduced to confirm, I daresay, the Freudian intimation about a " burning ambition ". Compulsion is also brought in as Hitschmann had done, but what is somewhat surprising is that Coriat is inclined to identify " the character trends of anal and urethral erotism " on the ground that they are both " furnished by the peripheral excretory zones or organs . . . which possess erogenous as well as excretory functions." [1]

However interesting the details, we have no basis for assuming that (a) the traits or tendencies exhibited by one in childhood are uncommon to most children, (b) that the later traits are in any way associated with the earlier games or play habits, (c) that they are all tied up with a specific pregenital character. Indeed, there is no scientific method shown in the grouping of the tendencies around either the urethral or the anal phase. Not only is the absence of a demarcation line a hindrance but we are confronted here as elsewhere in psychoanalytic writings with a plethora of assertions revolving around a vaguely formulated hypothesis.

ORAL-EROTIC CHARACTER

Character, as affected by oral eroticism in infancy and early childhood, is associated by Abraham and Glover with a self-assurance and optimism, if the early circumstances were satisfactory, while, if frustration as a result of deprivation had supervened, the character formed would be of the pessimistic, depressive type or even sadistic. Those in the first category will be most generous and some, under different circumstances, will almost choke their beneficiaries with their altruism, while those upon whom deprivation in infancy has left a mental scar will, in their unconscious vindictiveness, act stintingly toward others. As an illustration of the trait to withhold from the partner, Bergler [2] adduces the case of

[1] I. H. Coriat: " The Character Traits of Urethral Erotism." *Psychoanal. Rev.*, 1924, vol. vi, p. 426.

[2] E. Bergler: A Clinical Picture of Psychogenic 'Oral Aspermia'. *Intern. J. of Psycho-Analysis*, 1937, vol. xviii, p. 230.

ejaculatio retardata, apparently oblivious of the fact that such a state is a desideratum to her under the circumstances, and in no sense represents a stint for the partner.

The trait of undue independence, as well as degrees of spurious masculinity, is also laid at the door of oral eroticism. In fact there are so many characteristics, associated by one or another psychoanalyst, with oral eroticism that the remotest suggestion of any of the processes or organs involved in eating, or even talking, coupled with looking, or linked to reading, will yield an oral erotic trait.

Thus, aside from the ordinary speech difficulties which form the core of the conglomeration, and, of course, volubility, as well as rigid silence, one must reckon with the curiosity trait derived through displacement of hunger in the mental sphere, so that one might become a *voracious* reader (the application of " oral " to the eyes reveals a regression to the stage when visual perception and ingestion represented the same aim to the infant). In addition, there are the peculiarly oral-sadistic tendencies and idiosyncrasies observable in attitudes assumed in smoking, kissing, drinking, etc., with all sorts of variations due to such mechanisms as sublimation or reaction-formation. Again the *passive*-oral attitude, which is related to the pacification while breast-feeding, is quite different from the *aggressive* attitude of dominating the situation, which the adult develops, by way of reaction, to his erstwhile state of helplessness.

Karl Landauer [1] feels that there is an oral-anal character which derives from the regulations imposed upon the young child when allowed to sit down to table with the parents. The toddler discovers that he is expected to observe certain rules in regard to eating just as he was required to do while on the stool. " He must deal with a certain quantity at a given time and place and not otherwise. The feeling that eating is

---

[1] K. Landauer : " Some Remarks on the Formation of the Anal-Erotic Character." *Intern. Journal of Psycho-Analysis,* 1939, vol. xx.

an obligation is especially marked in depressive cases, in which oral and anal factors intermingle."

Landauer sees a number of differences between the eating regimen and that of defecation : (a) In the latter, the disposition may be to orderliness alone ; the former carries with it a tendency toward pedantry. (b) Since the training for the stool is undertaken by the mother or nurse, a maternal superego evolves as against the paternal, which is a result of the frequent intervention of the father in oral training at table. (c) In anal training, the negative reaction is only one of " I can't ", which translates itself into rigidity, with defiance as the sequel, while if a child is compelled to take nourishment against his will, he might clench his teeth (producing an attitude of rage) or spit out the food, as if in scorn.

Perls, in an earlier paper, has even gone to the length of extending the food-taking processes to intellectual activities. Thus there are people who will receive their reading assignments from others ; others will browse about for themselves in pastures free or forbidden. Again, there are the individuals who will disgorge their reading at the first opportunity, and those who will ruminate and assimilate, just as in the digestion of food.

Conflicts and Ambivalence. Coriat particularly has insisted upon that pre-genital stage of the child's life which is fixated at the oral level, the result of a conflict brought about by resistance against the possible betrayal through speech of certain repressed thoughts. According to him, the conflict between the superego to regress and the libidinal desire to utter obscene words is at the root of stammering.[1]

Abraham[2] sees two stages in the oral libido ; a sucking and a biting phase. " Thus the formation of character in such a child begins with the influence of an abnormally pronounced

[1] I. Coriat : " The Oral Erotic Components of Stammering." *Intern. Journal of Psycho-Anal.*, 1927, vol. viii, p. 57.

[2] K. Abraham : *Selected Papers on Psycho-Analysis* (English trans.), 1927, p. 398.

ambivalence of feeling." As against the pessimistic colouring of a specific anal character, which Abraham thinks " goes back to a disappointment of oral desires in the earliest years, those whose sucking at the mother's breast has been pleasurable and undisturbed and overindulged build up an optimistic and care-free attitude, as if they will always be provided for."

.   .   .   .

" A character thus rooted in oral erotism influences the entire behaviour of the individual, as well as his choice of profession, his predilections, and his hobbies." As an instance of this type is cited the neurotic official who does not care to mount the ladder of success but instead wishes to be secure in his humdrum life.

Those who have had an ungratified sucking period, on the other hand, will be constantly demanding in later life. They will request, plead, insist, and become importunate, even to the point of cruelty. In their sadistic phase they might be considered to be something like vampires.

But that is not all ; through the mechanism of displacement in the oral sphere, the " take " may change to a " give " urge, so that some individuals will yield to a volume of speech, which they must impose on their auditors in the belief that what they have to say is all-important. Even if we have followed Abraham through all these winding paths, we certainly must pause before he turns this displaced oral tendency into a " neurotically exaggerated need to urinate, which often appears at the same time as an outburst of talking, or directly after it."

With all the scores of articles dealing with oral eroticism, there are still some apparently unexplored nooks and crannies which may bear a definite relation to the oral region, and such unobserved activities or perhaps only a *laissez-faire* policy in a strictly deterministic system must at once strike us as suspicious and symptomatic of repression.

Smoking a Lost Opportunity. Let us take one instance that little has been made of in the psychoanalytic literature, viz., the smoking habit. Smoking, because of its acquired nature, and its relatively recent spread, should have received a good deal of attention on the part of Freudians. Not being a universal need, it presents more evidence of idiosyncratic behaviour and opportunities for motivational interpretation, particularly along dynamic lines. Thus whether one readily falls into the habit or resists it, whether cigarette, cigar, or pipe is preferred, the type of cigarette, cigar, or pipe used, the kind of tobacco one is addicted to, the manner of smoking (with or without holder), the inhaling and exhaling differences, the alternation of activities, such as sipping and puffing, and a hundred and one other considerations are relevant to the whole elaboration of the genital doctrine, in which the oral, anal, and urethral components occupy such an important place. We may even wonder whether smoking is exclusively an oral activity, inasmuch as the puffing, more or less rhythmic too, as well as the fumes which it *emits*, suggests anal processes as against the *ingestion* of food. The protrusion of the cigarette, cigar, or pipe also might indicate penis-substitution, or intrenchment against castration. The spread of smoking among women might especially argue for such compensation, certainly as much as bearing a child serves as a palliative of penis envy.

Smoking, however, has been treated very cavalierly in the literature. Would it be, perchance, because Freud himself was, unfortunately, an incessant smoker and most of his faithful followers identified with him ?

When we reflect that the various forms of silence rated a long article,[1] in connection with the oral libidinal levels, it is all the more surprising that smoking should have been so

[1] R. Fliess : " Silence and Verbalization." *Intern. Journ. of Psycho-Analysis*, 1949, vol. xxx, pp. 21–30.

neglected in this frame of reference. If silence could be anal erotic, urethral erotic, as well as oral erotic, one might expect at least all that of smoking.

What then do we learn from the psychoanalysts about smoking ? There may be more on the subject in the hundreds of volumes published within the last forty years, but only two articles, both of which appeared about thirty years ago seem to pre-empt the issue of smoking.

Brill [1] thinks that smoking, whether indulged in to a neurotic degree or even more moderately, is a regression to an infantile autocratic gratification or a contribution to it— a species of masturbation ! and yet he considers the smoker more normal than the non-smoker who is to be viewed, according to Brill, with suspicion !

Hiller [2] in a syllabus-like article shows that tobacco and smoking can symbolize almost anything : phallus, feces, semen, flatus, but the real reason for starting to smoke, according to him, is that it represents a substitute for the weaning which, in itself, meant castration (penis = mother's breast).

Phallic Character. The phallic-narcissistic character which W. Reich introduces is shot through with highly negative traits. The male (the female counterpart is rare) is haughty, if not arrogant, over-confident in himself, exhibitionistic toward women, and sought by them because of their external virility, which does not correspond to their orgontic potence. Their contempt of the female sex is related to their active homosexuality, and at the root of their trouble is the identification of the ego with the phallus, which swells their pride and serves them as a weapon of power rather than as a mediator of love.

[1] A. A. Brill : " Tobacco and the Individual." *Intern. Jour. of Psycho-Anal.*, 1922, vol. iii, p. 442.

[2] E. Hiller : " Some Remarks on Tobacco." *Intern. Journ. of Psycho-Anal.*, 1922, vol. iii. For the above reference, I am grateful to Dr. Ernest Jones.

Reich claims that frustration and disappointments during the period when they made special efforts to win their love objects, through phallic exhibition, were the cause of this character development. Nevertheless, he tells us that " it is not by accident that this type is most frequently found among athletes, aviators, soldiers, and engineers. One of their most important traits is aggressive courage, just as the compulsive character is characterized by cautious hesitation and the passive-feminine character by an avoidance of dangerous situations ".[1] But, if it is no accident that individuals of a certain build or constitution belong to this type, is not Reich conceding that this hereditary factor at least tells part of the story, and that if we make an honest effort to examine the other so-called characters derived from the stunting of the libidinal organization, we might discover that there too, constitutional factors play an important part, but we shall revert to this matter in the general critique of the psychoanalytic approach to the study of character.

The Genital Character. To one who is not familiar with the psychoanalytic outlook and doctrine, it would sound nothing short of a poor joke to hear that the *most finished character is genital*, i.e., after the pre-genital levels (the oral, the anal or urethral with their various components and combinations) have normally developed into the ordinary sexual impulses of adolescent and adult life.

Abraham has probably given us the best description of this character, which has freed itself from the immature behaviour, the various complexes, the ambivalence, displacements, resistance, etc., which are to be associated with the pre-genital levels. Such an individual will be a balanced man or woman and keep in stride with the environment ; and while, at times, certain undesirable features stemming from the pre-genital period will burst through, pointing to the mutability

---

[1] W. Reich : *Character Analysis* (3rd ed.), 1949, p. 202.

of character, homeostasis, if the term may be injected here, will not be long in asserting itself.

The genital character is an integrated and synthetic unit since, according to Abraham " From the early oral stage it takes over enterprise and energy ; from the anal stage, endurance, perseverance, and various other characteristics ; from sadistic sources, the necessary power to carry on the struggle for existence ". [1]

Abraham was one of the first to recognize that psycho-analysis is not to confine itself to the task of treating neurosis but must turn its attention to the problem of character deformities, although at the time he was writing, in 1924, he felt that " we are not in a position to make any general judgment about the therapeutic results of his character analysis ; that we must leave to the future ". [2]

It was W. Reich who, later, made it his business to tackle these characterological problems, although in so doing, he began to stray from the Freudian fold, and it is problematic, too, as we shall see later, whether he has met with the success he congratulates himself on attaining.

In addition to the characters stemming from the varieties of libidinal organization, there are cited in the literature the usual pathogenic characters : hysterical, compulsive, impulsive, etc., but it would seem that the classification here is horizontal whereas the libidinal characters were considered from a vertical point of view, and specific features are stressed in the one division while others would be singled out in the other. Certainly a good deal of material belongs to both and the overlapping and even repetition are among the defects of the exposition.

Universalized Reactions Hardly Character Types. Out of the psychoanalyst's workshop, Freud has added several

---

[1] K. Abraham : *Selected Papers on Psycho-Analysis*, 1927, p. 415.

[2] K. Abraham : *Loc. cit.*, p. 417.

character types based on his observations of unusual reactions.[1]

In the one case, we have the individual who will not accept the physician's prescribed regimen ; he must be an exception and justifies his attitude on the ground that he has endured so much in the past. Freud quotes extensively from *Richard III* in order to prove that the great bard possessed the insight which is conveyed to us, viz., that those who regard themselves as wronged by the world will seek to take it out on others. But Francis Bacon in his essay on " Deformity " has already told us this, as we shall see in another chapter (p. 373) and in regard to the universalizing of this tendency, inasmuch as we all feel that nature has stinted us in one or another respect, is Freud not thereby dissolving the force of the term " type " ; since to belong to a particular type means to be different in that one respect from others ?

His second character type concerns those who collapse on attaining their goal. Neurosis sets in as their dream is about to be realized. Cases are cited and Ibsen's Rebecca in *Rosmersholm* as well as Lady Macbeth are adduced as instances to show that the awakened conscience which leads to the mental disorder is bound up with the parent fixation and incest motive. If that is the case, we again have no special type, but rather a special phenomenon or situation consequent upon a general tendency.

The third character type which Freud reveals is the criminal who perpetrates his misdeed because his guilt feeling, stemming out of the unconscious, is seeking a rationale or justification. Here we are reminded of the reversed sequence in the famous James-Lange theory of emotions according to which we see a bear, we run and we are afraid. Thus it is with the chronic guilt-feeler. He feels like a miscreant but does not know

[1] S. Freud : " Einige Charaktertypen aus der psychoanalytischen Arbeit," *Imago*, 1916, vol. iv, later incorporated in his *gesammelte Werke*, vol. x (London), 1946.

Y

why ; and so in order to balance his guilt feeling, he commits a crime, in order that the guilt could be established. In other words, we might say that here the " crime fits the punishment ". Naturally Freud does not claim this for the conscienceless criminal. It is the too sensitive person, perhaps whom James would have called the " tender-minded " that is apt to act thus.

At any rate, one would scarcely call these " character types ". Perhaps " types of reaction " is a more appropriate label. The psychodynamics of such action may be accounted for psycho-analytically or otherwise, but whether we are in the sphere of character, when such behaviour is described, seems doubtful, unless character becomes a synonym of personality.

It is true incidentally that in psychoanalysis as a general rule the term character is employed generically even where the issue is strictly one of personality. Orthodox psychoanalysis practically ignores the latter term, perhaps as a result of compensation, since during the earlier stages, virtually nothing had been said about character.

Morality vs. Love. The issue of morality is broached in connection with love and character development by Ernest Jones,[1] who ponders on the situation when a moral attitude toward others takes the place of an attitude of love that would ordinarily have been expected. It is thought that in these individuals the id impulses must first pass through considerable modification in the superego before they can be directed toward others, and since morality is a species of sadism, that particular attitude is closely related to it.

This substitutive process has several consequences. Many who fall into this category are regarded by their fellows as hard-hearted and intolerant, and themselves never enjoy life

[1] E. Jones : " Love and Morality : A Study in Character Types." *Intern. J. of Psycho-Analysis*, 1937, vol. xviii, p. 1.

normally. Others suffer from an obsessional neurosis because of an inner protest against this moral substitution, the revolt manifesting itself in conflicts as to duty : Of this revolt there are two types, one emanating from the id, which is more conscious and corresponds to a hysterical reaction against performing a task that may be considered a duty imposed ; the second emerges from the superego and is unconscious, and more of the obsessional kind. Here " the person consciously wishes to perform his duty and is dismayed at finding himself prevented by some unknown agency from doing so . . . With the obsessional there is self-reproach at not being more ' good ' . . . With the hysterical there is self-reproach at not being more loving or at not being able to love at all ".

What is of some consequence in Jones's conclusions is the fact that " the cause of all these differences would seem to be partly constitutional, one type evidently having a more obsessional disposition and the other a more hysterical one and partly an economic one concerning the quantity of sadism present and the age at which this gave rise to insoluble conflict ".

The admission of a constitutional cause pops up here, in spite of the psychoanalyst, and should be placed on record together with other such instances which pass the " censor " ; for they may accumulate into a telling case on behalf of the non-libidinal view of character.

Weakness of the Pregenital Theory of Character. If the pregenital organization of traits has been dwelt on at length, it is in order to forestall the criticism that only a small segment of psychoanalytic doctrine has been singled out for discussion, as one reviewer contended when the book first appeared. Indeed, he thought that I ought to have given an exposition of the scores of mechanisms and submechanisms which psychoanalysis has either discovered or invented, but this is a volume on character, and not on psychoanalysis ; and psychoanalysis has already received more than its due share, considering the wide scope of the subject before us.

From what has been quoted and cited, the impartial reader will gather that most of the descriptions of the libidinal types, fixated at one or another stage of the genital development, are labored and based on perhaps no more than a hint from Freud, or a play of words or a simile. Sometimes, a lieutenant, here and there, will deviate from the doctrinal schema in some specific details. Thus Abraham does not appear quite satisfied with the norms set up by the libidinal organization. Women especially, he thinks, assimilate their characters to their husbands (if that were really so, the number of divorces would be fewer) ; then there are regressive changes or even a progressive development, while in cyclic disorders, as also in obsessional neurosis, there is a transfer from the oral to the anal-sadistic level.[1]

Again, if, as Abraham points out, there are considerations of class, race, nationality, etc., which affect the individual character, then we might well wonder to what purpose the definite and often emphatic statements are uttered in the last analysis. The glib transition made by all psychoanalytic writers from one genital level to the other, and the fact that at any level there are all sorts of possible divisions or combinations, and that many acts may be considered from different angles, render it impossible to achieve anything like a degree of likelihood, let alone certitude, as to what really happens.

We have now to take up the general question as to what extent the genital theory of character-formation is valid. For my part, it is difficult to accept such an all-embracing set of tenets. Proof, in the scientific sense, is unavailable, and from the very nature of the case seems impossible.

We must first espouse all the postulates in regard to the

---

[1] K. Abraham : *Selected Papers* (English trans.), pp. 412–413.

genesis of eroticism through oral, urethral, and anal (perhaps even muscular and cutaneous) channels during infancy, and then it is required of us to equate these various steps, often in combinations, at times side-steps and step-backs, with character types or constellations of traits, depending on the kind of components, and the stage at which the fixation has taken place, all of which we can only guess at, although it is presumed that as the analysis proceeds, definite cues point the way to retracing the early occurrences.

Moreover the universality of these occurrences is highly improbable. When we consider the multitude of different conditions obtaining in the rearing of children, whether through disparate cultures, early death of one or both of the parents so that the child did not know them, or the substitution of a nurse for the mother to bring up the child, adoption by foster-parents, and finally the decline of breast-feeding in the more civilized countries, particularly in college-bred families, the Freudian view becomes more problematic. We shall have occasion later to add to the list of difficulties, if not definite disconfirmations, in surveying the whole issue, but the curious part of the genital construction of character is that the master himself was rather skeptical about the relationship and not even confident about the anal component of character, which he himself propounded.

Doubtful Procedures. Let us quote from Freud in this regard " Naturally we expect to find that other traits of character will also turn out to be derived from pregenital libidinal formations either as precipitates or as reaction-formations ; but we cannot as yet demonstrate this ".[1] This was originally published in 1933, a few years before he died ; and there is no evidence that Freud has had the opportunity or the inclination to change his mind on that proposition. It will be noted that the term " demonstrate "

[1] S. Freud: *New Introductory Lectures on Psychoanalysis*, London, 1933, pp. 132-3.

applied in the instance of the anal-erotic character, is somewhat of an overstatement, because the minimum of proof would require first the establishment of the pregenital doctrine, with its various components, and secondly the correlation of such a specific type as the anal with the possession of the triad of traits, viz., parsimony, orderliness, and obstinateness, in a marked degree. Although I have read almost all I could lay my hands on [1] in the psychoanalytic literature on this subject, I have found no plausible *descriptive* account of the data, let alone a scientific welding of the facts. Freud himself does not evince the zeal in this particular sphere of characterology that he does in arguing out the unconscious guilt theory, to take one example, and the incest doctrine.

As a sample of the vague analogy or loose association in use even in Freud's own writing, the following passage may be cited for the benefit of the impartial. " A similar and perhaps even firmer connection is to be found between ambition and urethral erotism. We have found a remarkable reference to this correlation in the legend that Alexander the Great was born on the same night that a certain Herostratus, who, from a craving for notoriety, set fire to the famous temple of Artemis at Ephesus   It seems that the ancients were well aware of the connection there is between urination and fire and the putting out of a fire." [2] That the links of this chain of evidence are deplorably weak will be perceived by anyone who is not overawed by the authority of Sigmund Freud.

Of Freud, however, it must be said that he at least makes an attempt to relate facts. Regrettably this cannot be said of the majority of the epigones, both Freudians and para-Freudians, who merely set down a series of statements or conclusions arrived at on the basis of verbal or temporal

[1] I rather hesitated to employ this harmless phrase, lest psychoanalytic critics jump at the opportunity of discovering the unconscious hostile impulses against their empire.

[2] S. Freud : *New Introductory Lectures on Psychoanalysis*, London, 1933, p. 132.

associations, which are of course subjective, at times even whimsies, thought to support the psychoanalytic system of postulates. Their observations are valuable, indeed, while their interpretations are too flimsy even for a schoolman of the Middle Ages.

PSYCHOANALYTIC DEFINITION OF CHARACTER

During the early years of psychoanalysis, character was scarcely referred to, and even as late as 1930 the term was used in a biological rather than in a moral or ethical universe of discourse. " By a character-trait," Alexander wrote in 1923, " we mean a certain stereotyped attitude in life ; those people whom we call neurotic characters show this stereotyped attitude in the whole rhythm of their lives, at the most decisive moments and most important turning points.[1] Among the first to broach the subject was F. Alexander, but he, too, spoke of it as if it were a mode of reaction associated with rigidity. Of course the mechanisms of character-formation were, as we have already seen, but the different steps in genital development.

Fenichel, two decades later, was more explicit on this point. As he would have it, " the term character stresses the habitual form of a given reaction, its relative constancy. . . . Anticipatorily it may be stated that this relative constancy depends on a number of factors ; partly on the hereditary constitution of the ego, partly on the nature of the instincts, against which the defense is directed ; in most cases, however, the special attitude has been forced on the individual by the external world." [2]

In another passage he speaks of character " as the habitual mode of bringing into harmony the tasks presented by internal demands and by the external world ", and is thus " neces-

[1] F. Alexander : " Castration Complex in Character Formation." *Inter. Journ. of Psychoanalysis*, 1923, vol. iv, p. 15.

[2] O. Fenichel : *The Psycho-Analytic Theory of Neurosis*, N.Y., 1945 (Norton), pp. 467–8.

sarily a function of the constant organized and integrating part of the personality, which is the ego "—a neat way of leading up to the Freudian treatment.

According to Freud, " the permanent character traits are either changing perpetuations of original impulses, sublimations of them, or reaction-formations against them." Sublimation may be considered as a sort of successful repression, i.e., an inhibition of the undesirable impulse by its diversion into a channel which will yield socially productive results, whereas the class of reactive characters, which subdivides into the phobic or withdrawing, on the one hand, and the masking type, found in reaction-formations, on the other, will be the ones to get little joy out of life, and will be generally beset by anxieties and irritations which will interfere with their efficiency.

CHARACTER AND TOPOGRAPHY OF THE MIND

Perhaps a closer contact with character is derived from the so-called topographical interpretation of behaviour, according to which the human psyche is divided into an id, an ego, and a superego. Georg Groddeck apparently supplied the first clue to this tripartition through his *Buch vom Es*, in 1923. The same year there appeared Freud's central thesis on the *id*, *ego*, and *superego*, according to which the first represents the large reservoir of primitive impulses striving to gratify nothing but the pleasure principle, whereas the ego becomes a later development corresponding to the reality principle, an agency of the external world with its restrictions and impositions, while the superego, a rebound from the id, becomes a sort of watch and ward official, making it difficult even for the ego.

It is Freud's belief that in infants and young children, only the id, i.e., those blind, reckless impulses exist. Character, then, is out of the question at that stage. The ego emerges in the child's dealing with others, playmates, teachers, and operates through perceptual channels, steering the individual away, on a realistic basis, from noxious influences.

The ego may be considered as an experiential governor over the id, developing out of the impact of the environment, through a long chain of modifications. Its growth takes place over a considerable period, and apparently goes on even in adult life, if I understand the following quotation from Freud aright ; and thus the assumed *force majeure*, so to speak, of the primal incidents during infancy and early childhood, must be viewed in a different light when we read that " The character of the ego is a precipitate of abandoned object-cathexes and . . . contains a record of past object-choices . . . In women who have had many love affairs there seems to be no difficulty in finding vestiges of their object-cathexes·in the traits of their character ".[1]

It is, however, in the superego that the core of character, in the ethical sense, is disclosed. In fact this *ego-ideal*, which is an extension of the ego, alas, to its own sorrow, by means of manipulations as a result of the sequelae of id occurrences (e.g., castration complexes and guilt feelings out of incest and sadistic impulses) is the unconscious counterpart of conscience. Now whether we are conscience-stricken or not, the superego may contrive to afford us anguish and misery in other ways, through anxiety, compulsion neurosis, and guilt feeling which we do not associate with any particular misdeed. The superego, in a word, is the ego turned in upon itself, the tail of the mythical fish which is constantly flagellating itself.

" The superego retains the character of the father, while the more intense the Oedipus complex was and the more rapidly it succumbed to repression (under the influence of discipline, religious teaching, schooling, and reading) the more exacting later on is the domination of the superego over the

[1] S. Freud : *The Ego and the Id* (English trans.), 1927, pp. 36–7.

ego—in the form of conscience or perhaps of an unconscious sense of guilt." [1]

In other passages, Freud argues with characteristic eloquence that this unconscious guilt-feeling manifests itself in the guise of a compulsive imperative which imposes " thou shalt's " and " thou shalt not's ", redolent of the Oedipus and castration complexes which had been repressed.

From Id to Ideal. It is not altogether clear why the mind, which is not spatial, should be divided topographically, as if the id or superego could be located somewhere, but no doubt the *placement* is only figurative. The id would naturally suggest the lowest region, and the superego the highest, although it, no less than the id, resides in the unconscious, while the ego dwells as a none too firm arbiter in between. Perhaps according to the older tripartite division, the id would represent the *affective*, pure and simple ; the ego, the *cognitive* part of human nature (reason) and the superego the *volitional*, with an affective base. Thus while the ego supplies us with the intelligence to curb the id impulses, the superego imposes its will on the whole structure. The ego can only part company with the id, consign its cravings to the unconscious limbo, but the superego exercises a punitive authority which is in keeping with conscience and character.

The discovery, or perhaps the recognition of the superego must have been gratifying to Freud ; for the tirades which had been directed against his frank naturalism must have begun to wear on him, so that he could now turn on his tormentors with an air of subdued triumph, as if exposing his obtuse philistine critics.

" Psychoanalysis," he writes, " has been reproached time after time with ignoring the higher, moral, spiritual side of human nature . . . But now that we have embarked upon the analysis of the ego, we can give an answer to all those whose

[1] S. Freud : *The Ego and the Id* (English trans.), 1927, pp. 44-5.

moral sense has been shocked and who have complained that there must surely be a higher nature in man : ' very true,' we can say, ' and here we have that higher nature, in this ego-ideal or superego, the representative of our relation to our parents. When we were little children, we knew these higher natures, we admired them and feared them ; and later we took them into ourselves.'

" The ego-ideal, therefore, is the heir of the Oedipus complex and thus it is also the expression of the most powerful impulses and the most important vicissitudes experienced by the libido in the id." [1]

Let us however pursue more closely the Freudian conception of character, and the gulf between it and that evolved in this volume will become patent.

Therapy vs. Character Building. Freud, as is well-known, was primarily concerned with treating and curing patients. As a physician he cared little about the morals or character of those who consulted him, except in so far as the ill effects interfered with the therapy. His business was to relieve the patient, and therefore he was far more interested in the symptoms and their formation than in traits as such. Recognizing that the neuroses originated in the conflict between sexuality and the ego, between the *amo* and the *veto*, he and his immediate coadjutors delved in that direction, especially when they found the neurosis more accessible.

Later it was noticed that the ego instincts had been neglected, and more attention was now given to those than in the past, until emphasis began to shift to the ego, and with it to character, which seems to stand out like a thick wall that must yet be negotiated before some new excavation can be done. It was only during the last dozen years of his life that Freud reckoned with this newly discovered framework ; and as a matter of fact, thanks to the new insight, psycho-

[1] Op. cit., pp. 47–8.

analysis began on a new course. It was no longer a matter of ferreting out repressed complexes but looking into the resistances which held these repressions as in a vice. And here Freud came to grips with the problem of character. From then on more of the psychoanalytic literature is devoted to the subject, while some of his disciples who have diverged recently from the orthodox party line have made character, as we shall see in another chapter, the crux of their study. Indeed, it was the inability to see eye to eye with Freud on fundamental questions of character interpretation and morality which precipitated the rift.

To what extent Freud himself was influenced in this direction may be gleaned from his writings shortly before his death in which he states : " Every analyst of experience will be able to think of a number of cases in which he has taken permanent leave of the patient *rebus bene gestis*. There is a far greater discrepancy between theory and practice in cases of so-called character-analysis. Here it is not easy to predict a natural end to the process. . . . The business of analysis is to secure the best possible psychological conditions for the functioning of the ego . . ." [1]

It is evident then that he thought the ego, including the superego, far more inscrutable than the id, and felt that this region was destined for future investigation.

THE PITH OF FREUD'S ETHICAL RELATIVISM

Whether Freud, constituted as he was, could have changed his pessimistic outlook even if he had not been subjected to the humiliating outrages because of his ethnic origin as well as his unconventional psychology, even before the Nazis raided his quarters in Vienna, is doubtful. Certainly he had no faith in human values ; as for respect for moral origins, his libidinal doctrine is its very nemesis. If our ethical conduct depends

---

[1] S. Freud : " Analysis Terminable and Interminable." *Intern. Journal of Psycho-Analysis*, 1937, vol. xviii, p. 403.

wholly on whether our libido has been arrested at the oral, anal, or urethral level or has been developed to the genital point, where sexual intercourse is performed satisfactorily, there can be no standards possible of assessment; and character can be the result only of fortuitous, even if determined, events in the past. Characteristics, in the biological sense, would be a better name for it. Freud has imbibed at the font of the enlightenment philosophy, and a nondescript and indifferent relativity has been the outcome. In a little book scarcely ever referred to, he has delivered himself of the following discourse, significant in this connection.

" If we call a person's individual capacity for transforming his egotistical impulses under the influence of love his cultural adaptability, we can say that this consists of two parts, one congenital and the other acquired, and we may add that the relation of these two to each other and to the untransformed part of the emotional life is a very variable one.

" In general we are inclined to rate the congenital part too highly, and are also in danger of over-valuing the whole cultural adaptability in its relation to that part of the impulse life which has remained primitive, that is, we are misled into judging people to be " better " than they really are. For there is another factor which clouds our judgment and falsifies the result in favor of what we are judging.

" We are of course in no position to observe the impulses of another person. We deduce them from his actions and his conduct, which we trace back to motives springing from his emotional life. In a number of cases such a conclusion is necessarily incorrect. The same actions which are " good " in the civilized sense may sometimes originate in " noble " motives and sometimes not. Students of the theory of ethics call only those acts " good " which are the expression of good impulses and refuse to acknowledge others as such. But society is on the whole guided by practical aims and does not bother about this distinction ; it is satisfied if a man adapts his conduct and his actions to the precepts of civilization and asks little about his motives.

" We have heard that the outer compulsion which education and environment exercise upon a man brings about a further transformation of his impulse life for the good, the change from egotism to altruism. But this is not the necessary or regular effect of the outer compulsion. Education and environment have not only love premiums to offer but work with profit premiums of another sort, namely rewards and punishments. They can therefore bring it about that a person subject to their influence decides in favor of good conduct in the civilized sense without any ennobling of impulse or change from egotistic into altruistic inclinations. On the whole the consequence remains the same ; only special circumstances will reveal whether the one person is always good because his impulses compel him to be so while another person is good only in so far as this civilized behavior is of advantage to his selfish purposes. But our superficial knowledge of the individual gives us no means of distinguishing the two cases, and we shall certainly be misled by our optimism into greatly overestimating the number of people who have been transformed by civilization." [1]

Freud's philosophy of life is contained in compact form in these two paragraphs written during the first World War. It is in keeping with his system as a whole, sounding as it does, a pessimistic note, with a mildly cynical undertone accentuating its grimness. There is of course nothing new in this account of human nature. Virtually all the French moralists, as we have seen earlier in the book, were of the same mind.

Naturally, the gist of the disquisition is acceptable, so far as society goes, but what is society ? And which society has Freud in mind—contemporaneous society or posterity ?

[1] S. Freud : *Reflections on War and Death*, 1918 (English trans.), pp. 23–6.

If the latter, then it most assuredly will come to light whether a person was actuated by sordid or noble motives in performing some benefaction. Moreover, a single enlightened individual might set society right by examining the record of the benefactor. On a purely libidinal scheme of character, we must avow it is impossible to establish the moral quality of the motive, but who could express misgivings as to the motives of a Francis of Assisi, General San Martin, Jehudi Ashmun, Romain Rolland, Albert Schweitzer, Peter Kropotkin, Catherine Breshkovsky, and thousands of obscure men and women whose life of self-sacrifice is in direct contradiction with Freud's above assertions ? I, for one, do not anticipate that some day, it will be discovered that Albert Schweitzer spent forty years of his life treating jungle natives at the equator, although he could have lived in luxury in balmy climates, because of an originally sadistic impulse which turned into the opposite, *via* a reaction-formation, in order to throw the ego, and all of us at the same time, off the track.

FREUD ON CONSCIENCE, TABOO, AND ANXIETY

In the following account we have a sample of Freud's fascinating and suggestive but not always factual reasoning. It is quite germane to our topic, because it deals with the genesis of conscience, which is so closely related to character ; for the one is the mentor and inspector, so to speak, of the other. Character without conscience would be no less inconceivable than conscience without character. But how does Freud envisage the relationship ?

Unless we are mistaken, the understanding of taboo also throws light upon the nature and origin of *conscience*. Without stretching ideas we can speak of a taboo conscience and a taboo sense of guilt after the violation of a taboo. Taboo conscience is probably the oldest form in which we meet the phenomenon of conscience.

For what is " conscience " ? According to linguistic testimony it belongs to what we know most surely ; in some languages its meaning is hardly to be distinguished from consciousness.

Conscience is the inner perception of objections to definite wish impulses that exist in us ; but the emphasis is put upon the fact that this rejection does not have to depend on anything else, that it is sure of itself. This becomes even plainer in the case of a guilty conscience, where we become aware of the inner condemnation of such acts which realized some of our definite wish impulses. This same character is evinced by the attitude of savages towards taboo. Taboo is a command of conscience, the violation of which causes a terrible sense of guilt which is as self-evident as its origin is unknown.

It is therefore probable that conscience also originates on the basis of an ambivalent feeling from quite definite human relations which contain this ambivalence. One component of the two contrasting feelings is unconscious and is kept repressed by the compulsive domination of the other component. In the first place the character of compulsion neurotics shows a predominant trait of painful conscientiousness which is a symptom of reaction against the temptation which lurks in the unconscious, and which develops into the highest degrees of guilty conscience as their illness grows worse. Indeed, one may venture the assertion that if the origin of guilty conscience could not be discovered through compulsion neurotic patients, there would be no prospect of ever discovering it. This task is successfully solved in the case of the individual neurotic, and we are confident of finding a similar solution in the case of races.

In the second place, we cannot help noticing that the sense of guilt contains much of the nature of anxiety. The psychology of the neuroses taught us that when wish feelings undergo repression their libido becomes transformed into anxiety.[1]

A Linguistic Lapse. This little linguistic excursion is characteristic. Freud has connected the word *Gewissen* (conscience) with *gewiss* (certain), and would have us believe that our conscience stems from that which we know for certain, viz., our primal guilt—the incest impulse !

Had he consulted his Kluge, he would have found that the *ge* in *gewiss* (certain) is a relic of the past tense (in other words, that which *has been known* is " certain "), while the *ge* in the noun *Gewissen* is just a conformation of the Latin *con*. Evidently two different concepts and formations, *gewiss* and *Gewissen* are treated by Freud as one.

Conscience—and it takes no philological insight to perceive it—is that which we know in *common with others* to be right or wrong. Both the *ge* and *con* signify " collectiveness " or " community " (cf. *gemein*, *Geschwister*, etc.) ; and the formations of *con* and *scientia*, as well as *ge* with *Wissen* are no doubt modelled after the Greek σῦν and εἰδέναι, i.e., " to know together " (*with the rest of the world, that right is right and wrong is wrong*).

It is not *individual certainty*, as Freud contends, which connotes conscience, but *collective knowledge*. Freud, because of his preoccupation with his basic *motif*, has been lured by a distant sound, off-key, and thus has been harping on it, without doing his theory any credit.

Strange Interludes. While perusing the psychoanalytic literature we often have the feeling of reading Franz Kafka. First, the events seem to take place in a realm of ideas (or perhaps better " ids "), and proceed without rhyme or reason, in many instances. One tries to get to someone in charge, but such is invisible. All sorts of annoying trifles happen, each more bizarre than its predecessor, every step taken by the

---

[1] S. Freud : *Totem and Taboo* (English trans., new edition), pp. 114–15.

z

groping individual leads him nearer to his doom, and yet a grain of common sense, a direct approach to any public medium could have cut short the dénoûement, and saved the day ; but that would be too commonplace.

The chief stumbling block in the psychoanalytic treatment of character is, of course, that we are operating in the dark with only an occasional fire-fly illuminating the area for a brief moment. The unconscious—and no one who has had some clinical experience, or even the reflective layman, can doubt its existence—is only inferable ; its mechanisms and contents are more speculative, that is to say, some, like repression and sublimation or projection and rationalization, are reasonably certain ; others, like displacement, fixation, etc., are highly probable, while others are just possible, and still others are only conceivable. Attempts made recently to test some of the Freudian mechanisms or complexes experimentally are footless, to begin with, since experimental proof rests on measurable entities or introspective reports. The unconscious is inaccessible for this purpose.

Before closing the psychoanalytic chapter, let me add that in Freudian psychology there are submerged or repressed trends which only rarely will come to the surface. One is, as we have had occasion to read, his sympathetic interest in the doctrine of acquired characteristics, which fits in with a collective unconscious. The second subdued trend is the part which heredity plays in his personal belief. At times the professional ego in him cautions us against seeking constitutional causes, but his superego will at other times drop a hint that does not gibe with the system he has built up as a whole. The pressure of the superego must have been great for him to give utterance to such an ultra-conservative and almost Jungian tenet, naturally overlooked by all his disciples. " It seems that the male sex has taken the lead in developing all of these moral acquisitions ; and that they have been transmitted to women by cross inheritance." That Freud, without actually announcing the fact openly, is disposed to accept the doctrine of acquired characteristics to explain certain sociological phenomena, like totemism, and thus cannot be said to be altogether averse to Jung's conception of the collective unconscious and its contents, in the form of archetypes, may be gleaned from several other utterances in various books as, e.g., the following :

> The experiences undergone by the ego seem at first to be lost to posterity ; but when they have been repeated often enough and with sufficient intensity in the successive individuals of many generations, they transform themselves, so to say, into experiences of the id, the impress of which is preserved by inheritance. Thus in the id, which is capable of being inherited, are stored up vestiges of the existences led by countless former egos ; and when the ego forms its superego out of the id, it may perhaps only be reviving images of egos that have passed away and be securing them a resurrection.[1]

Logic and Psychoanalysis. It is not the mechanisms and complexes, as such, that one feels bound to call in question so much as the continual criscrossing, the endless gyrations without apparent cause, except to explain, in the most circuitous manner some trifling observation which could be accounted for in simple fashion. The child is bisexual ; as a boy his love object is his mother ; he identifies with his father who is his rival, but he can identify with his mother and thus the father becomes the love object as he is on the way to homosexuality. *Now* the female component in him is at work, so that the mother is rejected. All this is only a humble beginning, comparatively solid. As the architecture proceeds on slender reeds, Freud, at least, on occasion tells us apologetically " I am putting forward nothing but a supposition.

---

[1] S. Freud : *The Ego and the Id* (Engl. trans.), 1927, p. 52.

I have no proof to offer ". And this is one of the laudable features of Freud's scientific integrity—that more than once does he express misgivings or at least uncertainty in building up his hypothesis.

This little disarming admission is lacking in the thousands of articles which fill the psychoanalytic periodicals. The glibness with which many of the interpretations are rolled off makes one wonder whether it is a case of " speaking with tongues " or " speaking with tongue in cheek ". After seeing the mechanisms shuttled back and forth a dozen times, we are at a loss as to the method employed in making these operations. I am well aware that living does not follow the dictates of logic or even common sense, but that does not imply that interpretations in regard to behaviour should steer clear of logic or the elementary canons of scientific thought. In one of his scores of enlightening letters, S. E. Jelliffe, one of the most competent of psychoanalysts and in his day the Nestor of American psychiatry, writes, in reply to my above complaint, " I think the Freudians do stick to a rule, i.e., the pragmatic rule—i.e., let $X =$ so and so, and see how the equation solves. If it does, O.K., then if not, X $=$ something else—the general practice being that it is the patient who is mulling over what X means, not the analyst. He lets the nebulae dissolve if they will ; if they don't, he just waits until they do—at least enough to steer ahead a bit and get a new sounding."

That were very praiseworthy, if actually carried out, but in my experience, the writers did not consult the patients, nor is there any evidence that they rejected any of their own equations. Even Ferenczi's oft-cited genital theory is hardly more than a tangled skein of conjectures, the coherence of which leaves much to be desired. All system builders claim to have been pragmatic, but, curiously enough, if we look into J. G. Fichte's *Wissenschaftslehre* (which Schopenhauer facetiously referred to as *Wissenschaftsleere* (" scientific emptiness "), we shall find many passages reminiscent of the psychoanalytic presentations. Indeed, there is a similar dialectic movement in German transcendental idealism and psychoanalysis, except that the latter immerses the abstractions in a sex medium. The technicality and the shuffling of concepts in the following passage will surely have, for some readers, a familiar ring—

" 1. In so far as the Non-Ego is posited, the Ego is not posited ; for the Non-Ego completely cancels the Ego. Now, the Non-Ego is posited in the Ego, for it is opposited; and all oppositing presupposes the identity of the Ego. Hence, the Ego is not posited in the Ego in so far as the Non-Ego is posited in it.

2. But the Non-Ego can only be posited in so far as an Ego is posited in the Ego (in the identical consciousness), as the opposite of which it is posited. Hence, in so far as the Non-Ego is posited in the Ego, the Ego also must be posited in it.

3. The conclusions of our first and second are opposed to each other ; yet both are developed from the second fundamental principle ; hence, that second principle is opposed to itself and cancels itself.

4. But it cancels itself only in so far as the posited is cancelled by the opposited, hence in so far as itself is valid. Hence, it does not cancel itself. The second fundamental principle cancels itself and does not cancel itself." [1]

Reviewing a youthful work of mine, Ernest Jones rated my stand on Psychoanalysis as ambivalent. Perhaps this is an adequate description even to-day. I like it for the great contribution it has made to the mental and social sciences, but I am not disposed to swallow whole every statement

---

[1] J. G. Fichte : *The Science of Knowledge* (English trans.), p. 75.

simply because a practitioner who has had a training course sets it forth.

Four Attitudes. There are four possible attitudes toward psychoanalysis. First there is, of course, the all-acceptance of the psychoanalysts themselves and their camp followers. Then there is the old-school psychologist or psychiatrist who is volitionally opposed to it, so that he would have no truck with it *ab initio* : This reaction of the *will* is to be ascribed to men like Münsterberg or Titchener, for whom Freud was primarily the upstart rival. The *affective* attitude will be found in religious and very conventional or fastidious circles, to whom the sex angle, complicated by the irreligious or irreverent views of Freud, is obnoxious, if not revolting. Finally, there are those who, like myself, are sympathetic in general, but entertain some *logical* scruples as to the conclusions drawn or interpretations arrived at. In principle, we can very well adopt many of the Freudian generalizations, but until such time as the training of psychoanalysts will include a rigid methodological discipline, such as is evinced in other sciences, and a greater degree of self-criticism, many of us will have to exercise caution about resorting to it as an oracle deciding on all phenomena in the human sphere. Characterology, especially, should be protected against its pronouncements and kept in a separate bailiwick, immune from its dogmatic impositions.

This does not mean that psychoanalysts should be expected to refrain from adding to the field of character. We are, in fact, beholden to them for the mass of observations on human nature.

They have called attention to bits of behavior which are prone to be considered by the majority of academic psychologists as too trivial to mention, or for that matter, to take cognizance of. It is, however, the Procrustean operation as applied to these observations which must irk us. Whether the data are historical, sociological, or belonging to the domain of art, we always can be certain as to the trend of the explanation, but the formula cannot be as simple as all that in a frightfully complicated world, which has evolved through centuries, even aeons. A master key may fit many locks but not all which can be devised.

Since the issue between psychoanalysis and my own position was raised by one of the most prominent British psychoanalysts in his lengthy review of *The Psychology of Character*, when it first appeared, it would seem expedient to reproduce a passage from the review in which he attempts to meet my objections and to thresh out the points anew ; for they are actual to-day as they were about twenty-five years ago. It is interesting to note, too, that my critic, to judge from his most recent works, has veered somewhat from his original stand, and has become engrossed in the very problems which Freudians were wont to brush aside or gloss over. At the same time I must admit that the Unconscious means more to me now that it did to the young author almost wholly committed to laboratory results.

" As has been the case with so many other psychologists," my critic observes, " Dr. Roback is manifestly afraid of the Unconscious and will only resort to it when all other explanations have failed. This is the old principle of Occam's razor applied to science through the modern formula of ' safety first', but here as elsewhere, safety first may often be dangerous in the long run. And the danger inherent in the otherwise sound maxim ' *entia non sunt multiplicanda praeter necessitatem* ' is that in the endeavor to avoid superfluous ' entia ' one may often under-estimate the ' necessitas ', i.e., unduly simplify the facts to be explained. It certainly seems that Dr. Roback has to some extent committed this mistake, for it is clear to the psychoanalytically trained reader that he fails to take account of the complexities and intricacies of the

human mind which demand . . . the concept of the Unconscious. Thus although a whole chapter is devoted to
Compensation, there is very little real appreciation of Displacement, Overdetermination, and Ambivalence." [1]

My reply is : the *necessitas* has to be at least pragmatically
proven, before we can afford to build entirely on the hypothesis, ignoring at the same time possibly many other
necessitates, e.g., constitutional, perhaps even chemical,
determinants. In the case of the physical sciences, the
necessity of an ingredient becomes evident in experimentation, and as we keep adding new variables, we always, at the
same time, keep reducing the number of outmoded variables,
so that simplification and elaboration go on side by side.

Is this true of psychoanalysis ? Since Freud has originated
the system, the number of manipulations has become legion.
Almost every new article complicates the system. I shall not
speak of the dissidents and the para-Freudians, but the very
faithful disciples proceed to make new permutations and
combinations. If this should go on for another fifty years,
then the number of *necessitates* to deal with in psychoanalysis
alone will take on Gargantuan proportions. If all of them
must be considered before we can venture to evaluate character
then we might as well not begin, because before long, we
should find ourselves amidst utter confusion.

What is more, the general tendency for psychologists to
espouse many causes : psychoanalysis, cultural anthropology,
physiology, and sociological data will, in the course of a
generation, entangle us in a hopeless mess from which it will
be impossible to extricate ourselves. The fact is I do not
believe in over-simplification, but in operating with reasonably
certain parameters. Rather than gambling on unknown
premises through mystifying manipulations, savoring of
Talmudical *pilpul*—no doubt necessary under a theocratic

[1] J. C. F. : *Intern. J. of Psycho-Analvsis*, 1928, vol. ix.

form of legislation, which must be shown as emanating from the Bible—I prefer to take it for granted that (*a*) what appears logical to most intelligent people who are conversant with the clinical data, and not only to orthodox psychoanalysts, is acceptable for the time being, and (*b*) to negotiate only one set of principles at a time. Perhaps the maxim that nature abhors a vacuum needs revision to-day, but we can rest assured that science abhors a babel of hypotheses that can never be established, unless verbal association is a method of proof.

As to the second cavil of my critic, viz., that while devoting a whole chapter to the mechanism of compensation, I fail to deal with " the complexities and intricacies of the human mind ", I have fully explained my reasons for the seeming disproportion. Compensation is more fundamental, more universal, and more accessible to the " naked eye " than most, if not all of the other mechanisms in psychoanalysis. The fact that Jung, Adler, Stekel, and Rank resort to it constantly, that the older psychiatrists and physiologists have made ample use of this concept, that it has been commonly referred to in essays since the days of Montaigne, and even in antiquity, and has been recognized abundantly by the man in the street should be sufficient to make its status clear. Most of the other mechanisms are more problematic, e.g., introjection ; or else are species of compensation, like reaction-formation and sublimation ; or at least less integral or pivotal. Thus displacement as a mechanism, while important enough in wit, dreams, symptomatic acts, or neurosis does not enter in the evaluation of an individual's character. It has its place as a nut, a washer, a small cog, or a single spoke, but the wheel of character will not be affected by it in its course, one way or another.

If one cannot approach the subject of character except by means of this full panoply of the psychoanalyst, then it is quite possible that the protection is too heavy for such a quest. There is safety in such an outfit, but progress will be made with less accoutrement. If the whole of psychoanalysis must be traversed before one can reach any conclusion as to character, why must we not accord the same privilege to other systems or schools ? And the more extensive each individual approach, the less hope for attaining some common ground, which, after all, is our only salvation in a non-experimental science.

It is not my purpose to institute a general critique of psychoanalysis, except in regard to its bearing on our subject. The service its originator has rendered to our whole cultural outlook can be appreciated even by his chief adversaries. He has made the educated world more sophisticated, it is true, but he has also broadened and deepened our understanding of concepts which have never been fully analyzed because of their association with sex. The vast tower which has been reared by him and his collaborators may prove to be but pasteboard construction, but it is magnificent in its scope and colorful in its ornate details.

To him we are particularly indebted for a wealth of observations which he has endeavored to weld into a systematic interpretation of man and civilization. The dialectic skill which he displays in building up his pyramid of doctrines reminds us of the argumentation in Phaedo, Timaeus, and other gems of Plato. For a while we are prepared to subscribe to his conclusions, but Plato usually tried to prove one proposition at a time ; and everything would lead up to this one thesis, e.g., immortality. Freud, however, no sooner arrives at one result than he turns either about-face or, at least, at right angles, and thence to some new-fangled conclusion, and so on indefinitely, with the result that eventually the steps become altogether too complicated for us ; yes, and even too fast for our more deliberative pace, particularly if we belong to his obsessional category, rather than to the hysteric class, and we begin to falter, and then we start wondering whether what Freud has devised is not a stupendous fairy tale which appeals for the very reason that so many are enthralled by thrillers and detective stories of the most lurid sort. It might be paradoxically said that Freud has supplied the more or less literate world with an escape from reality.

On the other hand, whether we accept his whole psycho-rama [1] or not, he has furthered our knowledge in many respects, and he has permanently shaped the course of psychology more than anyone else in its history. Many of his principles I can countenance, even to the belief that there is a death instinct, which a number of his faithful followers are chary about sponsoring, but perhaps his greatest handicap is his strict determinism. He must find a reason for every deviation, which causes him to lead us on from one turning to another until we are lost in the labyrinth. It is evident that he cannot plead the cause of all the exceptions which he wishes to bring under the general rule, with equal cogency. Had he only on occasion admitted that somehow there is a snag here or there which he does not undertake to explain, he might have won over more adherents.

Considering the plethora of mechanisms at his disposal, each one of which assumes protean forms, e.g. projection, displacement, identification, sublimation, ambivalence, reaction-formation, to mention only a few ; taking account of his constitutional bisexuality, active and passive function, the principle of duality, and then the frequent and ready switching from the anal to the oral, oral to urethral level of eroticism (or vice versa), or sadistic to masochistic impulses, through self-direction ; and last but not least, giving free rein to the opulent and iridescent play of symbolism at his command, then small wonder that anything can be turned into anything else, and black can take on any colour in the

---

[1] I have already used this as the title of a book, in 1941, so it is not an entirely new word to be set off by quotes.

spectrum. Thus Freud may be likened to an organist sitting down before a huge organ equipped with half a dozen manuals several pedals and a large number of stops which he pulls and pushes every minute or so as he improvises. Of course, this may still be art, while Freud's function is to discover truth, in addition to treating the ill ; and you cannot improvise reality.

On Freud's behalf it may at least be said that *si non è vero, è ben trovato*. That, however, does not apply to most of the epigones, who look to his magic wand or baton for the cue. The merest suggestion will call forth a polygraphic contest. Sometimes, the disciple oversteps the confines of his discipline, and then he must either turn back or else he is outside the fold, and can no longer be recognized as a stalwart. There was a certain justification in Freud's exercise of almost dictatorial powers in a sphere which permits of so much speculation. Since his death, however, only the tradition can hold the orthodox together, and there has been evinced a greater tendency to stray from the path outlined by the master. Nor is there anyone invested with the authority to call into question the wobbly interpretations of some psychoanalysts, much less to bring them to book. Indeed, while in all other sciences, and particularly in psychology, controversies are rife and even experimental investigations are impugned, there has been remarkably little disagreement among Freudians. The divergents, of course, are forming coteries of their own.

Although much has appeared of late on some phase of character in this psychoanalytic literature, the contribution offers a very meagre morsel for the chief reason that it is made up of haphazard interpretations of behavior bolstered by nothing but verbiage. The bare observations are in themselves interesting enough, but the shuttling of trains of terms back and forth only bemuddles the issue. We realize that psychoanalysts must carry on and not stop with Freud, but if this verbalization in writing goes on for another fifty years, in the absence of evidence, the tower of psychoanalysis will become a veritable Tower of Babel. The indisposition or else inability to reason out a conclusion, as Freud was wont to do, is nothing short of appalling. In other words, a mere symbol, an association, a metaphor, a *soupçon* would be sufficient for most writers around which to weave a theory. When recourse is had to other fields of knowledge (philology, history, folk-lore, etc.) in order to lend support to the new deduction, the information is often garbled, misinterpreted, or at least questionable. Freud himself has erred in that respect, particularly in the selection of his authorities to suit his fancy.[1] This natural foible on the part of scientists may perhaps be called " natural selection " too, but the rigorous demands of science would bid us sift our selections, as Charles Darwin has done, with the possibility in view of self-criticism. To be sure, a single individual could not cope with problems imposed by such intellectual explorations, but experts should be called in to offer their seasoned opinions. I have found the supporting " evidence " from forensic fields, in many instances, ludicrous.

[1] A. A. Roback: *Psychorama*, chapters on Freud's *Moses and Monotheism* (Sci. Art.), 1942.

CHAPTER XVII

THE RIVAL SCHOOLS OF JUNG AND ADLER

I. ANALYTIC PSYCHOLOGY

It might be possible to find a common denominator for Freud's, Jung's, and Adler's schools in the label " Depth Psychology ", but psychoanalysts will not countenance the two latter under the head of psychoanalysis.

Persona and Anima. Jung's psychology derives mainly from Freud, but it is more mystical and betrays an Eastern source. Analogies may be found between the ego and Jung's *persona*, that phase of our personality which adapts itself to the world at large, as well as between the id—superego and the *anima*, that unconscious reservoir, both individual and collective, which harbors both depths of depravation as well as the potentialities of exalted idealism, depending upon the incubation of an age-long inheritance of ancestral experiences. Both angel and fiend are fashioned in the *anima*, which for man is represented in the misty form of a woman—a sort of sensitive mental plate upon which present experiences will mingle with those of past generations forming a hazy composite and influencing his life.

The *persona* and the *anima* are always in conflict. When the former usurps all the power, the individual becomes a petty realist, when the latter is all-dominant, he becomes a visionary. The art of normal living consists in achieving a happy balance between the two energy reservoirs.

JUNG'S PSYCHOLOGICAL TYPES

Jung's well-known classification of psychological types into introverted and extraverted individuals has received considerable recognition not only in educated lay circles, particularly journalistic and literary quarters, but even among psychologists. But that is as far as the latter will go with him. The breaking up of the original dichotomy into eight sub-divisions does not lend itself to ready acceptance, and, furthermore, the compensatory principle which he introduces to explain the vast majority of cases that elude the ordinary classification, while plausible in theory is scarcely applicable ; for, granted that there is a primarily conscious introverted type with a complementary unconscious trend of extraversion, and conversely a conscious extraverted type with an unconscious trend of introversion, our utmost ingenuity will be taxed in discovering the criteria in the first place, and secondly in reaching an agreement as to which fit whom. Illustrating with instances from literature and history, on which the Neo-Platonist of psychoanalysis draws so energetically, is not a wholly satisfactory method ; for, as in the case of the illustrations to be found in the various books on character analysis, they are *ex post facto* constructions, and out of innumerable possibilities one is apt to select just those which best suit the particular theory advanced.

Interplay of Conscious and Unconscious. The reciprocal interplay between the conscious and unconscious elements in one's personality is, in my opinion, the most interesting feature of the doctrine. In other respects, especially in the use it makes of thought, sensation, feeling and intuition as bases of the sub-divisions, it resembles the classifications of the French school.

But let us see how Jung develops his system of types.[1] First of all, he recognizes that there are two different sorts of attitudes in people, (a) the " extraverted ", which means that the libido (i.e. the psychic content and intensity) in such a person is directed outward, and (b) the " introverted " where the libido is turned inwardly.

Attitude of the Extravert. The extravert " tries to do or

[1] C. G. Jung : *Psychological Types* (Eng. translation), 1923.

to make just what his milieu momentarily needs and expects from him, and abstains from every innovation that is not entirely obvious, or that in any way exceeds the expectation of those around him ''. But on that account, he often neglects the subjective needs until they make themselves felt in neurotic symptoms, and hysteria is most frequently associated with the extravert *in extremis*, manifesting itself in various physical disorders. Coming to meet the emergency which so far takes place in the realm of the conscious, is the compensatory reaction from the unconscious, which in the case of the extravert, is of an introverted nature, and a series of phantasy symptoms resulting from the introversion of psychic energy now supervene.

Characteristic of the Introvert. The introvert, on the other hand, is inclined to disregard objects and the opinions of other persons, almost distrusting them. He is safely intrenched in his own feeling of security. In childhood he is shy, inhibited, takes a long time to become oriented, and develops later in life than does the extravert. The subjective in such persons is all-powerful, and they are willing to oppose the world if they happen to cherish a preconceived notion.

As in the case of the extravert, a compensatory reaction sets in from the domain of the unconscious to offset this exaggeration of the superiority illusion. The consciously under-valued object assumes tremendous proportions in the unconscious and causes the introvert to shrink in dread. Wishing to overpower the object, he spends his energy in adopting protective measures to no avail. When the conflict reaches the saturation point, the introvert succumbs to the form of neurosis called psychasthenia.

It should be noticed that the majority of people go to make up a third class, viz., the less differentiated normal man, the source of whose motivation can scarcely be determined offhand, as his introversion or extraversion is not sufficiently accentuated.

Varieties of Main Mechanisms. So much for the main divisions or rather, as Jung is anxious to explain (thus rectifying a former mis-statement of his) mechanisms. We must now remember that the mind consists of a number of psychic functions. According to Jung, they are sensation, thinking, feeling and intuition. The first three functions require no explanation. The fourth is " apperception by an unconscious method or the perception of an unconscious content ". [1] It would be ideal if all the four functions were equally developed, but in actual life one function usually stands out at the expense of the others. Those of the sensation type content themselves with perceiving concrete reality. Reflection or feeling is wanting. Those who " cannot adapt themselves to a situation which they cannot comprehend intellectually " belong to the thinking types. Then there are individuals who simply ask themselves whether something engaging their attention is pleasant or unpleasant (feeling type). Finally the " intuitives " are those who " give themselves up wholly to the lure of possibilities and abandon every situation where no further possibilities are scented ".

We can readily see that a minimum of eight types is obtainable, when each of these four functions is coupled with one or the other of the general attitudes. In the condensed paper, bearing the same title as his chief work, Jung intimates that the classes may be increased at will, since each of the types represented by the four functions can be split up into three sub-groups, as, with regard to the thinking type, (a) the intuitive speculative form, (b) the logical, mathematical form, (c) the empirical form ; and so on for the other three chief function-types.

The distinction between the introvert and the extravert has struck many psychologists as valuable enough to adopt, especially as Jung has thrown some light on the *modus*

[1] C. G. Jung : " Psychological Types," in *Problems of Personality* (1925), p. 297.

AA

operandi of these two general attitudes.   The illustrations from his rich psychiatric experience are well chosen, but the question is to what extent the sharply drawn classes can be applied.   Had Jung made himself familiar with the attempts of Ribot, Lévy, Paulhan, Malapert and Ribéry, he would have noticed that they have reason just as much on their side ;   and when he pronounces his own classification as the most practical, one would like to be able to substantiate this confidence by the proof of application.   After all it is the power to convince others that furnishes the best recommendation for a theory, and that can be achieved only by the possibility of scientific application.

An American Variant.   Hinkle, the American follower of Jung, while claiming to have reached independently the same classificatory conclusions as the Swiss psychoanalyst, nevertheless arranges her introverts and extraverts into the subjective and objective types, the distinction between which in behavior and character traits, " is so great as often to be more apparent than the distinction between extravert and introvert." [1] The subjective type differs from the objective in the degree of emotionality and also by partaking of the quality of bisexuality.   Individuals of this type are more complex, more difficult to understand than the others.   The objective type, both introverted and extraverted, steers clear of complexities and subtleties.   The objective extravert is unimpressionable, not sensitive ;   the objective introvert is slow, takes no account of human relations and therefore lacks judgment.

In all, Hinkle finds six types, adding the simple extraverted and simple introverted to the above four.   She does not agree with Jung in putting all the stress on the distinction between " extravert " and " introvert " ;   and in opposition to him, she affirms that she discovered " a definite group of extraverts who were as tender-minded as the classical introvert, and

[1] B. Hinkle : *The Re-Creating of the Individual*, 1923, p. 171.

contrariwise, many introverted philosophers and scientists who were as tough-minded as the typical extravert ".

Sometimes I get the notion that writers on types will incline to make distinctions according to their likes and dislikes. Jung seems to favor the introvert ; Hinkle, who matches Theodore Roosevelt with Woodrow Wilson, the English against the Germans, and Darwin against Kant, seems to have a warm spot for the extravert, with the result that she re-casts the Jungian material into a slightly different mould.

Extraversion and Dissociation. McDougall, who in his systematic text-book of abnormal psychology, adopts the original simple classification of Jung into two types and favors Hinkle's sub-classes as against Jung's, nevertheless regards Darwin as a typical introvert, and throws his lot in with the introverts. His theory accounting for the type differences is of greater importance than the attempts at subclassification. Basing his conclusions on the fact that the extravert is more affected by drugs and stimulants, especially alcohol, and that he is far more susceptible to hypnosis, he associates extraversion with a constitutional disposition to dissociation, due in all probability to the activity of the hormones, in a manner which is not the same as in the case of the introvert.[1]

The empirical findings of McDougall as regards the effect of alcohol and suggestion on the extravert are, I believe, borne out in everyday observation, but his conclusion thereon would seem to militate against the general tendency to connect the introvert with dissociated states (schizoid, schizothymia, paranoia) and the extravert with periodic dispositions (manic-depressive states). Certainly in this case we should be compelled to distinguish between the dissociation of the extravert or hysterical individual and the split personalities of the extreme introverts out of whom the paranoiacs and schizophrenics are recruited.

[1] Wm. McDougall : *An Outline of Abnormal Psychology*, 1926, p. 442 ff.

II. ADLER'S SYSTEM

Adler's contribution to the study of character, as developed in his chief works, *Organ Inferiority and its Psychical Compensation, The Neurotic Constitution,* and *Individual Psychology,* and most recently in his *Understanding Human Nature* (1927) is woven around the now famous inferiority complex and its compensatory mechanism. The gist of Adler's doctrine is really contained in this compact statement : "All manifestations of neuroses and psycho-neuroses are to be traced back to organ inferiority, to the degree and the nature of the central compensation that has not yet become successful and to the appearance of compensation disturbances." [2]

Knowing, as we do, the tendency of all of Freud's disciples, both present and former, to assign to every person a fair share of such manifestations at least in some mild form, we may readily see why, according to Adler, all the various aberrations in man's conduct, from the serious offences down to the mere peculiarities in everyday behavior, would be linked with an hereditary, often latent, inferiority of a certain organ and its nervous superstructure. Character then, must be understood in such terms ; but though Adler's detailed interpretations and diagnoses are highly ingenious, they fail to connect the specific conclusions and inferences with the doctrine in general. In Adler's texture we may find threads from Nietzche (Will to Power—Superiority Goal) and Weininger (Male Attitude in Female Neurotics) in addition to the material which contains the warp and woof of psychoanalysis at large.

Adler's Favorite Theme—Inferiority. In one respect, at least, Adler differs from Freud in that although he makes considerable use of sex symbolism, like his erstwhile master, he nevertheless considers all sex manifestations requiring interpretations as preparatory steps to the illumination of a

[2] A. Adler : *Individual Psychology* (Eng. translation), 1924.

more fundamental tendency, viz., the *craving for completeness, security, superiority.* This theme runs throughout Adler's larger works and is repeated on nearly every other page. The sex details merely enter into the technique of Adler's broader outlook. (Freud's position has changed latterly in this respect too, since he is now willing to recognize the potency of the ego impulses.)

To be sure, Adler is always having in mind the neurotic, but from his description of the neurotic, we may take it that he means everybody without exception. I found in one of Adler's books a marginal note which struck me as highly significant, even if it is not likely that the young reader was aware of the profoundness of his quip. " The neurotic is like the normal individual, only more so," reads this comment. If we analyze this innocent remark, we shall see that it implies no more and no less than that every trait of character is the symptom of a neurotic tendency, but in the typical neurotic, the mark is more accentuated.

Main Objection to Psychoanalytic Schools. *Indeed one of our main objections to psychoanalysis of the patented sort is just this, that finding so little rationality in human behavior, it denies that there is any.* The barrier between good and bad, the desirable and the undesirable, the reasonable and the unreasonable, is thus broken down to start with, and thereafter we are to rummage among the *débris.* But such a scientific hide-and-seek game has its origin in the implicit belief, at any rate, of the bi-polarity of truth. Whether you have a predilection or an aversion for sex subjects you are troubled by the same motive. Jones, as we have seen in the quotation above, makes anal-eroticism responsible for a number of contrasted traits. Stekel, perhaps the most prolific of all the psychoanalysts, in linking the exaggerated fear of the dentist with a special sensitiveness in the region of the mouth, says about people thus afflicted " either they are gourmands or else very abstemious . . . either they love kissing or else find kissing intolerable ".[1] And since a case could easily be made out for either alternative, it is not difficult for psychoanalysts to prove that they are right.

The " Guiding Fiction ". Adler is a typical scion of the romantic school. " Both refractoriness and obedience are only attitudes which reveal to us the jump from the uncertain past into the protecting future as are all other character traits." In the course of his various disquisitions he has occasion to mention scores of traits, good, bad and indifferent. Each one is to him a *finger-post to the operation of the ego-consciousness under some sort of guiding fiction.* " Fictions, maxims, guiding principles then . . . form part of the mental character of all persons, especially of neurotically inclined children. And reduced to their nucleus, all of these formulae are as follows : Act as though you were a complete man, or wished to be one." [2] Alas ! to what menial use Kant's lofty categorical imperative has been put through Adler's misappropriation of Vaihinger's Kantian philosophy of " as if ". The woman acts as though she wanted to be a man. The man acts as though he wanted to be a superior male. " The feeling of insignificance, of weakness, of anxiety and helplessness, of ill-health, of deficiency, of pain, etc., produces in the neurotic actions of such a nature that he seems to be compelled to set up a defence against effeminacy, that is to say, to be obliged to act in a manly and forceful manner. . . . The neurotic individual draws constantly effective guiding lines for his volition, action, and thoughts in the form of traits of character in the broad chaotic field of his soul, in order to make his security complete. The guiding maxim is always " Act as if you were obliged to shift for yourself by means of one of these faults, of these deficiencies to gain through it a feeling of superiority." [1]

[1] W. Stekel : *Disguises of Love,* p. 78.
[2] A. Adler : *The Neurotic Constitution,* p. 315.
[1] Loc. cit., pp. 100–1.

There is no need of examining here Adler's inferiority doctrine which has been set forth in various forms by earlier psychiatrists, Koch, Anton and Otto Gross particularly, as we shall see in the next chapter. There seems to be a modicum of truth in the thesis as a whole, whether relating to psychic inferiority only or to organic inferiority, which Adler seems to think is at the bottom of the other. Certainly Adler has not convinced anybody by citing the case of Beethoven and one or two other composers who have had a hearing defect. A good many more composers have been afflicted with eye trouble (two of the greatest composers, Bach and Handel, became totally blind in later life. Schubert was very near-sighted, Halévy, Rimsky-Korsakoff, Bizet, Raff, Offenbach, Bruch, Rheinberger, Paine, Marschner, Mahler, and Hérold wore glasses, and others may be cited whose defective vision was marked, although their hearing was not known to be other than normal). According to the theory, they should have become oculists, ophthalmologists, or painters. And may we not be excused for thinking that the brain specialist must have been born with a defective brain in order to become interested in his field ?

Non-Sequitur in Adler's Doctrine. What is weakest about Adler's whole treatment is his uncritical acceptance of data to fit his hypothesis. Granting him the privilege of selecting his own material, we yet frequently fail to see the link between the facts cited (including the interpretations) and the all too oft repeated conclusion about the superiority goal. "*Non Sequitur*" is the necessary reaction of the reflective reader. More than once, too, Adler implicates himself in the fallacies celebrated by the ancient logicians. To give one instance : Adler in many passages, implies that women are inferior to men (" One of the facts which, thanks to my method of viewing the subject, I was able to explain, concerns the less well known inferiority common to all girls and women, which is due to their feminine rôle in contrast to the masculine ") [1] yet in a later chapter we are told that the disparagement of women and the conviction which would deny them equal rights are reflections of the neurotic tendency in man to assert himself in his dread of the other sex.[2] Woman is inferior, yet he who thinks her so exhibits an inferiority complex.

Adler reminds us of a man trying to mop up a huge platter, containing drops of various liquids, with one wholesome crumb, shoving it about in all possible directions with his little finger. Adler entertains a different opinion of his achievement. " Our study has shown," he writes in his conclusion, " that man's character-traits and their principal function in the life of the individual are manifested as expedients, in the nature of guiding lines for the thinking, feeling, willing, and acting of the human *psyche*, and that they are brought into stronger relief so soon as the individual strives to escape from the phase of uncertainty to the fulfilment of his fictitious guiding idea. The material for the construction of the character-traits is contained in the psychic totality, and congenital differences vanish before the uniform effect of the guiding fiction. Goal and direction, the fictitious purpose of the traits of character, may be best recognized in the original, direct, aggressive lines. Want and difficulties of life lead to alterations of character, so that only such constructions find favor as stand in harmony with the individual's ego-idea. In this manner are formed the more cautious, the more hesitating character-traits which show a deviation from the direct line, but examination of which reveals their dependence upon the guiding fiction ".

Types should be Differentiated. The answer to this is that our author has described one character type only, viz., the neurotic ; and even assuming that all mortals are neurotic, it behoves us to ascertain the different sub-varieties and modes

[1] Loc. cit., p. 213.
[2] Loc. cit., pp. 386 ff.

of apprehending them. For his synthetic picture of this ubiquitous type we are beholden to Adler, but one feels that there are degrees and shades of neuroticism ; and furthermore that by comparison, there are *more* and *less* normal people whose traits interest us as such.

In this respect Freud has at least tackled the problem and has attempted to differentiate between the " character trait " as such and the " neurotic character trait ", the former being marked by the absence of any miscarriage of repression or of the return of the repressed. In character formation, repression does not come into play, or else it easily attains its goal, viz., the substitution of the repressed impulses, by means of reaction-formation and sublimation.[1] The processes of character-formation are therefore less transparent and less accessible to analysis than those of neurosis.

Also one feels that certain traits are more significant than others, but Adler, in common with all the other psycho-analysts, is inclined to make a mountain out of a mole-hill, in order to bolster up the general theory ; and exploiting the rich mines of symbolism at its command, the army of psycho-analysts is able to draw out the most harmless mannerism into enormous proportions without the fear of actual disproof ; for only facts and theories making use of facts can be dis-proved. Symbols are immune from conviction just as they cannot compel conviction in another sense.

Subsequently Adler has shifted the stress from organ inferiority to the " style of life " and environmental happen-ings. The child, to begin with, is active and aggressive, but difficulties arising in the immediate surroundings may modify or even reverse the original trait.

Just as in psychoanalysis character stemmed from the libido in all its peregrinations, so in Adler's system character issues from the goal of superiority.

---

[1] S. Freud : " The Predisposition to Obsessional Neurosis," 1913, *Collected Papers*, vol. ii, p. 129.

Traits of character are only the external manifestations of the style of life, of the behavior pattern, of any individual. As such they enable us to understand his attitude towards his environment, towards his fellow men, towards the society in which he lives, and towards the challenge of existence in general. Character traits are instruments, the tricks which are used by the total personality in the acquisition of recognition and significance ; their configuration in the personality amounts to a " technique " in living.

.   .   .   .

Traits of character are not inherited, as many would have it, nor are they congenitally present. They are to be considered as similar to a pattern for existence which enables every human being to live his life and express his personality in any situation without the necessity of consciously thinking about it.[1]

For Adler character traits are artifices for the purpose of gratifying one's desires. Thus a child is not lazy from constitution, " but is lazy because laziness seems to him the best adapted means of making life easier, while it enables him at the same time to maintain his feeling of significance." [2]

It is difficult to see how laziness can maintain a feeling of significance, but lazy people will no doubt grasp at Adler's dictum on their behalf and make of it an honored quality.

Adler repeats himself many times in his eagerness to impress us with the fact that traits are not inherited. Laziness is, to be sure, not inherited, but is it not possible that genes which later cause the child to acquire a lazy disposition are inherited ? And how does Adler explain resemblance of character traits in parents and children ? He simply assumes that the child, in his " striving for significance, seized upon the example of those individuals in his environment who are

---

[1] A. Adler : *Understanding Human Nature*, English trans., 1927, p. 143.

[2] Op. cit., p. 144.

already significant and demand respect, as an ideal model." [1]

It is probably nearer the truth to say that we are born lazy, but that our needs and ambitions create the drive for directed action. Adler believes that all children are happy buoyant, optimistic, until some accident occurs to thwart them. The pessimists are those " who have acquired an inferiority complex as a result of the experiences and impressions of their childhood ". That, too, is a whale of a generalization. Pessimists often are hereditarily linked. What is more, there is just as much inferiority feeling in the happy-go-lucky optimist as in the anxious pessimist. " An individual who cannot sleep well has developed but a poor technique of living " is another dictum of Adler's. But that might be said about any function of man, e.g. digestion and peristalsis.

Adler divides character traits into two classes : the aggressive and the non-aggressive. Among the first are included vanity and ambition, jealousy, envy, avarice, and hate, while the non-aggressive type comprises seclusiveness, anxiety, faint-heartedness, uncouth behavior, although it is not apparent why biting one's nails or drilling one's ears is a non-aggressive trait. It strikes me as rather aggressive, both as an expressive movement and as an offensive act. Adler would have us see in such manifestations a disinclination on the part of such individuals to coöperate. Again, the individual is supposed to indulge in such objectionable habits as a defense mechanism, i.e., blaming his uncouthness for his lack of success. " What couldn't I do if I didn't have this bad habit ? " Possibly there are such people, too, but unfortunately, most who are given to habits of this sort do not realize their badness ; they seem to be blissfully innocent in this respect.

In Adler's exposition, there is also a miscellaneous class of character traits some of which do not seem to fit in place here. Here we have cheerfulness (is it not really a mood or a temperamental frame of mind ?) stereotypy, juvenile immaturity, submissiveness (which I should think belongs rather to the non-aggressive traits), imperiousness (which should have had a place with the aggressive traits) martyrdom ideas, religiosity, and emphasis on principle, which Adler ties up with pedantry, as if principles were fads or trifles.

In the above presentation we have a brief condensation of Adler's views as set forth in the second half of his *Understanding Human Nature*, the part which is somewhat pretentiously labelled " The Science of Character ". Character is thus only a device engineered by the universal goal of superiority. In fact, the traits are only tricks, and the status of the vaunted individual in his *Individualpsychologie* is rather precarious when all that represents an integral whole is the " goal of superiority ", not the character of man.

III. STEKEL

If Stekel's brand of psychoanalysis is not discussed here, it is not because of any neglect but rather for the reason that Stekel was more of an eclectic and although perhaps the most brilliant interpreter of all of Freud's disciples, he had never established himself on a wholly independent footing, as did Jung and Adler. If the others were composers, good or indifferent, he was more the great virtuoso in execution. It may be said of him, however, that his polyphonic interpretations of dreams, in which he excelled, did make allowance for a characterial phase, which he called the *functional*, as opposed to the *materialistic* content that involved the pure id ; and thus Silberer's distinction of *anagogic* (elevating) and *catagogic* (" gutterward ", if such a coinage is permissible) found its way in his psychological outlook, drawing Freud's barbed shafts in consequence.

Stekel's voluminous works, most translated into English,

many of them written in a sparkling feuilletonistic style attracted wide attention. He also succeeded in gathering around him, in Vienna, a score or more of professionals who looked upon him as their mentor, among them, Emil Gutheil and Anton Missriegler. The group, for some time, even published a bulky annual *Fortschritte der Sexualwissenschaft und Psychanalyse*, which contained many articles of a psychosomatic nature, but Stekel was, as his autobiography (edited posthumously, in 1950, by E. Gutheil) would imply, no organizer of movements, nor even a systematizer, but a detailist, so that his school, if such it could be considered, did not last even during his lifetime. This, however, might be mentioned, in passing, that at a time when Freud had not yet bothered looking into the moral problems besetting his patients, Stekel, in his own therapy, was, to some extent, concerned with the ethical character of those who consulted him. Had his views been brought together under some label, as Jung's or Adler's, Stekel might have made more of a stir with textbook writers. As it is, scarcely any one alludes to him, in spite of the library of wisdom he has published over many years, and up to his voluntary death in England, after fleeing the Nazis.

A Mental Hygiene Slant in an Adlerian Perspective. It may not be just to catalogue Myerson's popularly written *Foundations of Personality* under the psychoanalytic rubric, since the author is far from identifying himself with either the Viennese currents or the Swiss eddy of the stream. Nevertheless, through the sociological style which permeates the book, an unmistakable Adlerian coloring is noticeable, though Adler is not anywhere in the volume mentioned by name. Myerson's account is too eclectic to allow of systematic incorporation. Its point of view is therapeutic. With *adjustment* as its watchword the presentation is an extension of the mental hygiene movement. The backbone, however, of the discussion is distinctly a version of the *inferiority doctrine*, lacking the organic substrate, which is fundamental to Adler's system. The character types which Myerson mentions such as the " hypokinetic " and " hyperkinetic " (designations much in use now among eugenicists and mental hygienists, and signifying merely less energetic or more energetic than the average) "ambivalent" (a term employed by Bleuler to designate those who are drawn in two different directions), " explosive " (used by James in connection with the will), " anhedonic " (a word coined by the French school and applied to persons who take no pleasure in anything) and others, like the psychiatric types (cyclothymic, monothymic, hypochondriac, paranoic), are in reality not applicable to character with reference to particular constituents. Hundreds of different types could thus be drawn up. Such an inventory would be faulty because of overlapping, particularization, duplication and other violations of logical and systematic classification. But perhaps Myerson is not concerned with theories and classifications of character or personality, but is rather interested in assembling useful data for the benefit of the layman.

Eclectic Affiliations in the United States. White[1] in America, has approached the problem through the psychoanalytic avenue more directly—though in a highly eclectic way—claiming that character is merely the resultant of an interplay of unconscious factors in which conflict plays the most important part ; the resolution of this conflict then becomes the desideratum of man. And to that end White places at our disposal all the mechanisms of Freud's, Jung's and Adler's schools, interwoven with a number of other factors. Van der Hoop's exposition of the theories of Freud and Jung, under the somewhat misleading title *Character and the Unconscious*, is based on the same presuppositions as those which White has set out with.

[1] W. A. White : *Mechanisms of Character Formation*, 1921, also "Individuality and Introversion," *The Psychoanalytic Review*, 1916, vol. iv.

Kempf, both in his *Autonomic Functions and the Personality* and *Psychopathology*, particularly in the latter work, harps *ad libitum* on the psychoanalytic theme, but his own contribution, viz., the linking of the autonomic functions with the affective side of man and his temperamental make-up, brings him into position with the seekers of character determinants in physiological and especially chemical processes ; and though not primarily concerned with the glands, he suggests a definite location for some of the Freudian and Adlerian mechanisms (even if he falls short of making actual specific connections). Thus he affords a sort of synthesis between the mental approach of the psychoanalysts and the physical approach of the endocrinologists.

A host of Freudian writers may be mentioned as authors of observations on this topic. Many of these observations display an insight into what is ordinarily called human nature. Some of the writers give evidence of penetration in special fields, such as Adler and Stekel in their descriptions of various sorts of neurotics and Pfister in his accounts of children's peculiarities, but on the whole, the psychoanalytic attack consists of sallies. It does not represent a carefully worked-out plan based on solid foundations, and for this reason it may be said that, while the intuitive scintillations are appreciated particularly from an artistic viewpoint, the scientific groundwork upon which they purport to stand cannot provide a foothold for the logically-minded investigator who must have his concepts clearly separated before they can be related to one another.

Minor Variations of the Psychoanalytic Theme. In addition to the more original and specific interlockings of character and psychoanalysis, as attempted by the greater satellites of the group, we have also a number of general and popular expositions in which the so-called new psychology is stressed as a key to the understanding of character formation. Burrow's paper [1] on this subject is a collection of odds and ends from the Viennese and Zürich schools revolving about the plea for psychoanalysis to appreciate the sense of obligation and the love of truth which are "fundamental in the neurotic character". Here we obtain a medley of Freudian, Jungian ("mother complex" "uterine sleep") and Adlerian terms all running smoothly into one another. The neurotic, as painted by Adler, differs in conception from that depicted by Burrow, whose picture is rather that of an angelic being than of a selfish and deceitful creature, as may be gathered from expressions like "possesses a nature full of gentleness" and "an abiding love of beauty", both phrases referring to the traits of the neurotic.

The article of Forsyth,[2] dealing with the growth of character in children, as illuminated by the psychoanalytic torch, and that of Long [3] which again is an appeal to the lay mind to heed the teachings of psychoanalysis, come under the same rubric. What may be said about most of this type of literature is that whoever has read a single book by an outstanding member of one of the three main schools has read all that the particular school has to offer.

CRITICAL NOTE ON DEPTH PSYCHOLOGY AS A WHOLE

One serious criticism which applies especially to the Freudian phase of psychoanalysis is the exaggerated importance attached to experience in the formation of character. While admitting that no individual is entirely immune to the effect of emotional stimuli, I should take occasion to point out that *since different people are affected differently by apparently*

[1] T. Burrow : "Character and the Neuroses," *Psychoanal. Rev.*, 1924, vol. i.

[2] D. Forsyth : "The Rudiments of Character," *Psychoanal. Rev.*, 1921, vol. viii.

[3] C. Long : "An Analytic View of the Basis of Character," *Psychoanal. Rev.*, 1920, vol. vii ; later reprinted as a chapter under the title "Sex as a Basis of Character" in her *Psychology of Phantasy*.

similar stimuli, it would be reasonable to maintain that character in reality precedes and determines the nature of the effect, instead of being the resultant of the multitude of experiences to which man is subjected.

If character is formed in such an utterly mechanical way, there is no reason why we should not attribute this quality to a radio apparatus or to a steam engine.

On the surface, Adler's type of doctrine would claim to escape this criticism, since his defection from the orthodox camp of Freud was due primarily to his hankering after a doctrine that would champion the cause of freedom against the extreme determinism of his master ; but on strict analysis it will be seen that, though the organ inferiority itself is held to have an hereditary basis, the compensatory reaction is a process developing out of the inferiority complex in relation to the environment.

Indeed toward the end of his *Neurotic Constitution*, Adler makes it plain that " the idea of a congenital origin of ' character ' is untenable because the real substratum for the formation of psychic character and whatever part thereof may be congenital, is metamorphosed under the influence of the guiding idea until this idea is satisfied ". The " subordination of the character traits to the guiding fiction " is also stressed elsewhere.

The psychoanalysts have undoubtedly done yeoman's service to the study of character, especially in its countless quirks and kinks.   They have ferreted out from hidden recesses curios which help us to realize that there is more in heaven and earth than a purely academic psychology ever dreamt of, but we notice that each individual worker, after making his find, elaborates the ore into a trinket to his own special liking. Owing to this particularized and individualistic treatment on the part of the psychoanalysts, the wise attitude would be to accept the facts gratefully and decline with thanks the interpretations which do not follow *logically*, or at all events, are not in accordance with common sense.

The members of the Freudian schools resemble excavators who are endowed with a special skill for unearthing valuable relics but who make the strangest hazards in explaining the history and nature of these relics.   It is for the trained archæologist and not for the working men to deal with the discoveries scientifically. The psychoanalyst apparently must belong to the intuitive function-type of Jung's classification ; for instead of keeping within the confines of empirical evidence, he chooses to soar into the heights of speculation and is beguiled by the " lure of possibilities ". Psychoanalysis is a boon until it over-reaches itself.   One safe guide in the acceptance of psychoanalytic teaching is the matter of agreement in the various schools. The more agreement with regard to a certain principle, the more apt is it to be sound ; the less agreement, the more likely is it to be extravagant.

CHAPTER XVIII

THE PARA-FREUDIANS

For the past twenty years, even many of those psychoanalysts who identified themselves with Freud's hidebound teaching were beginning to feel the need of *Lebensraum*, expansion along other than purely libidinal lines. An interpretative discipline will necessarily experience occasional revolts ; and psychoanalysis, in spite of the dominating personality of Freud, could not be an exception.

Cause of Secession. The earlier iconoclasts, Jung, Adler, Stekel were successful or fortunate enough, each in founding a school of their own, although Stekel might still be considered as a psychoanalyst, whereas the other two could not. As with creeds and cults, the farther we get away from the original dogmas in time, the greater discrepancy is there between the founder and his followers.

On this basis, one might wonder what psychoanalysis will be like in the year 2000. In some form or another, it will indubitably remain as a field of theory and therapy, but certainly, from present indications, one may predict that it will diverge considerably from the Freudian structure. Already there are about as many diluted as undiluted Freudians, and in time, the proportions will be favoring the former group.

The name by which the group has been known unofficially is " neo-Freudians ", but this appellation does not seem quite appropriate, in view of the fact that some of the neo-Freudians died before Freud, and most of them have been contemporaries of Freud. The adjective " neo " would indicate a lapse of time between the old and the new. For this reason I have chosen the preposition *para* with the force of " derived

353

from " or " alongside of ", as in *paradox*, to designate the relationship, and shall, therefore, employ the term *para-Freudians* instead of neo-Freudians, which is commonly used.

The name, however, poses less of a problem than the placing of the individuals who come into that category. We might begin with Otto Rank whose relations with Freud were not strained to the point of bitter hostility as in the case of Jung and Adler. The work of Melanie Klein, in the early thirties, has been regarded as a dent which paved the way for the new *para-Freudian* wall, although F. Alexander, Karl Menninger, F. S. Perls, and many others have lent a hand. At another psychoanalytic wall, Erich Fromm, Karen Horney, and Wilhelm Reich have been busily engaged loosening the stones and replacing them by some of their own choice—and the new *motif* is character in a sociological setting, with stress on the ego. Rank, who belongs to an earlier period, represents the regressive tendency in that his principle ontogenetically antedates that of Freud.

Birth Trauma. Otto Rank, the last of Freud's meteors to break away from the Vienna firmament, built up a world outlook on the basis of the birth trauma, i.e., that the fantasies dealing with the original separation from the mother are at the root of all the later deviations on the part of an individual, whether neurotic or normal ; hence the analysis, in reality, consists in a re-enaction of the process of birth, so that the primal anxiety of the fetus turned into infant, at long last, is dissolved after a period of analysis of shorter duration than was wont to be the case. But Rank displays great enthusiasm and ambitions in other directions too.

Taking into consideration the importance of the birth trauma, a new theory of character and types may be found which has the advantage over existing attempts of this kind of giving a far-reaching understanding of the *individual* determinants and consequently the possibility of influencing them. . . .[1]

Rank throughout his book on the birth trauma (certainly not his best) is constantly lauding the great insight of Freud while steadily inching away from the original foundations. Naturally such lip service could not be long tolerated by the hierarch of the system. Rank's high opinion of his discovery, and still higher hopes he held out for it, will be evident from the following passage which contains the gist of his ambitious doctrine.

We believe that we have succeeded in recognizing all forms and symptoms of neurosis as expressions of a regression from the stage of sexual adjustment to the pre-natal primal state, or to the birth situation, which must be thereby overcome. For medical understanding and for therapeutic intervention this insight must by no means be underestimated, although in reference to the theory of neurosis it may have remained unsatisfying, in the meaning indicated above, since it traces what is specific in the case, or in the symptom formation, to something so universal as the birth trauma. On the other hand, within the birth trauma, there is room and to spare for hereditary influences of the germ plasm as also for incidental individual peculiarities of parturition. Nevertheless, our concept attempts to replace the theory of different places of fixation, which are supposed to determine the choice of neurosis, by *one* traumatic injury (producing various forms of reactions) in a single place of fixation, namely the mother (parturition). There is then, according to our view, only one fixation place, namely, the maternal body, and all symptoms ultimately relate to this primal fixation, which is given us in the psychobiological fact of our Unconscious. In this sense we

[1] O. Rank : *The Trauma of Birth*, 1929 (Kegan Paul), English trans., p. 209.

believe we have discovered in the trauma of birth the primal trauma. There is, therefore, no need to ascertain the " pathogenic traumata " in single cases by the lengthy way of analytic investigation, but only to recognize the specific birth trauma in reproduction, and demonstrate it to the patient's adult Ego as an infantile fixation.[1]

The trouble with such a theory is that it is so nebulous that any conjecture stands a better chance of accounting for neurosis and character. Its universality, viz., the fact that we were all born, experiencing a great shock as we passed from the shelter of the womb to the " hurly-burly " of a strange world, is all that can be said in favor of it, but by the same token, it is all so diffuse and vague and inscrutable that even the high-pressure salesmanship of its originator cannot make much of an appeal to scientists, although a number of American social workers seem to have been impressed, largely through personal influence.

Instead of pointing out the specific weaknesses in this hypothesis, let me quote an incisive piece of criticism directed at Rank.

" The fact that the human being shares the birth process with other mammals, whereas a particular disposition to neurosis is the special privilege which he alone possesses, hardly speaks very strongly in favor of the Rankian theory. The principal objection to be raised against it, however, remains the fact that it hangs in mid-air, instead of being based upon verified observation. For no trustworthy investigation has ever been carried out to determine whether difficult and protracted birth is correlated in indisputable fashion with the development of neurosis—indeed, whether children whose birth has been of this character manifest even the nervousness of earliest infancy for a longer period or more intensely than others. If the assertion is made that

[1] O. Rank : Loc. cit., pp. 210–211.

precipitate births, those easy for the mother, may possibly have for the child the significance of a severe trauma, then *a fortiori* it would certainly be necessary that births resulting in asphyxia should produce beyond any doubt the consequences alleged. It seems an advantage of the Rankian aetiology that it postulates a factor capable of being checked empirically ; but as long as such a check has never actually been undertaken, it is impossible to estimate its real value." [1]

Let us, however, not rest here and adduce another series of objections to the all-embracing theory of Rank, objections which, it must be said, cannot easily be pushed aside.

Critique of Birth Trauma. " The detailed criticism of Rank's thesis is not our task, but merely its examination from the standpoint of its serviceability in the solution of our problem. Rank's formula, that those persons become neurotic who on account of the severity of the birth trauma have never succeeded in abreacting it completely, is theoretically open to the greatest possible doubt. It is not entirely clear what is meant by the abreacting of the trauma. If it is taken literally, one arrives at the quite untenable conclusion that the neurotic approaches more and more closely to a state of health the more frequently and the more intensively he reproduces the affect of anxiety . . . The emphasis upon the varying severity of the birth trauma leaves no room for the legitimate aetiological claim of constitutional factors. This severity is an organic factor, certainly, one which compared with constitution is a chance factor, and is itself dependent upon many influences which are to be termed accidental, such as for example timely obstetrical assistance. But the Rankian theory has left constitutional as well as phylogenetic factors entirely out of account. If one were to allow for the importance of a constitutional factor, such as via the modification that it would depend much more upon how extensively the individual reacts to the variable severity of the birth trauma,

[1] S. Freud : *The Problem of Anxiety* (Eng. transl.), p. 96.

one would deprive the theory of meaning and have reduced the new factor which Rank has introduced to a subordinate rôle."

Here we have good reasoning, common sense, and balanced judgment. If the reader will be curious to know who this trenchant critic, this modern Daniel, is that seems to hit the nail on the head in the direct manner of a scientist familiar with the canons of methodology, it might as well be divulged that the man is no less than Freud, and it must be said that here he appears in a new light. He is no longer the speculator, the concatenator of questionable data and linguistic associations but a realist who, had he only applied the same method to his own arguments, would have probably found much to revise and discard in his own system.

It is especially noteworthy that Freud should reject the birth trauma, which was first intimated by him, on the score of heredity and constitutional differences—the very factors which he himself belittles in building up his own edifice ; but such is life. The cogency of Freud's arguments can scarcely be denied. If only they could be brought to bear on his own case !

Play Phantasy as Indicators of Character. Melanie Klein's method in providing games for her child analyses, and observing their acts in detail, questioning them as well, is close to the projective techniques in vogue at present. Much is claimed for this type of analysis. Thus she contends that " The reason why we can foretell from the character and development of play phantasies in children what their sexual life will be in later years is because the whole of their play and sublimations is based on masturbation phantasies and finding an outlet for them, it follows that the character of their play phantasies will indicate the character of their sexual life in adult years, and it also follows that child analysis is able not only to bring about a greater stability and capacity for sublimation in childhood but to ensure mental well-being and prospects of happiness in maturity." [1]

In Klein's experience, constitutional factors play an important part in deciding the nature of the reactions. By the time Erna was between two and three years old " her character was already abnormal ", and that is traced to (a) strong sadistic tendencies, (b) precocious development of the ego , and (c) premature activity of her genital impulses— all this coupled with the fact that she had witnessed the copulation of her parents when she was two and a-half and again when she was three and a-half years old. [2]

Resurgence of Value Problems. Klein, however, who was trained by Abraham and Ferenczi did not stray too far from home. It was the group of Reich, Fromm, and Horney that introduced the sociological, and even Marxist, ideology into psychoanalytic theory ; and the problem of values which had been in the background or perhaps entirely submerged had again come to the fore with Fromm. The *total personality* instead of the atomized complexes and mechanisms also becomes a phrase looming large in the activities of the para-Freudians. Perhaps there was an Adlerian influence commingled with the impact of the Gestalt movement which favored the synthetic approach. Franz Alexander was among the first Freudians to stress the total personality [3] and, furthermore, to give due consideration to the somatic counterparts of the psyche, which Freud hardly deigned to deal with. Alexander, also, as we have seen, did make an attempt to define character and to bring it in relation with the overwhelming business of therapy.

The rebels in this domain did not speak their mind until the last decade, even if Reich was slowly developing a system

---

[1] M. Klein : *The Psychoanalysis of Children*, 1937, English transl. (Hogarth), 2nd ed., p. 163.
[2] Loc. cit., p. 87.
[3] F. Alexander : *Psychoanalysis of the Total personality*, 1935.

of his own, which he calls " character analysis ", but which seems far removed from the anagogic slant implied in the treatment of values and conduct. Fromm's books take up the issue anew and in a direct manner.

Social Trends in Psychoanalysis. Erich Fromm, who stresses the social aspects of character, may be considered a cross between Freud and Adler. With the former, he finds the oral- and anal-component instincts at the root of character, but, and here he might be said to veer toward Adler—not before the individual has had enough social contacts, primarily through the family—the immediate representative of society. It is this contact in various relations which re-activates and sublimates the original impulses, so important in the young child's life. The nubbin of Fromm's character structuration is the feeling of aloneness which necessitates getting together with others, either in submission to the strong, or else in domination over the weak. The mechanism through which these escapes from loneliness are effected is that of masochism and sadism—the mainsprings of social organization. The feeling of aloneness is, to some extent, reminiscent of the inferiority feeling as expressed in the sense of insecurity.

If the boy experiences setbacks in his experiences with others and is not strong enough to cope with them, and is offered aid or sympathy by close relatives, as well as guidance, he will allow himself to be led, and the " oral " phantasies of being fed and cared for will be the symbolic expression of the original oral attitude of infancy. On the other hand, if the hostility, maladjustment, or reverses he experiences happen to come to a youth whose anal component serves to make him later the exclusive and defiant individual to the point of exuding hatred, he will seek to domineer others, terminate his " aloneness " by ingesting or incorporating others into his enlarged system, as witness the Nazi youth.

Fromm's sequence of events moulding the social character

reminds us of the Virginia reel or some other such dance, where each of the dancers locks arms successively with a different partner in a brief grand right and left whirl, except that the whirls here represent historical eras, economic stages, religious and ideological phases, with the generations figuring as the individual partners.

While I am prepared to concede that no individual character develops in a vacuum, it is my feeling that the historical, economic, religious, and political effects on the individual have been overestimated by the sociologist, and that character—if worthy of the name—is not moulded so much as it moulds itself. If we are to make an inventory of possible influences, we might include the climate, the spots on the sun, the tides, the season of birth, as, indeed, Ellsworth Huntington has done, perhaps even the thunderstorms one has been subjected to, and a host of other situations. Possibly they all contribute their mite, but we don't know how even to begin assessing the part they play in relation to other influences. The psychological approach within the normative framework, however, does present a definite picture of character, and it is well that at least in one respect Fromm's view comports with that set forth in this volume, viz., the rejection of sociological relativism. He is apparently willing to espouse the regulative principles, so misunderstood by my critics, as we shall see later, as " an inherent trend of human nature ".[1]

In a more recent volume, Fromm attacks the relativistic attitude of orthodox psychoanalysis in unmistakable language. " My experience as a practising psychoanalyst has confirmed my conviction that problems of ethics cannot be omitted from the study of personality, either theoretically or therapeutically. The value judgments we make determine our actions, and upon their validity rest our mental health and happiness. To consider evaluations only as so many rationalizations of unconscious, irrational desires—although

[1] E. Fromm : *Escape from Freedom*, New York (Rinehart), 1941, p. 288.

they can be that too—narrows down and distorts our picture of the total personality. Neurosis itself is, in the last analysis, a symptom of moral failure (although ' adjustment ' is by no means a symptom of moral achievement). In many instances a neurotic symptom is the specific expression of moral conflict, and the success of the therapeutic effort depends on the understanding and solution of the person's moral problem." [1]

With greater zest the polemic is pursued toward the end of the book, where the Freudians are referred to as " the realists " in ethics. The point of view expressed is obviously that of the present work, which psychoanalysts would look upon as naïve and superficial. " The ' realists ' assure us that the problem of ethics is a relic of the past," Fromm writes. " They tell us that psychological or sociological analysis shows that all values are only relative to a given culture. They propose that our personal and social future is guaranteed by our material effectiveness alone. But these " realists " are ignorant of some hard facts. They do not see that the emptiness and planlessness of individual life, that the lack of productiveness and the consequent lack of faith in oneself and in mankind, if prolonged, results in emotional and mental disturbances which would incapacitate man even for the achievement of his material aims." [2]

Looking Upward. To a certain extent, the para-Freudians, at least the most influential group, is inclined to the hormic, the anagogic interpretation of instincts and impulses. Hence, the purely genetic account of the libido in a mechanistic framework, on the basis of a repetitive principle, takes a subordinate place to the goal of the ego. In this respect, there is a resurgence of Adlerian motives in the direction of the total personality and its lack of security. We have seen that Fromm tends that way, and in this secession from the orthodox centre, he is effectively supported by Karen Horney whose

[1] E. Fromm : *Man for Himself*, 1947 (Reinhart), p. viii.
[2] Loc. cit., p. 249.

critique of Freudian tenets is forcefully set forth in several books, but principally in her *New Ways in Psychoanalysis.*

Like Adler, though without accepting certain of his premises, she stresses environmental factors. " Among the environmental factors, however, that which is more relevant to character formation is the kind of human relationship, in which a child grows up. Freud is almost wholly committed to the individual episodes which have taken place in the course of the child's instinctual development. It is apparently a question of libido *vs.* a sense of security which is ever threatened because of the basic anxiety of the child, or the infantile adult who has never grown up, stunted as he is by his repressed hostility which is projected into others and results in his neurosis."

Of greater relevance to our subject, however, is her stand on moral problems and value judgments, which are left severely alone in psychoanalysis. The analyst's imperturbable tolerance is regarded as one of the indispensable conditions which enable the patient to become aware of and eventually express repressed impulses and reactions. She questions seriously the possibility of such tolerance. Even the patient senses that this neutrality is pretense. " My own opinion," she avers, " is that an absence of value judgments belongs among those ideals we should try rather to overcome than to cultivate." And again, " Our knowledge of cause and effect in psychic ailments should not blind us to the fact that they do involve moral problems. . . . The moral problems are an integral part of the illness." [1]

That moral problems deal with the character of an individual requires no special pleading ; and furthermore, such character cannot be said to be the mere passive outcome of oral or anal libidinal impulses polarized into guilt feelings, while a helpless ego serves as the doormat upon which these mechanisms and

[1] K. Horney : *New Ways in Psychoanalysis*, 1939 (Norton), pp. 300, 301.

complexes fight it out ; and the sooner the Freudians revise the doctrine of libidinal development in the light of character exigencies, the more consonant will be their general position with contemporary findings and the requirements of methodology.

Horney, like Fromm, is not chary about introducing the issue of standards in psychoanalysis. In 1927, the present author called forth either a frown or an amused smile in some quarters when the same stand was taken. But let us follow Horney's argumentation on the subject.

> Another aspect of the imperative nature of these standards is what Freud calls their " ego-alien " character. What he means by this term is that the individual seems to have no say in the matter of the self-imposed rules : whether he likes them, whether he believes in their value, enters as little into the picture as his capacity to apply them with discrimination. They exist unquestioned, inexorable, and have to be obeyed. Any deviation from them has to be carefully justified in the individual's conscious mind, or it is followed by guilt feelings, inferiority feelings, or anxiety.

> An individual may be aware that compulsory moral goals exist, may say, for instance, that he is a " perfectionist ". Or he may not say so—because his very insistence on perfection will not allow him to admit any irrational drives for perfection—but may talk incessantly about how he should be able never to feel hurt, how he should be able to control every emotion or cope with every situation. Or he may be naively convinced that by temperament he is " good ", conscientious, rational. Finally, he may be entirely unaware of having any such goals, not to speak of their compulsory character. In short, the degree to which a person is aware of these standards varies.[1]

---

[1] K. Horney : *New Ways in Psychoanalysis*, 1939, pp. 208–9.

Character Analysis. A para-Freudian of a different color is W. Reich who has long specialized in what he calls " character analysis ", but it is not character in the common understanding of the term. Character seems to be an earmark in his nomenclature ; and the core is the trait of resistance, which is likened to armor. While Fromm and Horney veer toward the right—the anagogic or uplifting slope—Reich is definitely of the left wing, and would be classed with the catagogic or naturalistic therapists, giving rein to the libido ; in fact, his chief objective is to improve the psycho-sexual apparatus and establish orgastic potency, which, to Reich, is the " prerequisite of full functioning ". It is evident that Reich has built around the genitality views of Freud who, it will be recalled, made the full genital development of the libido the essence of a decent or normal character.

Reich seems to believe that he has commenced where Freud left off, viz., at the analysis of character, such as Reich conceives it. Hence his large volume, which consists of a series of monographs, is labelled *Character Analysis.* Chief stress with him is not so much the bringing to the fore, i.e., into the conscious, of unconscious elements, as the breaking down of resistances—the character armor—in a certain ordered course and thus liberating the functional segments which alone could lead to the stage of orgastic potency requisite for normal living on a social plane ; and that is the consummation of the genital character.

Reich operates with all the Freudian mechanisms, and some even of the rebellious offspring (Rank, and in a modified degree, Adler) but the *ex cathedra* pronouncements, the involved manipulations of the various mechanisms are somewhat subjective, even though the long experience of the analyst and his undoubted ability invest him with a considerable amount of authority. Reich, like most of the para-Freudians, only more so, is deeply concerned with the socio-economic world situation. " It goes without saying, that a thorough knowledge of the mechanisms which relate economic situation, instinctual life, character formation, and ideology would lead to many practical measures, particularly in education, possibly also in practical mass psychology." Although this declaration is part of the 1933 preface, Reich is still collectively-minded, whereas Freud was an individualist, despite his sociological digressions (taboo, origin of clan, religion, etc.). Nevertheless, the former attaches more importance to individual differences in working out the salvation of the patient, considering his or her needs— biological in the first place.

Apotheosis of the Libido. Aside from that, Reich posits a somatic system, which is more speculative than real. Freud had, as is well-known, almost ignored the physiological in his efforts to establish the independence of the psyche (both conscious and unconscious). Reich speaks of plasmatic currents, orgone systems, lumination (which is the peak of excitation in coitus). He even thinks that this orgone, which he claims to have discovered, is of a piece with the cosmic orgone function, and that is why the action cannot be described in language. In order not to run the risk of misinterpreting him, the passage following will serve as an *ipse dixit* affirmation.

At a certain point, the natural law of the non-living substance must of necessity penetrate the living and express itself in it. This cannot be otherwise if the living derived from the non-living and returns to it. While the organ sensations, which correspond specifically to the living, can be translated into word language, those expressive movements of the living which do not specifically belong to the living but which derive from the realm of the non-living, *cannot be put into word language.* Since the living derives from the non-living, and since non-living matter derives from cosmic energy, we must conclude that there are *cosmic energy functions in the living.* The non-translatable expressive movements of the orgasm reflex in the sexual superimposition could, therefore, represent the cosmic orgone function.[1]

Reich, red-blooded and " red "-indoctrinated though he appears to be, is not devoid of the mystical ; for he believes that the orgasm is a bit of pulsating nature lived by the experiencing individuals. " The mystical ideas of so many religions, the belief in a hereafter and in a transmigration of souls, all derive from cosmic longing, and cosmic longing is functionally anchored in the expressive movements of the orgasm reflex."

The Jelly-fish as our Goal. In view of this fact, that the liberation of the orgasm reflex, after the resistances which lead to sexual stasis have been broken down, represents the genital, i.e., the normal character, it is noteworthy that the author triumphantly points to the approximation, under the most favorable circumstances of orgastic function, to the jelly-fish in its movements. " The expressive movement of the orgasm reflex, then, represents a most important present-day mobilization of a biological form of movement which goes way back to the jelly-fish." In this he sees a demonstration of unity with the lower organisms. That may be so, but we had all thought that *character* is one function which is infinitely removed from the characteristic of the jelly-fish, as common parlance, to boot, proves. It only goes to show that terms are helpless. They can be employed to suit the particular fancy of the employer, reminding us of the lengthy discussion between two Oxford dons, when after hours of wrangling, one of the interlocutors exclaimed, " Well, then, as I see it, your God is my Devil."

[1] W. Reich : *Character Analysis*, 1949, p. 393.

CHAPTER XIX

COMPENSATION AS A FUNDAMENTAL MECHANISM IN PERSONALITY

There is no concept which has shown such a fundamental bearing on all problems connected with personality as *compensation*. Only recently has the mechanism of compensation been studied empirically, that is to say, from actual observations in specific cases ; and much of the attention which this mechanism has attracted is due to the rise of psychoanalysis. In fact, if we were to look for a bridge which connects the two related fields, psychoanalysis and orthodox psychiatry, we should very likely find it in the compensatory process.

Another feature of the doctrine of compensation is that it is employed, although in different applications, by all the psychoanalytic schools, by Jung, Stekel and Adler, no less than by Freud himself. For that reason alone the doctrine must carry a great deal of weight. In the face of so much controversy which is rife among the schools, the principle of compensation seems to have established itself as beyond question, and furthermore of all the mechanisms stressed by the Freudians and their kin, that of compensation not only falls in best with the accepted findings of psychology but lends itself most readily to physiological explanation.

Explains Contradictory Behavior. This mechanism, even if we cannot yet put our finger on its *modus operandi* so as to be able to control it, has shed much light on the apparently contradictory behavior of most individuals. It has proved an asset in accounting for inconsistencies which might otherwise be taken for capricious conduct, if not deliberate hypocrisy. Even sheer caprice, we understand now, has its laws—or, at any rate, its hidden meanings ; and a considerable part of the puzzling antics which neurotics go through in life can at least tentatively be credited to compensation. The tenderness which seeks to cover up a streak of cruelty ; the generous dispensation of sound advice which many miserly people are known for ; the awkward forwardness of embarrassed or shy individuals ; the extreme cordiality of those who are given to a domineering paternalism ; even the undue interest which physicists and astronomers take in spiritualism—these several instances may be regarded as manifestations of this subtle mechanism which eludes the discernment of even the most sagacious, serving the supreme biological purpose of self-preservation in our highly complex form of civilization with its refined struggle for existence.

But because of its subtlety, the mechanism is also a liability in that we never can tell beforehand in what shape it is likely to occur. Indeed, we cannot say with certainty that we have a case of compensation at any time. It is thus possible to invoke this principle *ad captandum* and go astray in our interpretation, as when psychoanalysts generally profess to detect a repressed wish of death in what they consider an exaggerated devotion between parent and child or man and wife, often expressing itself in a feeling of anxiety for the welfare of the loved one.

Principle Needs a Guide. Unfortunately the very concept of compensation points to a logical contrast, and we have no other guide before us than the association of ideas to put us on the track of a possible mechanism. Evidently every exaggeration is regarded as a ground for suspicion, but who is to be the judge in a given case ? How can we gauge exaggeration in our world of relative estimates ? Must we assume that one with an exaggerated avariciousness is *unconsciously* generous and harbors somewhere in his inmost mental recesses a repressed generosity ? This were charitable of course on our part, but we are not warranted in drawing this conclusion when we lack empirical evidence.

With this question, we are really opening up a new line of inquiry which, however, must be only touched on for the present. It is this : if compensation is a reciprocal process, then if cruelty is compensated for by an unlooked-for tender-ness, and stinginess is covered over by a surprising good-naturedness, why can we not reason conversely that overt cruelty is a symptom of inner gentleness, perhaps repressed, and that extreme niggardliness points to the unseen diamond of generosity lying about somewhere in the unconscious ? Does the answer lie in the fact that the unconscious, as Freud held in his earlier and more consistent stage, has no room except for the animal impulses, and therefore cannot harbor morally desirable wishes, or is it to be found in the explanation that the organism will not compensate except for its own benefit, and therefore since generosity and gentleness are not repre-hensible, they do not have to be covered up, but where they are so marked as to handicap the individual in life, they surely would be expected to call forth the compensatory tendency ?

To my mind, it is simply a question of what is primary in the make-up of the person, coupled with the further issue of what is most useful to the individual in his competition with others. One who is by nature cruel or selfish will be more apt to compensate in his course of social adaptation than he who is considerate or lavish by nature. No reference is here made to the occasional *deliberate* reversals in consequence of bitter experiences. We must remember that compensation is avowedly an unconscious or subconscious mechanism. Thus we may envisage compensation as a biological principle ; and if psychology is to be ruled by a strict determinism as laid down by Freud, we shall at least do well to discover the determining factors. The unconscious motives in themselves require some-thing to call them forth, and that is *biological necessity* in the broad sense, including social demands too, since the individual's welfare depends on his place in society.

EARLY EXPONENTS

The impression must not be gained that until the advent of psychoanalysis, compensation in human affairs was not known.

The doctrine of compensation has had its exponents long before psychoanalysis was ever dreamt of. Emerson's inspiring essay on compensation bears testimony to this foreshadowing. Our poet-philosopher long ago cited the finding of physiologists to the effect that " a surplusage given to one part is paid out of a reduction from another part of the same creature. If the head and neck are enlarged, the trunk and extremities are cut short ". Indeed, he has set up compensation as a cosmic principle, which procedure rather weakened his case, and bares the possibility of a slight confusion in his grasp of the concept. When Emerson points out that " every man in his life time needs to thank his faults ", e.g. " if he has a defect of temper which unfits him to live in society . . . he is driven to entertain himself alone, and acquire habits of self-help ", we may take it that the compensation is simply forced through sheer circumstances, but is not an innate endowment coincident in origin with his defect, as we should infer from the previous case cited.

Still more does he swerve from the first interpretation, and herein his mysticism becomes apparent, when he declares that " every sweet hath its sour ; every evil its good. . . For every grain of wit there is a grain of folly. For everything you gain, you lose something, and for everything you have missed, you have gained something else ". If the law holds universally in such an absolute sense, then this is true simply because of *the inherent nature of things but not for psychological or physiological reasons.*

Emerson does not appear to have been acquainted with the work of Azaïs, whose *Des compensations dans les destinées humaines*, written in the first decade of the nineteenth century, passed through several editions during the author's life-time. In this book which was supplemented by *Du sort de l'homme dans toutes les conditions*, where the principle of compensation was applied in explanation of the fate of the outstanding historical figures of the seventeenth and eighteenth centuries, the author gives himself the pains of proving, by reviewing diverse conditions of man, that the balance of human destinies is one of the principal effects of the very cause which produced the equilibrium of the universe. Let us not dwell on this pious lucubration of an optimist who taught that no one has anything to complain of, and wrote a whole volume on it, without stumbling on the question whether anyone, because of this very balance of pleasure and displeasure, has anything to be particularly grateful for. Compensation had become for this author a sort of *clavis universalis*, yet nowhere does this philosophical pedagogue indicate that he has grasped the mechanism of compensation except to intimate that it is in the nature of things that every advantage should have its disadvantage and vice versa.

COMPENSATION UNDERSTOOD BY BACON

More than three hundred years ago, Francis Bacon came nearer the psychoanalytic conception of compensation in the statement that defects are principally covered under three cloaks, viz., (1) caution, (2) pretext, and (3) assurance. In this passage the allusion to rationalization in connection with compensation is quite patent, but the difference between him and the Freud-Adler schools is that whereas they regard these processes and mechanisms as wholly unconscious, Bacon makes this tendency to conceal and rationalize a studied art, and indeed enjoins it upon his readers as a precept to follow in order to advance themselves in the world, as if his readers had not already practised this precept since childhood, whether they were aware of it or not.

The cautious man—Bacon tells us—does not meddle in matters to which he is unequal, while the daring and adventurous spirit proclaims his faults by busying himself with things of which he has no understanding. Pretext is employed, according to Bacon, when " a man with sagacity and prudence paves and prepares himself a way for securing a favorable and commodious interpretation of his vices and defects ; as proceeding from different principles, or having a different tendency than is generally thought. For as to the concealment of vices the poet said well, that vice often skulks on the verge of virtue. Therefore, when we find any defect in ourselves, we must endeavor to borrow the figure and pretext of the neighboring virtue, for a shelter ; thus the pretext of dullness is gravity ; that of indolence considerateness, etc. And it is of service to give out some probable reason for not exerting our utmost strength, and so make a necessity appear a virtue. Assurance, indeed, is a daring, but a very certain and effectual remedy, whereby a man professes himself absolutely to slight and despise those things he could not obtain, like crafty merchants, who usually raise the price of their own commodities and sink the price of other men's. Though there is another kind of assurance, more impudent than this, by which a man brazens out his own defects, and forces them upon others for excellencies ; and the better to secure this end, he will feign a distrust of himself in those things wherein he really excels : like poets, who, if you except to any particular verse in their composition, will presently tell you that single line cost them more pains than all the rest ".

But even the unconscious phase of compensation, as viewed from the angle of Adler's " individual psychology " has been fully recognized by Bacon as his essay on " Deformity " reveals.

" Deformed persons are commonly even with nature ; for as nature hath done ill by them, so do they by nature ;

being for the most part, as the Scripture saith, ' void of natural affection,'　and so they have their revenge of nature.　Certain there is a consent between the body and the mind, and where nature erreth in the one, she ventureth in the other. ' *Ubi peccat in uno, periclitatur in altero.*' " . . .

" Whosoever hath anything fixed in his person that doth induce contempt, hath also a perpetual spur in himself, to rescue and deliver himself from scorn : therefore all deformed persons are extreme bold.　First, as in their own defence, as being exposed to scorn ; but in process of time, by a general habit.　Also it stirreth in them industry, and especially of this kind, to watch and observe the weakness of others, that they may have somewhat to repay."

Kant on Compensation.　Nor has the principle of compensation escaped the perspicacious mind of the great Koenigsberger.　In a little-known work entitled *Beobachtungen über das Gefühl des Schönen und Erhabenen*, Kant, in a footnote,[1] gives us the following bit of racial psychology, which is all the more marvellous, coming as it does from one who never left his native town.

" It has otherwise been observed that the English, though a very sensible people, nevertheless are easily inveigled to give credence, at least at the beginning, to something wonderful and preposterous that is boldly announced, of which there are many instances.　But a daring mental disposition, prepared through various experiences in which many remarkable things had yet been proven true, readily breaks through the trifling scruples which soon put a damper on the weaker and more distrustful mind, thus at times, and without any merit of its own, guarding it against mistakes."

Genius as Compensated Degeneracy.　The most sensational claim made on behalf of compensation was contained in Lombroso's　much　disputed　theory　developed　in　his *Man of Genius*, for what other than a species of this protean

[1] I. Kant : *Gesammelte Werke* (Prussian Academy ed.), vol. ii, p. 250.

doctrine is the contention that the cultural giant invariably exhibits symptoms of an epileptoid form of degeneration ? In fact Adler may be said to have drawn on Lombroso's work when he regards degeneracy as due to a failure in compensation, and genius as the result of a successful compensation, while neurosis he considers the outcome of an oscillation between two extremes, so that the neurotic is always living in a sort of purgatory which prevents him from attaining the mark of genius and yet saves him from sinking to the lower depths.

This brief historical survey of the principle of compensation makes it at once clear that such a doctrine was not necessarily bound up with mysticism, but was in keeping with the demands of sound observation. A long list of brilliant names, both in literature and philosophy, could be linked with this significant concept. Nevertheless there is no denying that Freud, Jung and Adler, though each has applied the concept to suit his own special system, have done much to firmly intrench the principle of compensation in a scientific foundation. Much that is obscure in one's behavior may be explained by this mechanism, *provided* the facts are sufficiently known and the interpreter has no " axe to grind ", and is above all blessed with a judicious mind.

But the psychoanalytic theory of compensation in general is not attached to any physiological mechanism.[1] We are led to believe that one phenomenon is due to some latent fact because there seems to be some connection, often only a logical connection—as that of contrast—between the two points at issue. The theoretical basis of compensation is yet to be justified. For this reason Anton's doctrine of compensation may be looked upon as an improvement on the psychoanalytic version at least in a limited sphere.

---

[1] Adler's compensation theory presumes to be physiological, even to the extent of throwing much of the weight on the peripheral organs, but his thesis is declaratory rather than explanatory.

PHYSIOLOGICAL THEORY OF COMPENSATION IN NERVOUS DISORDERS

Anton's starting-point is the reflection that in the struggle between the organism and the oncoming disorder, whether it be physical or mental, there are three stages : (a) the reaction of the organism by means of general symptoms, (b) the tendency of the organism to localize the trouble or to delimit its intensity, (c) in case the effort is unsuccessful and the organism is overcome, the general symptoms break out anew with increased intensity.

Anton's Explanation. What has happened ? It is inferred that two antagonistic forces are at work in situations of this kind. The one is a " restricting process " (*Eindämmungsprozess*) and the other a " compensatory tendency ". Whenever a cerebral function is impaired, there is a redistribution of function among the different components of the brain, so that there is actually a deviation from the normal operations of the cerebrum which now assumes a changed form.[1] This virtually means that a new brain type has been created. It stands to reason that such compensation can take place only at the expense of other parts of the brain with a lowering of resistance as its consequence. Excitability, fatigue, anxiety, and other like conditions follow in its wake. The re-cast brain,

[1] The whole theory as developed by Anton and Gross harmonizes well with McDougall's notion of " *vicarious* usage of freed nervous energy " with its accessory hypothesis of a common reservoir of freed energy and the further corollary that inhibition comes about through the drainage of energy from one point in the nervous system to another. The picture of the sluice-gate swinging open and allowing the dammed-up energy in the nervous system not only to flow freely through the efferent channels but to overflow even in subsidiary acquired channels may well be brought to mind in order to illuminate the Anton-Gross theory of restricting and compensatory antagonistic processes in the maladjusted nervous system. McDougall's view on vicarious usage and the integrative working of the nervous system as regards the liberation and distribution of nerve energy is set forth in several places but principally in his " Sources and Direction of Psycho-physical Energy," *American Journal of Insanity*, 1913, vol. lxix.

in order to adapt itself to the new duties, must call on reserve energy which it is forced to consume at a rapid rate, and in excess of the original appropriation, thus adding to the extent of the disorder, and often actually leading to cortical lesion. The "restricting process" exercises a selective influence on the new equilibrium, due to the compensatory tendencies, and differentiates certain specific symptoms. At this stage, the general miscellaneous symptoms are not in evidence, at least not until a new state of equilibrium is achieved through the compensatory process.

Compensation as Psychical Transplantation. Anton builds on a solid foundation. He cites profusely the work of neurologists which bears on the facts of compensation. Here are passed in review the experimental researches of Hitzig, Ewald, Gudden, Luciani, Dohrn, Russell and Sherrington. After all it is only one step forward from the neurological in surgery to the psychological. We know of the wonders of organ transplantation. Why not take it for granted that there is such a thing as *psychical transplantation* ? And that is indeed what Anton purposes showing, viz., that these transplantations take place in the personality sphere of individuals. The cowardice of neurotics, he believes, has its root in a defence mechanism.[1] Often neurotics are very irritable, but to prevent themselves from blazing up when provoked, they lapse into an attitude of apathy and become *blasé*. Hysteria is a sample of overcompensation in the sense that the effect of deep grief is forestalled by laughing spells.[2]

Instead of dealing with Anton alone in this brief exposition, it would be better to present a composite sketch of his doctrine

---

[1] G. Anton : "Über den Wiederersatz der Funktion bei Erkrankungen des Gehirnes," *Monatsschrift für Psychiatrie und Neurol.*, 1906, vol. xix. Gross slightly misquotes the title (" Grosshirnes " instead of " Gehirnes ").

[2] Wm. McDougall's theory of laughter may easily be looked upon as a piece of supporting evidence in this connection. Cf. his *Outline of Psychology*, pp. 165 ff.

of compensation as elaborated by his pupil Gross, since the latter provides it with a background and perspective which are not discoverable in the article cited, but which may have been suggested in the lecture room or through personal contact with his teacher. This synthetic view is more closely knit, even if it is not clear as to how much of it is grafted on to Anton's thesis.

SYNTHETIC TREATMENT BY GROSS

It is this theme of Anton's which his pupil Gross elaborates, intermingling it with the " sejunction " note of Wernicke and the powerful strain of the psychoanalytic band. Through the whole structure withal, there penetrates the *motif* of the primary and secondary functions, which, as we have seen in Chapter XIV, constitutes the key to the understanding of the main personality types.

Relation of Mental Breadth to Depth. The difference between the primary and the secondary functioning as conceived by Gross need not be gone into again except to say by way of a reminder that the latter is associated with a narrowed and deepened consciousness, whereas the former gives rise to the shallow and broad consciousness. What determines the depth or breadth of the mind? Gross holds that the number of *materially different thought items* which a mind can exploit in a given period of time marks its *breadth* ; its *depth* is constituted by the number of associations bearing on the same topic which can be exploited by consciousness in the same period of time.[1]   The greater the secondary function in a person, the deeper and more concentrated the mind, which is in all such cases characterized by a *contractive* force.

Individuals with a reduced secondary function exhibit a flattened consciousness. Their associations are diffuse. They

---

[1] O. Gross : *Über psychopáthische Minderwertigkeiten*, p. 29 ; also in his *Die Zerebrale Sekundärfunktion*, loc. cit.

lack the persistence to follow to its consequences a given trend of thought. When this condition is inherent from birth, we have the " hypomanic " or " sanguine " inferiority, which Gross prefers to designate as an " inferiority with flattened consciousness ". The incapacity to deliberate and to assign proper values to important particulars gives rise to that state which Gross calls affective uncriticalness (*Kritiklosigkeit*). Such patients are unable to unify their thoughts, to subsume the details under some plan. Yet on account of the ready flow of disparate associations and the quick reaction to their immediate environment, they are always at ease and because of their being continually under the sway of the primary function, they are bothered little by inhibitions (which involve as a rule a harking back to former ideas) and are therefore known for their presence of mind and daring.

Levelling of Ideas a Species of Compensation. Furthermore, the inability to cope with complexities of thought, the rapid succession of unrelated associations, the lack of insight and the uninhibited response to external stimuli all make for that state which Wernicke called the " levelling of ideas ". In the inferior with flattened consciousness, the tempo of the ideational flow is too undifferentiated to allow for the assignment of values to particular ideas. The result is an affective " equivaluation " of all groups of ideas, which is virtually an undervaluation of the more important ones. It is out of this class that the " moral insane " are recruited.

In the disposition of the secondary function which is the basis of those with the contracted consciousness, the processes take the opposite direction. Here it will be remembered, the associations all drift into one main current, perhaps with related outlets. Disparate spheres of ideas, especially if the intensity and the duration of the constricted force exceed the normal limit, do not fit into the family compact of ideas and form a group by themselves, hanging but loosely together. Thus this dissociated constellation produces a state of *sejunction* which manifests itself in the disharmonic personality type. The psychopathic person with contracted consciousness also displays the dominant stigma of inferiority, viz., affective uncriticalness, but it takes its origin in different conditions. The false evaluation of ideas in this case arises from the fact that in spite of the unity and persistence of thought, there is no opportunity *for comparison with other trends*, since by hypothesis, the individual with sejunctive formations (due to a highly constricted consciousness, which in its turn is the result of an intense and lingering secondary function) cannot dovetail the various materially different associations into his main theme, where particular moments are overcharged with an affective glow. Instead of the " levelling of ideas " and the relative undervaluation on the part of the inferior individual with flattened consciousness, we have " profoundness " and overvaluation going with the individual of excessive constriction.

I must not allow myself to dwell at greater length on Gross's conclusions which are replete with pregnant possibilities, but one instance of the application of his far-reaching doctrine will be in order.

Application to Cynicism. Cynicism is regarded by this author as the establishment of close associations between the attractive and the repulsive, a tendency which finds expression (and here Gross follows Freud and Stekel) in the infant's coprophiletic activities. The smutty joke is an example of the same phenomenon at a higher stage. The person with the primary function dominant can easily make the transition from the attractive to the repulsive, but he who is under the sway of the secondary function will find the process painful ; for the erotic associations will release one group of impulses, while the repulsive associations will set into play a defensive, and therefore an entirely different, group of tendencies, but the psychic mechanism of such an individual is, as we have seen, not able to effect this rapid adjustment. Hence the tendency toward cynicism is only rarely to be found among those with constricted consciousness but frequently with persons of flattened consciousness.

Biological Foundation of Theory. We may doubt whether Gross has really solved the problems which he has brought up, but in this respect he at least excels the Freudians ; his closely thought out theory rests primarily on a physiological basis and is moreover biologically grounded, e.g. when he attempts to show that through social conditions, the originally abnormal type of woman, helpless and inadequate to supply her own needs, has in the course of ages become the universally sought wife, and therefore the normal type, and perpetuated through natural selection, once social selection (on the part of men) has initiated this downward move.[1]

Finally, it may be added that Gross is with Lombroso inclined to consider every variation from the normal as a sign of incipient degeneracy. This applies also to our two extreme types, the inferior with an over-shallow consciousness and the inferior with an over-contracted consciousness. The former, however, is the relic of a *bygone* utility, while the latter is in embryo a *new* utility type, pointing to a new form of civilization. Both are at the mercy of the two opposing forces ; natural selection and social cultivation ; and their survival will depend on their capacity to help in the remoulding of the new form by contributing the raw material.

Compensation not a Cosmic but a Physiological Mechanism. It is a mark of scientific progress that the concept of compensation, as we understand it to-day, has a definite locus and has been transferred from the immeasurable expanse of cosmic vagueness to the plane of physiological and psychological observations of the behavior mechanism. The defect

[1] O. Gross : Loc. cit., p. 117 ff. Of course the author does not seem to realize that the social conditions, the preference for the psychically inferior, may also be regarded as a trick of natural selection ; otherwise how explain the universal craving of the male for the unserviceable female in the first place ?

of a system like that of Azaïs and Emerson is the *failure to differentiate individuals*, the deliberate effort to deal with cut-and-dried conditions. Contemporary psychology recognizes that compensation is a function of the individual's particular make-up and will therefore manifest itself differently in different individuals, though the circumstances be the same.

CHAPTER XX

Varieties of the New Movement. In the last decade or so, a number of German schools, under the sway of the *Geisteswissenschaften* (cultural sciences) have been' making steady advances toward one another until they consolidated into the *Struktur* movement that is at present rocking German thought and carrying away with it the *débris* of a once iron-clad systematic psychology, which,, however, is fortunately building up anew under more favourable auspices.

The vanguard of the *Struktur* movement does not form an even line ; for on the right there is the tendency to follow the lead of philosophy, as developed by Dilthey and Simmel, while on the left wing the ranks are cautioned by the experimental lieutenants of the *Gestalt* school to tread forcibly but circumspectly. The genetic school (*Entwicklungspsychologie*) of Krueger, and the structuralists proper, form the centre of the line. But perhaps it would be better to treat the allied schools of the movement as concentric rings with that of the *Geisteswissenschaften* as the most inclusive yet at the same time least distinctly outlined circle. The *Struktur* school constitutes the nucleus of the whole organization, and although we must not confuse the issues of these various schools, there is no reason why the several concentric groups cannot be treated together on the basis that the difference is more in the selection and concentration of the subject-matter rather than· one of method or fundamental presuppositions. While realizing, therefore, that the main discussion in this chapter concerns only remotely the more restricted *Gestalt* school, we may gather from intimations, such as Koffka s allusion [1] to some lectures on personality by Wertheimer, one of the leaders of the *Gestalt* psychology, that not all its representatives share the circumscribed view that we must preëmpt the problem of perception in all its diversified phases before we can venture forth on any other task.[2]

Earmarks of " Struktur " Psychology. What characterizes the *Struktur* psychology, which, as is well-known, should not be mistaken for structural psychology in contrast with the functional kind, may be regarded as the reaction against the older division of mind into elements, such as sensations, images, and feelings. It is the conviction of the new structuralists that, even assuming that such elements are entities and not mere fictions in mental life, then unless we have a key to the organization, in the form of a *meaning* (*Sinn*) for the relationship between each of the parts and the whole, we have made no step forward in our investigation,

---

[1] K. Koffka, " Psychical and Physical Structures " : *Psyche*, 1924, vol. v, p. 84.

[2] This is by no means intended to ignore the desultory studies undertaken from the *Gestalt* angle on memory, aphasia, paranoia, and the notable work of Koffka and Köhler on learning, but with the exception of the paper on paranoia there is little bearing on the problems of personality, will, affection, or temperament. Even in the section on character and personality in R. M. Ogden's *Psychology and Education* (1926) there is nothing to show that the *Gestalt* psychology has an independent approach to the problem. There is nothing said under that head which might not have been said in the same words by the traditional psychologist. This applies to the striking observation borrowed from H. Schulte (" Versuch einer Theorie der paranoischen Eigenbeziehung und Wahnbildung ": *Psychol. Forschung*, 1924, vol. v) that the symptoms of paranoia are often induced by lack of participation in social activities. The thought itself lends colouring to the *Gestalt* picture and is suggestive, but anyone with a strong leaning toward the social interpretation of the individual (Baldwin, for instance) might have given utterance to the belief that in the degree in which man " fails to enter into sympathetic contact with his fellows, he becomes suspicious ; and suspicion leads him to believe that others are conspiring against him ".

just as if we were to try to make out the behaviour of a
certain organism by examining its organs when dead.

The principal feature of the *Struktur* school, whether it
approaches the study of perception, after the fashion of the
Gestalt group, or dwells on the problem of personality, the
pièce de résistance of the movement consists in the emphasis
it lays on the complex as a totality. The parts or elements
receive their proper attention and evaluation only in the light
of the whole. For our present purpose, I think, we need not
consider the important difference between the *Gestalt* theory
and the allied *Struktur* doctrines, which, according to Koffka,
consists in the separation of mind and body in the latter,
while his own school regards personality as a natural
phenomenon, not a mental or spiritual fact.

It is highly significant that even *Gestalt* psychology,
which is a strictly experimental movement, must make
room for an artistic and intuitive current in the treatment
of personality. And this streak is especially noticeable in
the writings of the *Struktur* psychologists. The psychographic methods of William Stern are pushed into the background to allow for a life *cliché* as taught by Dilthey and
Spranger, whose philosophy concerns itself with the pulse of
life, not with congealed elements.

In contrast with the various analytic personality
investigators, Spranger in his *Lebensformen* and William
Stern in his *Die menschliche Persönlichkeit* set out to look
for a form of structure which would polarize a personality,
setting it off as a distinct entity. And it is noteworthy that,
at the risk of injecting metaphysics or even mysticism into
psychology, they and others of the school tend to recognize
the uniqueness attaching to personality in its value aspect.
As Erich Stern, one of the younger representatives of this
wider school, states it, " In what a man sees value, especially
in what he sees the highest value of his life, that value, in
fact, which makes life important to him, that is what we must

know, if we are to be capable of understanding his personality." [1]

Spokesman of the "Geisteswissenschaftliche Psychologie". Since Eduard Spranger is at present looked upon as the mouthpiece of the *Geisteswissenschaftliche* Psychology, we shall do well to become acquainted with the chief thesis of his *Lebensformen*. In this work, which has seen a fifth edition in a few years, the methodological procedure centres about the effort to establish fundamental types of individuality which might be recognized in a scheme of values.

It would not be possible to follow in all its intricate by-ways Spranger's carefully and lucidly worked out plan ; the upshot, at any rate, is that there are primarily four life-forms : the economic, the theoretical, the artistic and the religious, with two additional types in view of the social nature, of man—the social and the political. A Robinson Crusoe, argues the author, would have to recognize economic values ; he would be bound to reflect and to receive aesthetic impressions ; his awe-experience of a world course could hardly be denied him, but, concludes Spranger, perhaps with slight justification, he could neither love nor rule.[2] The two subsequent forms then are grounded in society, which invests the individual with the *power of love* and the *love of power*.[3]

The Six Forms of Life. We may consider, then, every individual as dominated by one or the other of these formal (*ideal*) types of value so that while a Kant is contemplative in all his being, Napoleon is the *Machtmensch* who lives for power only. Spranger is so positive in his antithesis between the two, *ab origine*, that he unhesitatingly declares " *Der Wissende im höchsten Sinne jedoch ist niemals der Handelnde* "

---

[1] E. Stern, " New Ways of Investigating the Problem of Personality " : *Psyche*, 1923, vol. iii (New Series), p. 364.

[2] E. Spranger, *Lebensformen*, 1925, 5th ed., p. 35.

[3] Loc. cit., p. 66.

(The man of knowledge in the highest sense, nevertheless is never the man of action).[1] Yet every individual not only has his dominant life-form, but also the other five forms as subordinate functions. The whole gamut is there only in a different modulation, determined by the particular clef. Or to take another simple analogy, which Spranger is not to be held responsible for, we may regard the different life-forms as a series of costumes taking on different colours according to the light that is thrown on them. The contemplative man will not lack the will to power but it will spend itself in theoretical polemic. He might possibly experience the urge to engage in affairs of the hour, but he will remain content in the feeling that he could attain power in the practical world if he only so desired. Again in religion, he will not resemble the man whose dominant interest in life is religion, but he will not totally lack the religious vein, which will find its outlet in an *amor intellectualis dei*, Aesthetically, the reflective man may be on a lower plane than the artist, but even here he will seek the beautiful perhaps in the forms of geometry or the uniformity of nature. Thus every life-form creates its own set of relationships. In matters of politics, the intellectual inclines toward radicalism or at least liberalism, while the man of action leans more toward conservatism.

Greater Specificity. But Spranger does not rest here. He speaks of further subdivisions of the life-forms according to the factors by which they are determined. The theoretical man may further be distinguished as an empiricist, an intellectualist, or, again, as a criticist. There are people who can encompass only inductive cases. They have no faculty for recognizing principles or laws to embrace the cases. In opposition to these there are individuals who adhere to rigid categories and become nonplussed when they cannot fit a given fact into the framework of their life theories

[1] *Loc. cit.*, p. 133.

and prejudices. It is rare to find him who can combine the perceptual and the conceptual so as to reach a *critical* conclusion.

Other subdivisions and dichotomies are undertaken, but these are all trite, even when we are reminded that a certain type of atheist may be regarded as most religious or that systematic scepticism is to be thought of as the purest manifestation of the theoretical individual.

Complex Types. In addition we are introduced to the complex forms of life, such as combinations of the economic and the theoretical or the aesthetic and the religious, as also of such derived types as technology, which usually though not invariably is in the service of the useful; law, which is an auxiliary to politics; and pedagogy, which is grounded in love and subserves the social end. Finally, toward the end of the book, Spranger does justice to the influence of the milieu in a chapter on historically conditioned types. No stone is left unturned in order to bring out the complicated ramification among the different types from the various angles of value.

Ethical Value Dominated by Chief Life-Form. That Spranger should have in his system of types omitted the ethical life-form strikes one as strange at the outset, but it is not long before we are enlightened on this point with the remark that there is no one system of ethics which could be regarded as a distinct life-form or function, as a specific value reference. Every particular life-form has its own one-sided, ethical ideal. The economic man favours utilitarianism; the theoretical life-form corresponds to the ethics of uniformity and principle. The Greek ideal of harmony with emphasis on the Golden Mean is embodied in the artistic or aesthetic character-type. Love of one's fellow-men is the ethical code of the social life-form, while the will " to power " represents the morality of the *Machtmensch*. Finally, the highest expression of ethical value, that which contains its essence, is to be found in the religious conception. This approach aims at nothing but bliss or beatitude which may be attained in one of two ways, either through affirmation of all positive life-values (expansive) or in renouncing them (reclusive). Indeed, all ethics partakes of both tendencies : the injunctive and the prohibitive.

Ranking of Values in Life-Forms. If we followed Spranger up to this point only, an important objection would naturally occur to us on the ground that the author is judging in terms of interests rather than on the basis of values. Value implies linear measurement. But the artistic form of personality is certainly on a par with the theoretical or the religious type. The forms are not commensurate ; and one form is just as valuable as any other in the scheme. Now, what affords to value its distinctive mark is the possibility of appraisal and contrast which it carries with it. In this case then the term *value* which is to serve as the touchstone, if not the dowsing rod, of personality, may be regarded as a misnomer. The question then reduces itself to this : Can we discover uniqueness by collating a number of interests and colligating them under some predominant bent of mind ?

As a matter of fact such was the criticism which appeared in my paper on *Character and Inhibition*,[1] where the discussion of Spranger's views is based on the original essay. But the latter has dealt with this question at length in his expanded work, arranging the several life-forms in hierarchical order. What determines their ranks in this system is their claim to objectivity and remoteness from material, temporal, or spatial (sensory and imaginal) attachments. With this for our criterion, we can easily surmise that the economic life-form, although the most urgent, would remain at the bottom while the religious type would top the list. Between these extremes may be placed, next to the economic form, the aesthetic type which is still moored to a world of sense

---

[1] A. A. Roback, *Problems of Personality*, 1925, p. 115.

and imagination, and the contemplative or theoretical ideal, since science converts the material into conceptions ; but it is difficult to assign a higher place to the one or the other ; rather are they to be envisaged as the feminine and masculine poles of the same type of value.   On the next plane, where the egocentric gives way to the social viewpoint, we have a similar polarity in the case of the social and the political life-forms, which approach the religious value-type only as they are removed from the utilitarian considerations of quantity and number, and are bound up with the more abstract idea of an *esprit de corps* (" *Kollektivmacht* ", " *Soziale Geist* ").

We have now come to the end of the brief exposition of Spranger's penetrating work which is replete with ingenious turns.   The religious or, at any rate, metaphysical direction of the reasoning is readily sensed, but far be it from us to condemn his system on that account.   Even if it is not always that he succeeds with his *constatations*, his methodical procedure compels our attention, and after we have pondered the question of fundamental types, we shall probably be impressed with the logic of his position.   Without attempting the onerous task of pointing out minor inadequacies or inconsistencies in a work of such scope and so rich in detail, I shall signify my willingness to accept Spranger's categories of personality after supplying them with a *genetic* foundation and a *dynamic* character.

Inadequacy of Spranger's Position.   Spranger's deduction of his fundamental life-forms rests on the differentiation of the mental acts (not in the sense of processes) or performances peculiar to man.   Whatever we do after a purposive fashion falls into one or another of these classes, but this sort of deduction lacks the apodeictic attribute because, excepting the case of the economic category, there is nothing to show the necessary connection between the constitution of man and the particular life-form.   The method which I should call *historical empiricism* is invoked to establish the primacy of the proposed system of life-forms, but we may conceive of an era in which the values will have an entirely different setting and significance.

Another reason why Spranger's life-forms are not identifiable with characters is the *static* treatment of the former. A life-form, as Spranger sees it, refers rather to what an individual is than to what he *does or can do*. There is a kind of fatality about the *Lebensform*, such as is not ascribable to character. It is true that our author evaluates the life-form just as we should appraise characters, but does this not hold also of our attitude toward different levels and varieties of intelligence? Do we not say that the bright boy ranks above the stupid and do we not admire talent and range abstract above mechanical intelligence? The question is not whether the person whose dominant interest is economic should be despised, but whether a man, born with such and such dispositions, on curbing them when brought face to face with an environment which calls them forth, should not be adjudged superior in that respect to one who has not given evidence of the same behaviour.

Supplying a Bio-Genetic Foundation for the Prime Life-Forms. There is, nevertheless, something glowingly familiar about the forms which Spranger has so minutely described, something which bids us take account of the logical *motif* that has selected these and only these out of numerous possibilities. It is as if we were beginning to recognize in the faces of adults before us the features of the sturdy youngsters we knew in our childhood days. Will it seem surprising then if we acknowledge at least a partial identity between the respectable life-forms and the unpolished instincts out of which they were hewn? Let us accept Spranger's prime forms or types of value and proceed to deduce them not transcendentally but from ·below, from their very mechanisms which are co-existent with our being, viz., the instincts.

Life-Forms Traced to Instincts. What did the economic viewpoint evolve from, if not from the need of food ? And is not the *Machtmensch*, the powerful politician, an embodiment of the instinct of pugnacity or combativeness, if not of self-assertion ? As to the contemplative man, the scientist and philosopher, we may recall that Aristotle said in his *Meta-physics* : " It was owing to wonder that men began to philosophize in earlier times just as it is to-day, wondering at first about the problems that lie close at hand, and then little by little advancing to the greater perplexities. . ." Nor is it difficult to appreciate that the underlying foundation of religion is fear in its derived and cultural stages (awe, reverence). The social life-form clearly corresponds to the gregarious instinct, but since Spranger makes out love to be the keynote of this form, we have ample provision for this in our instinctive make-up, without even requiring to introduce the tendency of sympathy at this point. There is left then the aesthetic value-type or life-form which at first blush seems to elude our method, but Spranger himself more than once in his book shows the connection between the artistic and the erotic impulses in man. " Humanity as an aesthetic life-form realizes itself only in eroticism," is the conclusion in one place.[1] Elsewhere he writes, " The prototype of the beautiful is for us the human— the human body, the human soul : for the man, the ' eternally feminine ' . . ." [2] Certainly the erotic and the sexual are not necessarily to be identified, but the distance is so close that the course of the evolution is patent. Other original tendencies may be resorted to in order to trace the origin of the artistic impulse, play for instance ; but since Spranger himself seems to favour the connection between the

[1] Loc. cit., p. 177.
[2] Loc. cit., p. 187.

erotic and the artistic, we may just as well accept the suggestion.[1]

Ethical System as Life-Form. I doubt whether Spranger is justified in referring the ethical life-form to a separate domain, for if the type of ethical reaction will be governed by the dominant life-form, so that the economic man will be utilitarian, the theorist inclined to the ethics of principle and the politician swayed by the right of might, etc., the same modulation holds for every other life-form. Thus religion for the artist and religion for the tyrant will mean two different things ; and their reactions in other value-planes will disclose similar variations.

For my part, I should assign an equally important place to the ethical system of values, and would look for the instinctive basis in sympathy and the consistency urge which I explain elsewhere in this book.[2] Morality of the conventional and unreflective kind is grounded in sympathy, but the life of the man of character who radiates acts which are almost of necessity ethical has passed through the sympathy stage on to the rational stem of consistency which has grown out of the original root as a result of the assimilation of ideas. Just as friendship is constituted by an intellectual core built upon an instinctive foundation, so the consistency urge is a rational outgrowth of the blind general tendency of sympathy.

My aim has not been to institute a strict parallelism between Spranger's life-forms and the instincts, but merely to indicate that granting the validity of his fundamental types of personalities, their basis is still to be sought in the instincts, the most important of which are at the bottom of his six forms. The instinct of self-preservation does not appear

---

[1] The fundamental difference between the theoretical man and the artist lies for Spranger in the fact that the one always considers everything as part of a system, while the other cuts out a slice of reality and contemplates it as if nothing else existed with which to connect it.

[2] See Chapter XXVIII.

as such in any of the enumerated forms ; as a matter of fact it is involved in several of the instincts, in flight and food-seeking at any rate, but there is no concrete manifestation of this inferred instinct apart from the tendencies which are directed toward and away from a given stimulus. It may also be associated with the mooted vitalic life-form which Spranger, at the instance of Scheler,[1] is inclined to adopt. As a life-form it would include the physical and vital (health, energy), but not necessarily the sensuous experiences of man, and might easily be interwoven with the higher forms of life.

The spirit of Spranger's school has made itself felt not only in his own and allied circles, but has independently registered its influence in more foreign quarters. Thus we find Th. Lessing inveighing against all descriptive methods in vogue for the study of character, and after enumerating the many different approaches to this field that to him are fatuous, he introduces the rather obscure concept of *Ahmung*,[2] with its sub-varieties, by way of a solution.

The more philosophical discussions of Jaspers, Pfänder, Häberlin, and particularly Max Scheler show points of contact with the *Struktur* doctrine, in that the interpretative note is underscored, but, since they have taken up positions on a plane where there is less resistance to their speculation than in the case of Spranger, we shall have to reserve the brief exposition of these writers' main ideas for another chapter.

Transparency. Let us not suppose that the interpretative and structural view of characterology is confined to the experts in the philosophical and psychological disciplines who have discarded the experimental bias. The identical word " transparency " which is made so much of in the technical articles by Lessing, constitutes the title of a vivaciously written essay in a popular magazine where the

---

[1] References to Scheler's work will be found in Chapter XXI.
[2] For the discussion on this view see Chapter XXI.

same thesis is put forth as is to be found in the writings of the *Geisteswissenschaften* schools.   People are transparent, claims Sarton, and he explains his meaning in this fashion :

Thus when I am talking with people, I hear at once two voices : the material voice uttering the symbolic sounds of the language which happens to be the vehicle of our thoughts—and another voice, immaterial and undefinable but, if you hear it at all, far more distinct and, to be sure, more trustworthy. And for all the world, these two voices may contradict one another ! For example, one speaks to me eloquently of his disinterestedness.   It is a mania with him : his words always are sweet and generous, yet I descry his ugly, selfish soul none the less.   Another called upon me and talked business and money all the time. He is very poor and as he has not the knack of making his great talent profit himself, he finds it very hard to solve the practical problems of life.   ' How much would the editor pay him ?   Was such a contract fair to him ? ' A stranger might have thought that he had no other interest in his work, but his soul belied his every word.   Any shrewd business man must see that as clearly as I did, and it would be easy enough for him to let my friend *talk* business, and at the same time to take full advantage of his complete lack of business instinct, to leave him with all the dream and the glory, and run away with most of the ' substantific marrow '.   This other man, dressed like a mendicant, speaks of humility and seems to enjoy his self-abasement.   Yet his immoderate pride is shining through every hole of his garment. . .

" ' Of all unfortunates,' remarked Stevenson, ' there is one creature conspicuous in misfortune.   This is he who has forfeited his birthright of expression, who has cultivated artful intonations, who has taught his face tricks like a pet monkey.'   But even this wretch of a snob is not as depersonalized as he seems. Hard as he may try to make others and himself believe that he is something different from what he really is, the snob is not less transparent for that. Once his snobbery has been pierced through, he is as unable to hide his real self as any professional actor. He may pose as an artist, but he will only succeed in proving to the real ones that he is not one of them ; he may impersonate any hero, but somehow the stuff he is built of will always show through.

" I never cease to admire the indelibility of human nature. It does not wear off. Whatever they may do, men are and remain what they are. They may deceive themselves ; they may deceive others, especially the short-sighted ones, those who cannot look from the proper distance. Thus the surface of the sea seems quite dark when you are very near to it, but if you climb into the crow's nest, you will see how clear the water is ; and the higher you go the deeper you see." [1]

No further explanation is given of the concept of transparency, and it would seem that this property, far from inhering in the object judged, rather is a quality attaching to the person making the estimate.

Since Lessing has made use of the same term, attempting to explain it at least through analogies, we may do well to pause on this subject a while longer. Displaying a scholastic penchant for making subtle distinctions although in his galloping tempo he takes a tilt at the schools of Meinong and Husserl, Lessing indicates that the transparency phenomenon is equivalent to what Brentano called " Intentional Inexistence ", i.e. the conceptual sphere to which the object points but which is not the object in its actual form. By way of analogy, light may either be reflected by an object or pass through it. In the latter case,

---

[1] G. Sarton, " Transparency " : *Scribner's Magazine*, 1925, vol. lxxvii.

we have the phenomenon of transparency. Thus also in the matter of character, psychology as a science is concerned with the classification of a given type. The " understanding " is thus of the general or the universal, but it is the phenomenon, the particular, which should be dealt with and grasped not conceptually but *intuitively*. For this task, the language which all science must resort to is inadequate, for it cannot go beyond the conventional restrictions of the symbol representing the object which, however, is above all a life embodiment, an actual thing. Character then, because of its essential uniqueness, asserts Lessing, must not be subsumed under psychology, but should take up a position of its own as *characterology* wielding a purely intuitive method. We must not merely *understand* in the sense that science endeavours to do, but *grasp* the individual.[1] It is not easy to render the various shades of difference which the author is so fond of dwelling on (*Begreifen* and *Verstehen*, *Wesensfühlung* and *Wesensverständnis*, *Begriff* and *Inbegriff*) but the comparison of Titian and Galilei serves to elucidate the main distinction. The former has scarcely been surpassed in grasping (*begreifen*) all the nuances of light and colour, although he had no understanding of the phenomena ; the latter, on the other hand, although he possessed the clearest understanding of light and was the inventor of the telescope, which it might almost be said made it possible for us to picture the universe, had no *Begriff* of the phenomena, for he was blind. The latter statement is scarcely correct, for the great physicist became blind only in advanced age, but the force of Lessing's illustration remains unimpaired.

Cultural Dominants. In Marcuse [2] we have a kindred spirit striking a cultural key-note in his discussion. A personality

---

[1] Th. Lessing, " Über die Möglichkeit universaler Charakterologie " : *Arch. f. System. Philos.*, 1917, vol. xxiii.

[2] L. Marcuse, " Die Struktur der Kultur " : *Jahrbuch d. Charakterologie*, 1926, vol. ii/iii.

or a character is to him one who bears the banner of civilization, or rather culture. But what is culture, if not the sum-
total of all the realized possibilities of the human psyche ?
Each era has its own *dominants of culture* which represent
the most intense psychological experiences of that particular
age. Now different people will contribute in various degrees
toward the formation and expression of these dominants.
Hence a character is to be graded in the hierarchial scale
of values according as it is a passive, a quasi-passive or active
element in these dominants.

Most people are merely the targets of circumstance and are
dependent on every new tendency, fad, and fashion. These
constitute the lowest layer of the cultural structure. Then
there are the so-called characters in fiction and their counterparts in real life who are dominated indeed by some one
exaggerated trait, but their dominant is merely psychological,
not cultural ; particular and not universal. In the one it
is avarice ; in another, it is jealousy ; in a third it is hypocrisy
—all individualistic dominants. The genuine, compact
character, however, is neither the slave of his milieu, nor the
tool of his own arbitrariness. A character is fully fashioned,
becomes crystallized only when its dominant has established
a universal relationship. And here Marcuse delivers himself
of a pregnant remark which might have been uttered by
Emerson : " A genuine character is a specific perspective
of the universe." The number of these perspectives is limited
and history varies them in ever fresh constellations. The
true man of intellect receives his impress of character as
he gives expression to the world perspective in him in
proportion to the following three important qualities :
(1) the comprehensiveness of the perspective, (2) the fructi-
fication of the perspective, and (3) the originality of the
perspective.

"**Holism.**" An unwitting approach to the *Struktur*
movement is made by Smuts in a review of the biological

problems involved in personality.[1] Emphasis is here laid on the creative function in the organization of the parts, a point of view which, as the author maintains, would do away both with mechanism and vitalism. What he calls " organic holism " develops into human personality. That Smuts is interested in the purposive side of man may be seen from his favouring the study of biography as the best means of establishing what he calls the science of " personology ".

SUMMARY

It is not necessary to make further expeditions into the realm of the *Geisteswissenschaften*. The illustrations that have been drawn upon are representative of the various angles in the movement ; and the first reaction on the part of those who have been schooled in the experimental sciences will probably be that the views of the *Struktur* psychologists, especially of the right wing, are obscure, that they are tinged with metaphysics and even religion. But an unbiassed mind will make allowance for these deficiencies as regards psychology and will probe into the value of the doctrine as a whole. Certainly there is a good deal of sound reasoning in Spranger's closely knit exposition. Meaning and value cannot be divorced from our concept of character, unless we choose to speak of it in the sense of biological characteristic. It does seem more significant to place a man in the economic or aesthetic category than to say of him he is slow or rapid, hypokinetic or hyperkinetic. The slow may accomplish as much as the quick and more, if ruled by a dominant purpose throughout life.

The problem of character cannot be formulated under the mechanical auspices of the physical sciences, but—and there is the rub—their method is far superior to that advocated by the interpretative psychology ; for it has greater claim to objectivity. How character can be intuited, merely grasped

[1] J. C. Smuts. *Holism and Evolution*, 1926.

EE

as a whole, and yet remain the subject-matter of a science has not been established by the votaries of the cultural conception of psychology. If *understanding* is all that can be resorted to in a given situation, then everything would hinge upon the prepossession and the mental calibre of the understander, and characterology becomes at best an art.

My own solution to this dilemma would rest upon the *combination of methods*, or rather the supplementing of the analytic method by interpretation. The problem, however, would still be a cultural one. To cite as an example, instead of dissecting Luther's character into the thousand and one possible traits and qualities which are merely so many *membra disjecta*, we might examine his instinctive make-up, analyze his voluntary inhibitions and only then are we warranted in training on his personality the X-Ray apparatus of understanding so as to reveal the underlying motives and tendencies from the viewpoint of life-purposes and values.

CHAPTER XXI

Lure of the Glands. For the last quarter of a century the interesting results obtained in experiments with the ductless glands have turned the thoughts of many a worker in the borderland territory between physiology and psychology to conjectural expectations as to gross mental changes in consequence of processes going on in certain glands. The astonishing transformation brought about as a result of operations on the sex glands and the thyroid, as well as the less spectacular findings of Crile, Carlson, Cannon, and others, in regard to the emotions as affecting and being affected by the humoral processes in the body, has been responsible for many a bold statement which scarcely bears examination.

The thesis of the endocrine enthusiasts, the most articulate of whom is Berman, sets forth that an individual's personality is regulated by the glands. According to this writer, " Character, indeed, is an alloy of the different standard intravisceral pressures of the organism, a fusion created by the resistance or counter-pressure of the obstacles in the environment. Character, in short, is the gland intravisceral barometer of a personality.[1]

Aside from the extreme haziness of such a definition, the essential mark of character is missing in it. Manifestly we cannot envisage character as a pressure. This were ludicrous. What the author, I suppose, means is that character depends on these various pressures, etc., but he has not told us what character is.

---

[1] L. Berman, *The Glands Regulating Personality*, 1921, p. 107.

Exaggerated Claims. In a more recent book by the same author we read, " It has been my observation that in physiological hyperpituitarism, at any rate, character stability and integrity are personality traits." [1] The most conservative of us are probably ready to concede that our personality would undergo slight changes in consequence of alterations in the functioning of the ductless glands. A treatment of the subject of character and temperament, such as Jastrow's, without the mention of endocrine secretion, must be regarded as deficient in that respect ; but to base character entirely on metabolism and the hormones is, in spite of Bertrand Russell's speculations with regard to the possibility of transforming emotional dispositions through physiological manipulation,[2] a mere romance of modern science.

The argument which weighs a great deal with Berman is this : that while " it had long been known that many disturbances and changes and even diseases of the personality occurred without any observable pathology of the nervous system . . . careful examination showed that no disease or disturbance of any of the glands of internal secretion happened without some corresponding and often striking change in the personality ".[3] If we really knew that the gland disturbance was the only factor involved in such changes, we should indeed have the key to the whole situation, but the erstwhile enthusiastic author himself, toward the end of the article admits that " no one is more aware than the writer of the limitations of our knowledge of the endocrine

---

[1] L. Berman, *The Personal Equation*, 1925, p. 225.

[2] Bertrand Russell, *Icarus*, pp. 53–4. Russell's tone in this booklet is hardly a serious one. It is rather in the vein of a *feuilleton* when he writes : " Assuming an oligarchic organization of society, the State could give to the children of holders of power the disposition required for obedience. Against the injections of the State physicians the most eloquent Socialist oratory would be powerless."

[3] L. Berman, " Anthropology and the Endocrine Glands ": *The Scientific Monthly*, 1925, vol. xxi.

glands ". Hence how can we tell except in the case of the gonads and the thyroid just how the over- or under-functioning of the internal glands affects the make-up of the individual ?

The " Index Incretorius." Certainly we need not go so far as Dumas [1] who annihilates the whole structure which Berman has erected in *The Glands Regulating Personality*, but we have the rather circumspect testimony of those who have made an extensive study in this field to warn us against taking too much for granted. Thus Josefson, who presents evidence of amazing results obtained with cretins by feeding them thyroid extract and introduces the significant term *Index incretorius*, yet does not commit himself on the question as to the part incretion plays in shaping the personality. Indeed he says quite plainly that " it is impossible to say " just what its rôle is, " as compared with other factors." " Every judgment of the endocrine function " is according to him " more or less subjective in the absence of knowledge regarding the average index " (*incretorius*).[2] Naturally, his conclusion that we should obtain a better understanding of personality types, if the endocrine formula were known, sounds like a truism. Nevertheless, it is indicative of the status of the subject as related to personality.

A Concrete Example. Another writer, Lipschütz, after summarizing Berman's undeniably stimulating book, is practically of the same opinion as Josefson. Commenting on Berman's diagnosis, or as I should be inclined to call it " endocrinograph ", or " incretograph " of Oscar Wilde, Lipschütz asks whether, granted that the endocrine anomaly of the famous Irishman did have much to do with his aberrations and ruination, the author of *Dorian Gray* " might not have been a great artist, even if he were not homosexual or

---

[1] G. Dumas, *Traité de Psychologie*, 1924, vol. ii, p. 113.
[2] A. Josefson, " Endokrine Drüsen und die Persönlichkeit ": *Ergebnisse d. gesamt. Medizin*, 1925, vol. vi, p. 387.

effeminate or thymo-centric ".[1]   What Berman might reply,
I suppose, is that Wilde would not have become the type
of artist he was, that he might not have developed a
scintillating cynicism, that his poetry might have had a
different flavour, and so forth, but of course all this hypothe-
sizing must remain fruitless, and therein lies the limitation
of a conjectural endocrinology.

Our Ignorance about most of the Gland Functions.   To
quote from an even more recent book by a physician, who
from his professional contact might be expected to emphasize
the relation of the endocrines to personality :

> It is one of the misfortunes of modern psychology, that
> the study of the action of the endocrine organs is one of
> such great complexity and difficulty.   Everyone is agreed
> that these structures are of great importance in the regula-
> tion of both the bodily and mental activity of the individual,
> but, in spite of a very large literature which has grown
> up, exact knowledge in this sphere is still very restricted.
> Certain works which have been published in late years
> purport to give a clear picture of the mental and bodily
> alteration dependent on the excess or diminution of the
> secretory activity of the various glands ; but many of the
> statements, especially in relation to mental factors, are of
> the nature of a priori probabilities, rather than of empirically
> proved facts and are consequently of a very limited value.
> The difficulties which beset the path of investigators in
> this field are largely due to the fact that the system of
> endocrines works as a whole, so that, if one drops out,
> certain phenomena are met with which may be the effects
> of deficiency of the given secretion, or of the compensatory
> over-activity of others.   Hence the exact function of one
> gland, or a pair of glands, is hard to determine.   Moreover,

---

[1] A. Lipschütz, " Innere Sekretion und Persönlichkeit " : *Jahrbuch
der Charakterologie*, 1926, vol. ii–iii.

two given glands may act in co-operation in one respect,
but in opposition in another. For example, the thyroid
and the pituitary are both katabolic in function, that
is, they convert potential energy into actual energy, and
sugar from the blood will be mobilized for immediate
use as fuel, if they are stimulated to activity. But the
mental effects produced by overactivity of the thyroid
are quite different from those consequent upon hyperpituitarism. In the former, the energy is dissipated in
fretful irritable emotionalism, while in the latter, it may
be used to foster a pushful ambitious efficiency.[1]

After reviewing all our knowledge about the functions of the
ductless glands, he is forced to admit " that our knowledge
of the exact function of these organs is woefully deficient,
and that if the future brings us a clear understanding of the
interaction of the nervous system and the endocrine glands,
many problems in the study of personality, and its multi-
farious reactions will be solved. For the present, however,
it is not fruitful to pursue this subject further, and we must
proceed to the study of higher mental integrations.[2]

The More Direct Issue Before Us. Hitherto Berman's
thesis was applied to personality rather than to character.
We must ask ourselves now in what way the dysfunctioning
of the endocrine glands could affect character as conceived
in the present book. We have already seen that illness,
and especially a chronic disease, might change one's disposition,
so that an ordinary cheerful person can be expected to turn
grouchy or morose. More than that, disease would be apt
to reduce one's inhibitions. There is a tendency in invalids
to pamper themselves, possibly by way of compensation
for their affliction. This induced quality, however, seems
to be of a mental origin, and therefore is not something

[1] R. S. Gordon, *Personality*, 1926, pp. 65–6.
[2] Loc. cit., p. 81.

which would materially affect the application of a character standard.

Connection Between Glands and Instincts. The only way in which it might be possible to link up character with the endocrine glands would be to show the actual connection between these and the mechanism of inhibition or the instincts. When the patristic philosopher Origen made himself proof, much to his later sorrow, against all sex impulses, he deliberately removed one instinctive source. Thereafter he could never be brought into a situation which required him to inhibit the sex impulse. But it is not only at this point in the contour of character that he had made himself invulnerable and therefore unappraisable (since inhibition is the basis of character) but in respect of all the complications which arise out of the sex impulse. So much of the character test then does not count for him. We must remember, however, that in his case it demanded an extraordinary inhibitory power in the first place to inflict upon himself the act, knowing as he did, what he was about to be deprived of for all time. Now without going into the subtle matter of the desirability of the result or its conformity with a rational principle, we surely ought to accord to Origen, in the face of his courage in undertaking the excruciatingly painful operation and determination to court his subsequent privation in addition, a marked degree of character.

The Case of Origen and Abelard Compared. With Abelard the situation is of course different, since his condition was forced upon him, and therefore his inhibition of the sex instinct, after the tragic episode which changed his life, falls outside the scope of character. The same conclusion holds for the eunuch and any person whose gonads function so feebly as to make inhibition of the sex instinct practically superfluous. Such an individual will be able to avoid other character lapses without any effort on his part. If a priest, he is sure never to break his vow of celibacy. Infidelity, seduction, and various other forms of generally condemned behaviour could never apply to him.

Similarly, if it should be discovered that the instinct releasing the fear reactions is governed by the adrenal glands, then an individual found with a marked deficiency in the supply of such hormones could not be compared with the normal person as regards (inhibiting) the instinctive tendency to escape from imminent danger.

Compensation in Glandular Make-up. In short, every instinctive tendency and complex (such as self-preservation) would have to be bound up definitely with the function of a particular gland in order to reduce character to glandular determination. But even if this were the case, the fact that with the exception of gross anomalies, the glandular constitution is, if not about the same in the general run of mankind, at least compensatory in its make-up, would make the even inhibition of instinctive tendencies equally difficult for all; since the favourable conjuncture of one set of organic conditions is apt to be offset by the defect in another group of conditions.

Another interesting line of attack to follow up is the examination of possible racial character configurations, for instance, whether the Germans, aside from their different national constitution, can show greater character in one respect while the French excel them in another direction— not that this would prove anything more than that, the whole make-up being different, the character-complex naturally would manifest differences too.

Are there Racial Differences in Character ? It seems to me, however, that there is no warrant for believing that there are racial differences in character, as the concept is developed here, although there seems to be ground for maintaining that there are racial endocrine differences—a thesis elaborated in a series of papers by A. Keith who sees in the European races the predominance of pituitary activity while the Negro type is adrenally centred and the Mongolian races governed by peculiarities of the thyroid.[1]

Noble Characters in All Nations. Is it not true, however, that a man of character, in the strict sense of the word, inhibits his instinctive dispositions in abeyance to some ruling principle, whether he be an Oriental or an American, whether he presents the characteristics of the Mongolian or the European, whether he is born of French, German, or English parents ? That races differ in many respects goes without saying, but these characteristics in the first place are not primarily character traits, secondly they are influenced in large part by the tradition of the locality (environment), and thirdly since true character is so rare (see Chapter XXXIV) it behoves us to consult rather the behaviour of the outstanding national figures than the doings of the masses who are seldom guided by principles.

" Ignoramus "—Our Present Plea. In a word, then, the Scotch verdict " not proven " will have to be brought out in the matter of drawing a parallelism between endocrine activity and character. That there is a wide field for research in this sphere is to be taken for granted, and experiments on human subjects, such as are available, considering the danger of the method, would prove at *least the effect of glandular functions on the affective side of personality.* The isolated cases known in the literature do not constitute sufficient evidence. It may well be that there are two types of people, the one more susceptible than the other to any glandular change. After the relationship between the endocrine secretions and temperament has been established we might proceed to devise some technique through which the more debatable question with reference to character may be investigated.

[1] A. Keith. " The Evolution of Human Races in the light of the Hormone Theory " : *Johns Hopkins Hospital Bulletin,* 1922, vol. xxxiii.

The most complete summary of the literature on endocrinology for our purpose is that of F. A. Beach, who adduces a good deal of evidence, as may have been expected, that mating and maternal behavior are affected by the hormones, although even in the sexual sphere, we learn not without surprise that normal sexual behavior is possible in male rats after the *vasa deferentia* has been totally removed, and that the loss of the uterus and vagina " does not prevent the exhibition of heat behavior in adult female rats ". In connection with maternal behavior, Riddle, cited by Beach, supposes it to result from the effects of prolactin upon the nervous tissue, at least in rats and fowl, which constituted his subjects. Riddle is of the opinion that " the hormones affect a neural state or function as yet unexplored ' adding a new element of consciousness ' ".[1]

One of the chief findings is undoubtedly that the specificity of the hormonal effect hinges upon the innately organized i.e., inherited central nervous mechanisms. Acquired responses, as, e.g., in learning, are not intimately bound up with glandular processes. The common denominator of the glands and the mechanisms which were referred to as innate or instinctive is the gene.

Again, it is noteworthy that although moods and cycles and instinctive behavior dealing with reproduction may be influenced indirectly through hormone action, personality as a whole, and particularly character, is outside its bailiwick.

[1] F. A. Beach : *Hormones and Behavior*, 1948, p. 261, and p. 278 (Hoeber).

CHAPTER XXII

THE BEHAVIOURISTIC DETOUR

Character as a Traditional Set of Reactions. If the problem of character presents so much difficulty to the traditional psychologist, the behaviourist, naturally, could not be expected even to attempt a solution, and, like the fox in the fable, denies the value of the object. At least this is the attitude of Watson, who may be taken as the spokesman of the behaviourists, and who is usually clear and consistent in his views.

In a footnote he tells us that " Character is generally used when viewing the individual from the standpoint of his reactions to the more conventionalized and standardized situations (conventions, morals, etc.) ".[1]

Apparently he makes short shrift of this term on the ground that it is an ethical and not a psychological concept. *Prima facie*, we might be inclined to apply in support of the behaviouristic contention the remark of James in his famous chapter on *Habit*, to the effect that there is, physiologically, no difference between a good habit and a bad one. But, as has been said earlier, a character is more than a habit. It is a system of tendencies which permits a considerable amount of predictability. And certainly one system of tendencies is far different from another system, while in many cases the tendencies do not hang together so as to deserve a unifying mark.

But it is possible to expose the *ratio ignava* of Watson's school in a more direct manner. The behaviouristic fallacy of giving an environmental turn to everything conceivable is apparent here as elsewhere. Whoever would say that a

[1] J. B. Watson, *Psychology from the Standpoint of a Behaviourist*, p. 392.

person like Herminia Barton in *The Woman Who Did* was
without character simply because she chose a path which
in the eyes of her community and indeed the world at large
was considered irregular ? Or, turning from fiction to
grim reality, would not the very judges who sentenced the
Irish patriot Roger Casement to the gallows testify to the
noble traitor's well-knit character ? Is it necessary to call
attention once more to the elementary distinction made time
and again between reputation and character ?

Not a Social but an Individual Fact. *Character is a relation
which holds not between a man and his community, but between
his reason and his own acts.* It is because character emanates
from one's own self that it transcends the community and
presents an objective problem. To be sure, in the last analysis
posterity is the judge, but its criterion is not what Watson
implies it to be, viz., conformity to conventionalized
situations, but the living up to one's own convictions in spite
of social pressure.

A mere acquaintance with the lives of universal heroes
will convince us that the man of character was usually he
who combated the prevailing notions of his time by word
and deed. Were the community in which he lived to be
asked about his character, the consensus would be decidedly
condemnatory. When, in response to Napoleon's captious
remarks about his music, Cherubini replied, " Your Majesty
knows as much about music as I know about battles," thus
bringing upon himself the disfavour of the redoubtable
Emperor, with the consequent humiliation and disgrace.
it matters little really whether or not Napoleon had an
ear for music or whether Cherubini's music was of a high
order or not. Still less does it matter what Napoleon's court
or his worshipful subjects would think of such *lèse-majesté*.
The remark of Cherubini will have to be considered for all
times, even if his operas and masses should pass into oblivion,
as an indication of the man's character.

We need not linger on this negative platform, which con-
fuses a psychological issue with the ethical judgments
surrounding it, and were it not for the fact that so many
psychologists find it expedient to dispose of a troublesome
subject cavalierly rather than to take account of it, we
should have passed over the behaviouristic denial in silence.

Majority of Behaviourists View Character Differently. It
must be said that the American psychologists who lean
toward behaviourism are not of the same mind as their
uncompromising leader. Many of them do in fact assign
a conspicuous place to character, taking it, however, in the
sense of characteristic behaviour. In this way they come
closer to carrying out the behaviouristic programme than
Watson himself.

It is in the sphere of personality that a thoroughgoing
behaviourism professes to build up a programme of
study ; and how is the concept of personality envisaged ?
It is regarded as an organization of habit systems,
socialized and tempered emotions, regulated instincts,
including all the combinations and interrelations amongst
these. Now are we to believe that an individual's personality
cannot be judged unless all the one thousand and one items
that enter into such a really aimless survey, as suggested by
Watson, are investigated ? Is it not true that we do make
reliable estimates on the basis of certain factors which we
deem more useful or significant ?

Awe and Sex Appeal as Determinants of Personality. The
behaviouristic reply would be to the effect that indeed we
do express opinions about the way a person impresses us ;
but these judgments are based on two factors, (a) awe, harking
back to a childish habit-system in formation at the time
when the child was impressed by authority (and yet Watson
is violently opposed to psychoanalysis) and (b) the sex element.
" When this element is strongest—that is, when the speaker
or associate (the stimulus) brings out those positive reaction

tendencies, the popular characterization is put in somewhat different words. The man or woman has a ' pleasing ', ' thrilling ', or ' engrossing ' personality. Friendships are almost instantaneously begun largely upon the basis of this element. It must be recalled that according to modern usage this kind of reaction tendency is aroused not only by members of the opposite sex but also by members of the same sex."

In his recent popular lectures the dominance appeal is underscored : " What do you mean by a commanding personality ? Isn't it generally that the individual speaks in an authoritative kind of way, that he has a rather large physique and that he is a little taller than you are " (apparently Watson loses sight of the stature of Napoleon) and here personality is defined as " the sum of activities that can be discovered by actual observation of behaviour over a long enough time to give reliable information. In other words, personality is but the end product of our habit systems ".[1] And yet we should have thought that even a child who has not yet had the opportunity of developing its habit systems possesses a personality, in some instances of a marked degree.

Theory Contradicted by Statistical Data. Soon the author is compelled to admit that " a statistical analysis of the factors entering into the formation of friendship found that the element of truthfulness was ranked first and loyalty second." [2]

My own questionnaire circulated among a group of several hundred persons, heterogeneous as to occupation, race, age, sex, and social status, revealed that the majority of people are attracted most by (a) an agreeable personality, which might include a number of qualities, (b) the trait of sincerity,

---

[1] J. B. Watson, *Behaviourism*, 1925, p. 220.
[2] J. B. Watson, *Psychology from the Standpoint of a Behaviourist*, p. 395.

and (c) general intelligence. Next comes honesty. It must be borne in mind, too, that to be attracted by a trait and to regard that trait as the essence of personality are two different things. We see then that neither the commanding aspect nor physical attractiveness stands out particularly among the elements that enter into the evaluation of personality.

How then can the hypothesis advanced by the ultra-behaviourist fit in with the facts disclosed by the results of his own questionnaire ? Here a concession is made and immediately thereon a qualification. " These are of course conventionally the correct answers and the ranking obtained was the one expected in a mixed crowd. When the questionary asked for other important elements, such items as sympathy, congeniality, and the like took a prominent place." But the issue has only been beclouded by such hedging and straddling. The inference which that paragraph implies is that although we say or think that truthfulness or loyalty has played a large part in our selection of friends, " the deeper reasons lie below the organized word level " and supposedly point to the influence of authority in the case of a commanding personality and to sex in the case of a pleasing personality. The " deeper reasons " in other words are those which will satisfy the demands of a thorough-going behaviourism.

Illustrations Refuting Watson's View. Need it be pointed out that the most likeable personalities in the history of culture, to take instances like Socrates and Moses Mendelssohn, both of whom seemed to have charmed even their enemies— neither exercised the alleged authoritative hold on those with whom they came in contact nor did they peradventure possess the physical attractions that could appeal to the sexual urge, no matter in how broad or derived a sense the word " sex " might be taken.

With reference to the first clause, it is true that in

appraising new acquaintances, we have nothing to go by except their features, facial expression, and other outward characteristics which we interpret as a result of previous associations, but that is not the issue. The question is whether the stimulus *immediately unlocks an old memory system without the interposition of more recent associations and judgments, or whether the external individual creates an impression on the strength of the accumulated experience of the observer*. It seems that the latter case is better borne out by the facts.

Putting the Cart Before the Horse. As usual, the behaviourist is begging the question. Instead of realizing that a person who commands respect does so by *virtue of those superior qualities which are ascribed to him* by those who come in contact with him, Watson apparently believes that there is some physical cue which touches off the submissive hang-over from childhood in the impressionable individual.

To show how this theory will not bear examination, let us suppose that the same individual who displayed an authoritative bearing was discovered to have been involved in an unsavoury dealing. In that event, the person would lose for most people that commanding quality which formerly instilled respect, although no change in manner, presence, expression, bearing, carriage, or gait could be detected on the part of those who were thus affected by the transpiration. Why was the halo dimmed ? The " unconditioning ", to employ this mechanistic terminology, could not have taken place so rapidly and so effectively as to counterbalance all the connections that have linked up the hero-worship memory of younger days with the commanding bearing or countenance of the individual in question. Nor is the change in attitude to be explained as a result of the publicity that was possibly given to the case ; for, in the first place, it is not necessary that the unwholesome facts be known generally ; even if they are confided to the one individual alone, the hitherto dominating personality will for the individual take on a different aspect. This is so common an observation that no illustrations need be adduced here. Secondly, we may gather that the undesirable publicity is of slight consequence in the actual estimate of personality on the part of independent observers, because where the condemnation is deemed unwarranted, the aura around the commanding personality is enhanced rather than diminished.

It is not to be understood that Watson's notion of personality comprises only the authority and sex elements that have here been discussed. What he claims is that in our loose usage of the concept, we stress in our rough estimates usually one of these two factors. He, on the other hand, analyzes personality into perhaps hundreds of qualities, evidently dwelling on none in particular so as to single it out from the rest.

OBJECTIONS TO BEHAVIOURISTIC TREATMENT SUMMED UP

The criticism directed against this view then was, (1) that the average man and woman have a better understanding of the problem than Watson gives them credit for, basing their judgments on more objective data than those alleged by him ; and (2) the mere cataloguing of an individual's behaviour will give us little more insight into the personality of the subject than the description of the locations and positions of certain stones would reveal their mineralogical properties.

Since Martin, who has exhibited a great deal of admiration for behaviourism and its apostle, nevertheless rejects the new materialism at this point, we can do no better than conclude this chapter with a review of his excellently stated objections to the discrete method outlined by Watson.

The Case Against Mechanism. " The behaviourist view of personality is a curiously mechanistic one. We are told that personality is merely the organism at work. Those who regard personality in any other way are said to be ' superstitious people ' who either have a romantic view of persons or are the victims of erroneous religious considerations. Personality as a whole is compared to a gas engine. The way in which a gas engine works is its ' personality ' and that is all there is to it. When the separate parts work together efficiently so that the engine runs smoothly, its personality is well integrated ; when not, it shows that the engine has a ' personality disturbance ' of some kind.

" The behaviourist attempt to give an account of personality means that he has to resort to what I want to call an additive process. Having first in his laboratory separated behaviour into a number of specific reflexes, inherited or conditioned, the behaviourist, in the end, seeks to reintegrate his subject by the simple process of putting his ' Humpty-Dumpty together again '. Now, of course, a unity so achieved must necessarily be artificial and of the *inorganic* type. The gas engine has truly an inorganic unity. One builds a gas engine by assembling parts, which in the state of nature may have been widely distributed in space. But the unity so achieved is merely that of a balance of forces.

" The unity of an *organism* is different. A tree begins its life as a single cell and grows out from that simple centre. Its unity is central and given. However great the ramifications of its roots and branches and leaves may be, there runs through it all, as a living organism, a unity which is very different from that of a machine. The structure of a machine is achieved from *within in* ; that of an organism from *within out*. No strictly mechanistic theory of organic functioning seems to me to take this fact adequately into account." [1]

[1] E. D. Martin, *Psychology*, 1925, p. 278.

CHAPTER XXIII

Applied Atmosphere in American Approach. Not much time or energy has been spent in the United States on theoretical discussions of character. Here the subject, as might perhaps be expected, took on an applied form, and the question asked by investigators was not so much : What is character ? as, How can character be judged ? But owing to the want of delimitation, and therefore the possibly loose usage of the term, it was thought best to centre attention on the larger field of personality which would comprise all traits and qualities of a non-intelligent nature. Temperament, attitudes, interests, emotions, instincts, moral judgment, sentiments, and true character traits are all treated as of a piece, and individuals have been subjected to more or less promiscuous experiments and tests presumably on the principle that with a great deal of mining some gold will probably turn up.

The empirical approach to the study of character is not to be belittled, and some of the experimental methods devised bespeak a considerable amount of ingenuity applied in such a manifestly elusive sphere. At the same time, it is doubtful whether the combined efforts of all the experimental investigators have established half a dozen new facts or have placed the subject in a new light.

Various Methods. In their excellent report on such measures of character, May and Hartshorne [1] speak of " about one hundred tests either standardized or in the form of

[1] M. A. May and H. Hartshorne, " Objective Methods of Measuring Character " : *Ped. Sem. & Journ. of Genetic Psychol.*, 1925, vol. xxxii.

definite proposals ", and the writers set themselves the task of analyzing this collective battery under the following heads according to the technique or method employed : (1) The Order of Merit Method, (2) The Scale of Values Method, (3) The Multiple Choice Method, (4) The True-False Method, (5) The Cross-out Method, (6) The Distraction Method, (7) The Information Test Method, (8) The Comprehension Test Type, (9) The Recognition or Identification Test, (10) Performance Tests, (11) The Association Test Method, (12) The Physiological Method of Expression.

· Of the four classes into which these tests have been divided, viz., those claiming to measure (a) ethical, moral, social, and religious discrimination, (b) character and personality traits, such as aggressiveness, caution, confidence, etc., (c) interests, attitudes, prejudices, etc., and (d) instincts and emotions, only the second class properly falls within our range, although the others help as settings. Even in their careful and business-like classification of the tests according to the claims of the devisers, May and Hartshorne have not been able to offer definite contours or boundary lines. One wonders why altruism is an attitude any more than caution or conformity ; and herein lies the weakness of the purely empirical school. To take this very illustration : is altruism a stand or attitude one takes *intellectually*, or is it a *practice* incorporated in one's conduct ? Is prejudice a matter of character or of intelligence ? Similarly F. H. Allport has never given any reasons for regarding insight as a personality trait rather than an intelligence function. Still more questionable is Chassell's classing originality under the head of character and personality. Either all the intelligence factors are components of personality, or else originality belongs with the other functions of intelligence.

Knowledge and Action Not Comparable. After the same fashion of reasoning, we must rule out moral discrimination and judgment from our consideration, since the knowledge of right and wrong, though a *sine qua non* of character, does not afford any guide for the actual possession of character. To know what to do and to do it are two totally different things.

As for those tests which purport to measure interests, attitudes, prejudices, social relations, as also instincts and emotions, it may be said that their bearing on character in the proper sense varies from a very slight to a fairly considerable degree, but in no way do they strike the nucleus of the problem.

Actual Character Tests. There remain then the tests which constitute class (*b*) of May and Hartshorne's list, and these, after allowance is made for the questionable classification (due mainly to the claims of the devisers) reduce themselves to about a dozen, comprising such as measure incorrigibility (Cady), conscientiousness (May), honesty (Franzen, May and Hartshorne, Slaght), honour, reliability, and truthfulness (Voelker, Raubenheimer, Knight, Sinclair), fairmindedness (Watson). Even these have not all an assured symptomatic value. It is doubtful, for instance, whether conscientiousness may be measured by an information test such as May proposes.[1] On the other hand, the Voelker series of tests [2] presents situations that are true to life, and although it is debatable on moral grounds whether persons may be subjected, even in the cause of characterology, to devices which are bound to be prejudicial to many of them, there is no denying that these actual performance tests are more likely to gauge the individual's traits than any other tests. To the question : Will the individual refuse credit not due to him ? or, Will the subject refuse help when he has been told to work independently ? Voelker obtains the answer by placing the subjects in circum-

---

[1] M. A. May, " The Psychological Examination of Conscientious Objectors " : *Amer. Journ. of Psychol.*, 1920, vol. xxxi.

[2] R. F. Voelker, " The Function of Ideals in Social Education " : *Teachers College Cont'ns to Educ.*, 1921, No. 112, pp. 78–80.

stances, unknown to themselves, which call for an act that decides the question for the examiner. Thus in the " over-change test " the examiner arranges with the storekeeper to overchange the subject who is sent to a given place for a specific purchase. Similarly to test the subject's trust-worthiness, the latter is told to keep his eyes closed and assemble parts of a board, a performance which experience has shown to be practically impossible without the use of the eyes.

It is true that not all the situations are of a uniform simplicity and Voelker was obliged to eliminate several tests in which the responses were all the same. Thus the " stealing " test was discarded because all of the subjects had a perfect score, that is to say, gave evidence of no temptation to steal the attractive puzzles that were scattered about before them, or else they were afraid of being detected.

Voelker's subjects were practically all boy scouts and camp girls. Since both groups are as a general rule not permitted to accept tips, he was able to test their resistance in declining a tip when it was offered them by a stranger. Other questions that were answered by the tests are : Will the subject do a test exactly as ordered ? Will the subject work at a test against distraction ? Will the subject return borrowed property according to promise ?

Technique of the Voelker Tests. An illustration of the technique employed in the administration of these tests is afforded by the " tracing and opposites test " by means of which cheating could be detected. This test is given on a prepared four-page folder, perforated at the fold and con-taining on page 1 a list of words beside which the opposites are to be given ; pages 2 and 4 are blank while a piece of transparent waxed paper is fastened with a clip at each corner upon page 3, in such manner that the figure and the typed instructions are perfectly legible. Page 3 consists of a jagged figure for tracing.

The technique of this test is as follows : A folder is placed before each subject with face side down, and page 4 (blank) up. At a given signal, the folders are opened and the subjects trace the figure on page 3 according to instructions, one minute being given for this work. When the signal is given to stop, the folder is closed so that page 4 is down and page 1 is up. The subjects are then instructed to write their names at the bottom of the page, and then to write as many opposites as possible within the space of two minutes.

When the time is called one of the examiners asks for the Tracing Test for the purpose of correction. The *examiners* then proceed to teár off the Tracing Test at the perforation (including the waxed paper which is still attached by means of the clips), the first page being left with the subject. The assistant examiners leave the room at this point, while the chief examiner reads the correct opposites, giving the subjects the opportunity to mark their own papers. Care is taken to create lax conditions during the process of correction, the subjects being encouraged to ask questions. The examiner goes to the window or arranges to have some one call him to the door. The subjects are thus given ample opportunity to cheat.

A comparison of pages 1 and 3 will reveal whether or not the subject attempted to cheat by adding words or making changes during the process of correcting his own paper. The waxed paper will show a perfect tracing of all the words which the subject wrote originally. The examiner, of course, had provided each of his subjects with a hard pencil.

Scoring : The subject scores 10 if he has made no attempt to cheat ; he scores 0 if he cheats.

Modifications of the Original Tests. Voelker's series of character tests has formed the basis of subsequent batteries. In studying incorrigibility in delinquent children, Cady [1]

---

[1] V. M. Cady, " The Psychology and Pathology of Personality " : *Journ. of Delinquency*, 1922, vol. vii.

has modified but slightly the Voelker method and used five tests, measuring trustworthiness in a motor task, honesty in scoring one's own paper, overstatement, moral judgment, and tendencies to instability, as brought out by the Woodworth questionnaire. The last two tests are not strictly speaking within the scope of our subject, for the responses involved knowledge or discrimination rather than action.

Raubenheimer has made a different selection of tests, borrowing ideas from Fernald, Voelker, Franzen, and Cady. Only two of his battery—the book checking and the overstatement tests—are true character tests. The others like activity preferences, offence ratings, reading preferences, and one or two more of this sort cannot be regarded as touching the core of our problem, although in dealing with individual cases they may throw some light on the development of particular traits in a certain direction.

In the extensive investigation of gifted children which Terman directed,[1] Raubenheimer's tests were given both to a group of selected children and to control groups. Six tests were used with two forms for the overstatement test. The first variety is a modification of Knight's book-titles test which consists of a number of titles of works, some of them fictitious, the examinees being asked to check all the titles of books that they had read. The other variety of the same test brings to light overstatement in knowledge claimed.

A Measure for Trustworthiness. The Cady trustworthiness test which is based on the Voelker original calls for the insertion of crosses in circles with eyes shut. This of course affords a temptation on the part of some to cheat. In another form of the test, a similar task is set by asking the children with eyes shut to run their pencil around several squares, one inside the other, without touching the sides " more than just a little ".

[1] L. M. Terman *et al.*, *Genetic Studies of Genius*, 1925, vol. i, p. 485 ff

In the Voelker-Cady-Knight-Raubenheimer tests considerable ingenuity is displayed on the part of the devisers to ward off suspicion of the purpose of the procedure.

Characterial Age. One of the interesting results in Raubenheimer's work is the curve obtained for levels of character development both among the gifted and control groups as also among the boys and girls, showing that the " gifted child of nine years has reached a level of character development corresponding roughly to that of unselected children of 14 years ", and that the " gifted girl makes a better average score than the gifted boy ". The data really open the way to the establishment of a " characterial age " scale analogous to the mental age scale. We may readily gather that the tests devised by the several investigators are suitable for making " comparison of groups with respect to certain important character traits ", but as to the value of the tests in helping us to orient ourselves in the central problem of character, its elements, criteria, genetic antecedents, we may, without seeming captious, profess a profound doubt.

Tests for Honesty. The most methodical test that has yet been developed along Voelker's lines is that of May and Hartshorne for measuring the tendency to cheat among 300 children.[1] The considerations which the investigators have taken into account so as to insure a high degree of validity for the tests can hardly be found fault with.

Seven different tests were used, the series being arranged according to difficulty ; e.g. it is easier to cheat where a check mark in pencil is to be erased or added than where a sentence is to be erased or added, or where something is to be changed in ink. Motivation of course is a significant factor, and the warning that the answers will count induces some of the children to cheat, while others will remain unaffected by the information.

---

[1] M. A. May and H. Hartshorne, " First Steps Toward a Scale for Measuring Attitudes " : *Jour. of Educ. Psychol.*, 1926, vol. xvii.

A sample of the technique of these tests is given below :
The series begins with

an information test consisting of 28 items steeply graded in difficulty. Instead of underlining the correct answer, the pupil is required to encircle it in *ink*. He is told to guess if he does not know. In fact, he is not allowed to hand in his paper until he has guessed at every answer. These papers are taken to the office where a duplicate of each is made. A day or so later the original papers are returned to the children with answer sheets and they are instructed to grade their own papers. Each child has previously been supplied with an ink eraser in connection with his school work.

In order to cheat on this test it is necessary for the child to erase a circle drawn in ink and make another. This is rather difficult. It is not easy to make a clean job of it. By comparing the corrected paper with its duplicate in the office, it is possible to see how much cheating has gone on.

Results and Recommendations. Aside from the interesting and carefully evaluated results, e.g. that eighty-four per cent made at least one change in their papers and that the brighter pupils do not cheat so readily as the poorer ones, May and Hartshorne suggest that their scale may be extended in scope so as to be applicable to various situations in games and play. Another scale might be worked out for situations involving money or business transactions. When the several scales are placed side by side and compared at each level we should have " a measure of the whole complex of behaviour tendencies called dishonesty. The same procedure could be followed in constructing scales for other tendencies. Both positive as well as negative trends would be included. Situations involving all kinds of attitudes would be selected and graded. The outcome would be a general scale with many symptomatic situations at each level. A total character score or index might be obtained from the general level reached on the scale, or a more detailed picture of the relation of these trends to one another and of character as a whole might be revealed in the profile or some statistical coefficient."

Paradox of American Workers. The only flaw which can be pointed out in the preceding research by May and Hartshorne is one of central importance. The concept of character remains with them psychologically unanalyzed. It is one of the paradoxes of the American character testers that while they move in a mechanistic and moderately behaviouristic atmosphere, they yet are content to busy themselves with virtues and vices (honesty, dishonesty, trustworthiness) instead of attempting to pick out the psychological warp and woof of these traits—their *genetic motives*.

Varieties of Dishonesty. Dishonesty is a term which embraces types of behaviour of a wide variety. Its most common form is manifest in money matters, but surely this is only one species of dishonesty. Will it be denied that dishonesty is possible in the intellectual sphere ? He who " doctors " up the results of an experiment, or even shuts his eyes deliberately to the negative cases, so as to prove his pet theory—he who pretends to have made a new discovery, whereas the essentials were furnished him by others, is strikingly dishonest, although the man in the street will perhaps not realize the nature of the defect, at least not to its full extent. When Voltaire, as is reported, in order to call attention to a new work of his hit upon the ingenious idea of scathingly reviewing his own book under a pseudonym so as to take the occasion afterwards of defending himself against the severe critic, he assuredly was indulging in a bit of subtle dishonesty which must be sharply condemned in spite of the humour attaching to the situation. Now Voltaire's conduct in pecuniary affairs was, so far as I am aware, not objectionable.

Others again are social climbers and will say and do such things as will further their courtier ambitions. They may be careless about money matters to their own disadvantage, let alone making capital of someone's unwariness, but they are determined to get on socially at all costs.

Analysis of Dishonesty. Indeed I should go so far as to suggest that all undignified opportunism is dishonest, and the fact that it is so commonly resorted to does not invalidate this judgment. By opportunism, I do not mean of course making use of every opportunity that presents itself, which is a legitimate course to take, but angling for opportunities, by " pulling strings " as one expresses it colloquially. If an author arranges with a brother author for each to praise the other's works in print, or if he asks an admiring friend to write a glowing review of his book, he has already laid himself open to the charge of dishonesty. Similarly, if an editor, through some ulterior motive, sends an opponent's book received for review purposes to the author's harshest critic to be reviewed, he has engaged in a bit of underhand tactics which should come under the head of dishonesty.

Different Instinctive Sources of Dishonesty. It is patent, however, that not all the illustrations of dishonesty are actuated by the *same psychological springs*. The acquisitive instinct operates in some cases; in others, the instinct of self-aggrandizement is at the bottom of the overt trait. There are cases to be explained by an intense or persistent congenital pugnacity and feeble inhibitability coupled perhaps with an inadequate consistency urge.

My contention is then that unless we discover the psychological bonds of the various forms of behaviour designated by a term like honesty or dishonesty, the most consummate technique will be of no avail, and we should be groping about in the underwood of virtues, vices, propensities, and what-not, without getting into the open of the psychological arena. No psychological textbook will find a place in its pages for the discussion of such traits as dishonesty or trust-worthiness. In our practical world these virtues and vices are of paramount importance, but until they are placed *psychologically* with reference both to the circumstances (stimuli) and the original nature of man (instinctive tendencies) we should let them rest in their ethical and legal domains.

The Downey Will-Temperament Tests. The series of tests devised by Downey do not approximate the life situation as do Voelker's but may be regarded as of a symbolic type. The three phases of the personality pattern under which, according to her, all the traits of the will-temperament may be included are (*a*) the speed and fluidity of the reaction, (*b*) the forcefulness and decisiveness of the reaction, and (*c*) the carefulness and persistence of the reaction. In the first category we find such tests as speed of movement, freedom from load, flexibility, speed of decision ; in the second— tests of motor impulsion, reaction to contradiction, resistance to opposition and finality of judgment. The third group of tests purports to gauge motor inhibition, interest in detail, coördination of impulses, and volitional perseverance.

Proceeding from the premise that the various patterned forms of activity as revealed by temperament are determined by (*a*) the amount of nervous energy at the disposal of the individual, and (*b*) the tendency of such nervous energy to discharge immediately into the motor areas, or contrariwise to find an outlet only after a considerable detour, she seeks to ascertain by means of her tests the " general level of activity or impulsion, the degree of inhibition and the modes in which impulsion and inhibition function in an individual ".[1] Motor activity in the form of handwriting exercises constitutes in the main the locus of her measure, with distraction as an essential condition. Her most reliable test, however, is probably the contradiction or suggestibility test which involves going through a miniature life situation and requires

[1] J. E. Downey, *The Will Temperament and its Testing*, p. 59.

little symptomatic transfer from the result in the test to the diagnosis of trait.

In a practically complete survey of the literature dealing with the Downey will-temperament tests, May sums up the value of these tests as follows :—

Critical Estimate of the Downey Tests. " One of the most common methods of character study is that of analysis into traits. Can character traits (assuming that there are such things) be studied profitably by the WT [1] tests ? Perhaps they can, but the above results seem to show clearly that the Downey tests do not measure any easily identifiable traits. It is very doubtful if these handwriting exercises will correlate highly with anything that could be regarded as a character trait. Whatever else they measure, they do not measure traits.

" Character is commonly regarded as conduct. Do the WT tests measure conduct ? About the only data we have on this point are those of Clark and he found a negative correlation between WT score and the conduct-response score of delinquent boys. But he also found a slight positive correlation (0·29) between change in conduct-response and WT score. Conduct is a complex social affair and one would hardly expect to find it correlated with simple handwriting exercises.

" Character may also be regarded as the predictability of behaviour. Can behaviour be predicted by these tests ? The results seem to show that academic success is in some instances better predicted by a combination of WT tests and intelligence tests than by intelligence alone. But when we consider the rather high correlation between some types of intelligence tests and the WT tests we wonder how much of the prophecy is due to intelligence and how much to temperament.

[1] The letters WT are here used as an abbreviation for " will-temperament ".

" While it is true that the WT tests will not foretell what any person will do in a given situation, yet the general nature of his reactions may be predicted. For example, Downey would say that the will-profile will foretell whether or not an individual's responses will be strong or weak, deliberate or impulsive, aggressive or its opposite, and so on. This type of prediction is very desirable and it seems that the WT tests have definite value at this point." [1] Collins, in her preliminary report on the Downey tests, administered in Scotland, offers much the same criticism, and while she admits that the series does differentiate " the strong character from the weak, the careful from the careless, and the quick from the slow ", she finds fault with the tests on the following grounds : (a) they are time-consuming (not an adequate objection), (b) too much depends on the personality of the experimenter, (c) the scoring is at times puzzling, (d) the real character is to a certain extent occasionally masked by practice in handwriting.[2]

There appears to be agreement on the satisfactoriness of the " reaction to contradiction " test but, as Collins remarks, " if the subject has the slightest idea of the object of the test, it entirely loses its value."

We must infer then from the statements of those who worked with the Downey will-temperament tests on a comprehensive scale that they are not yet safe guides in the hands of the tester, although their service in bringing out individual differences is to not be disputed.

Aggressiveness Tested by Distractibility. Distraction as a condition figures chiefly in the tests of Moore and Gilliland [3]

---

[1] M. A. May, " The Present Status of the Will Temperament Tests " : *Jour. of Applied Psychol.*, 1925, vol. ix, p. 50.

[2] M. Collins, " Character and Temperament Tests " : *Brit. Jour. of Psychol.* (Gen. Section), 1925, vol. xvi.

[3] H. T. Moore and A. R. Gilliland, " The Measurement of Aggressiveness " : *Jour. of App. Psychol.*, 1921, vol. v.

employed to measure aggressiveness. It is not so easy to accept the conclusion of these writers that the shifty eye, together with certain response words in a free association test is the indication of a lack of aggressiveness, but even less satisfactory is the general notion which they attach to this trait as " personal force ", " initiative ", or " assurance ". One feels that initiative is one thing and aggressiveness another, that personal force may emanate from a leader, but it need not be confused with the importunateness or insistence of sales managers. The value of aggressiveness will thus depend on motives and purposes, not on mere persistence or " push ".

Debatable Assumptions. In the majority of personality tests devised by American investigators, the main assumption is open to question. Thus when Ream asks a number of subjects to check first a number of traits generally considered desirable and then to re-scan the list of pairs, checking the one trait of each pair which more nearly describes the individual, he is taking it for granted that he is measuring self-consciousness " on the thesis that the highly self-conscious individual will be proportionately slower in making subjective personal judgments than in making non-personal decisions ".[1] But this assumption is far from being obvious. The two judgments are not at all on a parity as measures of decision. To know which of two traits is more desirable is a fact usually acquired in education or in one's intercourse with people, but to place oneself in respect of this trait requires some weighing. The score may measure caution, scrupulousness, or other traits equally well if not better than self-consciousness. Perhaps a self-conscious person is apt to be more careful or deliberate or more conscientious, but such a parallelism or correlation still does not justify us in saying that our results are a measure of self-consciousness.

[1] M. J. Ream, " Group-Will Temperament Tests ": *Jour. of Educ. Psychol.*, 1922, vol. xiii, p. 11.

THE RELIABILITY OF THE TESTS

This leads us to the intermediate question on our way to the discussion of the validity of the tests, the question of how consistently a test will bring about a certain response or as May and Hartshorne define it " the similarity of responses made on different occasions ". Only two tests are mentioned as having been subjected to the procedure of self-correlation to establish their consistency value—and of these the Downey tests offer a low correlation, while that of the Woodworth Personal Data Sheet is very high. But it should be pointed out that the latter is not strictly a performance test and allows for the operation of association and memory to a considerable extent. We might accordingly expect a more or less uniform score.

Another method to determine the amount of uniformity in a set of responses, viz., intercorrelation among a number of tests which claim to tap the same trait, produced no better results. Speed of decision, suggestibility, confidence, are not adequately measured by any one of two tests, and the authors of the survey already referred to very properly conclude that " the response to one situation is not a reliable measure of a complex trait. Many situations must be used and many responses given ", but I am not sure that it is altogether a matter of the number of items and that " the greater the number of items, the more reliable is the test ". It seems as if the variety of the items is even more important than their number, and furthermore a sharp line must be drawn between the verbal tests (questionnaires such as the Pressey X–O tests, the various ethical judgment tests and the personal data sheets) and the conduct tests. For the measuring of intelligence a verbal test is quite in place, but in the realm of personality testing, it affords but an indirect clue.

Moral Judgment Tests Not Character Tests. That the various ethical discrimination tests are in reality intelligence tests of a special kind is the conclusion of several investigators who worked with them. Quadfasel,[1] for instance, examined 770 children with the Fernald test as employed by Jacobsohn, and the only positive results he obtained were in connection with the ability of the children to judge between various degrees of right and wrong. The experimenter doubts in fact whether these tests throw any light on the temperament or the moral sentiment of the child, as Sander [2] claims. There is a considerable body of literature on this subject of moral discrimination in children, but even Fernald, with whom this method originated, declared expressly that " Morality or moral stamina may not, as yet, be measured successfully by tests ".[3] Fernald, of course, had not anticipated at that time the possibilities of reproducing life situations, which skilful investigators soon afterwards discovered. What he had in mind was the verbal test which required a judgment response with reference to behaviour questions.[4]

A Behaviouristic Caution. Symonds makes some appropriate remarks on the generality and specificity of a given test. " The line of most progress," he says, " is in the attempts to measure very specific traits or habits. Of

[1] F. Quadfasel, " Die Methode Fernald—Jacobsohns, eine Methode zur Prüfung der moralischen Kritikfähigkeit—und nicht des sittlichen Fühlens ": *Arch. f. Psychiat. u. Nerv'ten.*, 1925, vol. lxxiv.

[2] H. Sander, " Die experimentelle Gesinnungsprüfung ": *Zt. f. angew. Psychol.*, 1920, vol. xvii.

[3] G. G. Fernald, " The Defective Delinquent Class: Differentiating Tests ": *Amer. Jour. of Insanity*, 1912, vol. lxviii.

[4] A confirmatory statement of the inadequacy of the interpretation of fables as a test of character is contained in an article by Lowe and Shimberg, who conclude that the results " make us suspicious of all tests having as their underlying principle the assumption that moral judgments offer a reliable estimation of moral integrity. We are convinced that verbal judgments of moral situations are an index of the individual's intellectual and social apperceptions and not his moral character " (" A Critique of the Fables as a Moral Judgment Test ": *Jour. of App. Psychol.*, 1925, vol. ix, p. 59).

course every test does this—it measures a very specific response to a very specific situation. But the test maker blindly interprets this as a general reaction." He gives instances of two different kinds of traits. Thrift, e.g. " seems to be a bundle of more or less loosely connected special habits —habits with regard to and conservation of materials, earning, saving, spending, and repairing ", while neatness according to this writer constitutes a different kind of trait. " It is the individual's response to a single element in a number of different situations. I have elsewhere called such a trait a confact (cf. concept), to use a word which may acquire a connotation in harmony with behaviouristic notions. A confact is a conduct response (as opposed to a mental or verbal response) to a common element of various situations. It is these confacts that workers have been interested in. . . But the confact must be tested in more than one situation." [1]

The " Confact " Does Not Tell the Whole Story. The distinction between the two types of traits is not quite clear to my mind, but the new concept introduced is a useful one as an intermediate station between the specific response and the trait to be established, since after all it is the trait which we are desirous of placing. I have a feeling that these very " confacts " will in their turn be largely determined by the interests and motives of a given individual, so that a person might be neat and tidy about his or her personal appearance and yet manifest a sloppiness and carelessness about belongings. I have often observed the curious fact that clear thinkers have their desks all littered up with various papers, while many of those who have their papers systematically arranged in the tidiest fashion are muddle-headed. Of course there is a comparison here of intelligence and personality traits, yet the contrast is striking and calls for explanation ; and the explanation seems to lie in the

[1] P. M. Symonds, " The Present Status of Character Measurement " : *Jour. of Educ. Psychol.*, 1924, vol. xv, p. 493.

coöperation of two factors, viz. the rôle of the driving interest and compensation.

We may again turn to the refreshing reminiscences of the late Anatole France, who is describing a social *faux pas* in his seventeenth year, for a state of mind which gives evidence of this duality—a problem so perplexing and one not so rare to meet with as the grand old man of French letters supposed : " What put the coping-stone on my imbecility was that my mind was as daring as my manners were shy. As a general rule, the intellect in young people is crude and undecided. Mine was rigid and inflexible. I believed that I was in possession of the truth. I was violent and revolutionary, when I was alone. When I was alone, what a blade, what a slashing fellow, I used to be ! I have changed a deal since then. Now, I am not overmuch in awe of my contemporaries. I try to make myself as snug as possible between those who have more brains than I and those who have less ; and I trust to the cleverness of the former. On the other hand, I am not without misgivings when I come to look myself in the face. . . But I was telling you about something that happened to me when I was seventeen. You will readily imagine that such a blend of shyness and audacity made me cut a most ridiculous figure."

HOW VALID ARE THE CHARACTER TESTS ?

Hitherto the constancy value of the tests was examined, but now supposing the individual tested does react uniformly, how far are we warranted in inferring the possession of a particular trait from the results in a given test ?

May and Hartshorne have dealt with this question briefly but rather incisively. Five methods of validation are enumerated : (*a*) validation by correlation with ratings, which is the most common and at the same time the most objectionable method, (*b*) validation by correlation with other objective evidence, (*c*) validation by differentiation where a test separates the examinees into distinct groups with but a limited number in a middle class to be wholly disregarded, (*d*) validation by age gradation, such as is true of various suggestibility tests, and (*e*) validation by sampling. All these methods have their drawbacks. The two writers point out that ratings are poor criteria, and even if reliable, we are not certain that the rating is on the same quality which the test purports to measure.

To validate one test by correlating it with another test is to assume that the latter is a standard of comparison, which of course it is not. Validation by means of correlating a test with an actual behaviour record is a sounder method but the behaviour record of an average person, let us say the average student, will probably not contain anything noteworthy, with the result that recourse will be had again to ratings. On the other hand, the behaviour record of delinquents would prove an adequate standard, provided the facts could be disentangled. We must remember that in delinquency, one misdeed leads to another, and the mosaic of crime is often complicated.

As to validation by differentiation, a method which has been exploited by several investigators, May and Hartshorne think it marked by two difficulties in that it " is almost impossible to get two homogeneous and yet contrasting groups " and also because it does not give any information regarding the efficacy of the test in the middle ranges, which are untouched by the segregation of the extremes into two groups, such as aggressive and non-aggressive, timid and bold, etc.

We may omit the method of validation by age gradation for the present, as the characteristics measured by it, like suggestibility, have a greater claim to being considered under the head of intelligence. This applies to all of the tests validated by this method—judgment of relative values, ethical discrimination tests and social perception tests.

They tap knowledge and experience rather than character or conduct.

The Most Reliable Tests. There remains then one other method, that by *sampling*, which consists in "selecting from life-situations certain sample or representative items as test material". Trow's confidence test is offered as an illustration by May and Hartshorne, and their conclusion is that the validity of such tests, as in a large measure of all other character tests, depends on their "symptomatic or transfer value", i.e. "how symptomatic is this test performance of performance in a multitude of life situations"—a conclusion which seems almost self-evident.

Difficulty with Life Situation Tests. Travis in his "Diagnostic Test of Character" (which involves the order of merit technique), given to ten psychopathic patients, used four methods in an attempt to validate the results, (*a*) correlation with associates' estimates, (*b*) correlation with teachers' ratings, (*c*) correlation between intelligence test scores and character test scores, and (*d*) correlation between the results of a test and the case histories and analyses. Only the latter he found to be of service in validating a test of this kind.[1] But the chief difficulty is to devise such tests as approximate the life-situation and at the same time could be scored without complications. The problem is somewhat similar to that presented by animal psychology and to a certain extent solved by the greater facilities, equipment and technique gained in the course of time—the task I am referring to is that of studying the animal in its natural environment and yet controlling conditions to the extent of observing the responses in a variety of situations.

VALUE OF THE AMERICAN EXPERIMENTAL APPROACH

At times it appears as if the American studies of character traits by means of tests were a hit-or-miss affair, lacking the

[1] R. C. Travis, "The Measurement of Fundamental Character Traits": *Jour. of Abnor. & Soc. Psychol.*, 1925, vol. xix.

theoretical basis to begin with. The results are not apparently of the same type that we obtain in experiments on perception or in intelligence testing, but the investigations do seem to bring us closer to a general conception, and in spite of the different starting points, there is a surprising uniformity at least with regard to the negative phase of character testing, so that new paths must be beaten out. We know, for instance from Trow's work that confidence is not an integrative trait which manifests itself uniformly with regard to various situations, but that a person may display confidence in judging lines, without exhibiting the same trait in ethical discrimination and vice versa.[1] Similarly, Filter [2] found that speed of decision cannot be measured by any one test of a group purporting to measure this characteristic. Both Otis [3] and Brown [4] drew a like inference for suggestibility, and the theoretical question now arises : Why this variety of response with a single trait ? Are we mistaken about the label, that is to say, are we confusing a number of different traits by treating them under one head, or is each particular response conditioned by a separate setting, so that one could hardly talk of a trait at all, but is under the necessity of referring to a " reaction under such and such conditions ? " A standpoint like this would be fatal to the study of character as a branch of science. It would imply that we could never tell anything about a man's possible behaviour until it has become manifest ; and that the situation, not the personality or mental constitution of the man, is of paramount importance in prediction. But we do know that the same situation

[1] W. C. Trow, " The Psychology of Confidence " : *Arch. of Psychol.*, 1923, vol. x, p. 40.

[2] R. O. Filter, " An Experimental Study of Character Traits " : *Jour. of App. Psychol.*, 1921, vol. v.

[3] M. Otis, " A Study of Suggestibility in Children " : *Arch. of Psychol.*, 1924-5, vol. xi.

[4] W. W. Brown, " Individual and Sex Differences in Suggestibility " : *Univ. of Calif. Publications*, 1916, vol. ii, p. 425.

elicits different reactions from different people, hence it is the personal organization which counts.

General Function or Syndrome ? To some extent it is true that certain traits are not sufficiently discriminated. Credulity and suggestibility are often mistaken for each other, although I know of not a few instances of non-suggestible people who are credulous and of uncritically sceptical individuals who are unusually suggestible. This, however, does not close the issue. The fact still remains that certain personal traits will reveal themselves differently even for the same person. Does this point to an anomaly ? Before we give up the puzzle, let us ask ourselves whether a given trait like confidence, boldness, or generosity must be envisaged as a general function, or whether it is bound up as a syndrome, to borrow a word from psychiatry, with various tendencies and interests ; and the mechanism of compensation is only one way of accounting for seemingly contrasted and therefore surprising responses on the part of an individual. May it not be that a person's confidence in a certain sphere is due to his strength in that province, and conversely, his lack of confidence with regard to other things is ascribable to his weakness therein ? But compensation, in Adler's sense (see Chapter XVII) implies a developmental affair—the want of the one function has been compensated for in another direction and vice versa. It seems even more likely that we are born with predispositions for some things and not for others, or rather for certain classes of things. The fearless and original Pascal keeps his mind airtight in matters of religion. The temperate Frederick the Great stifles all sentiment to the point of wanton cruelty when he is on the battlefield.

Empirical Analysis Needed. Is it not the *relationship* of the objects or the situations that we must look to for an explanation of the seeming anomaly ? And by this I certainly do not mean the fact that every situation has its own response. If, let us say, a social situation is of an entirely different texture from an abstract situation, then we should not be astonished to find that the same individual will be confident with regard to the one and not with regard to the other. Rather than deny the existence of such inborn dispositions, it would be more sensible to differentiate these dispositions on an empirical basis. Generosity is one of these dispositions in point. Does generosity refer only to material giving ? In the popular sense it is doubtless so taken, but we may query such a narrow use of the word. I have come across misers who would be most generous with their energy and in fact give hours of their time when they would be unwilling to part with the value of ten or fifteen cents. On the other hand, there are men of moderate means who would seldom lend a hand to assist anyone with a difficult task but would generously offer to pay for such work. Some there are who are liberal with funds but niggardly in imparting information, and the converse type is not rare.

The absurdity of making out an inborn trait to be the result of tradition or environmental influence is too palpable to refute and even to mention, were it not for the fact that such views are put forth by a certain species of American psychologist every now and then. All such environmental explanations will be found lamentably wanting in soundness, and when carefully examined will be seen to betray a restricted knowledge of the facts and a circular procedure of inference as is illustrated in the footnote below.[1]

Character Testing on a Comprehensive Scale. Out of forty

[1] R. E. Leaming actually attempts to explain the ready wit of Irish children by saying that the youngsters cultivate it because of the premium set on it by the adults in the Irish community, and at the same time corroborate this conclusion by tracing the money-mindedness of Jewish children (though her data are anything but adequate, distilled probably through the medium of her own prejudices) to the very dubious fact that the " Jewish group hold the ability to make money up as a measuring stick by which the success of each member of the group is measured ". " A Study of a Small Group of Irish-American Children " : *Psychol. Clinic,* 1923, vol. xv, p. 36.

tests which were administered by Lentz [1] to groups of boys alike in age and intelligence, but far apart in conduct, only seven yielded results that were worth checking up. Accordingly six other groups consisting of 242 delinquent and non-delinquent boys were given the tests with no significant differences except in the case of two of the battery. These consisted of a questionnaire and a daily contribution test.

Social Differentiation as Standard. In casting about for a criterion that could be applied as a standard, Lentz found none which could answer the purpose as well as that of social differentiation in terms of delinquency and non-delinquency. The procedure then comes under the " differentiating " class, and the objections raised in a previous section against this method in general hold naturally of this investigation also.

Let us see what the two promising tests are. The first is really a questionnaire consisting of questions on the social conditions of the family, personal likes and dislikes, interests, and activities. This is scarcely a character test in any real sense. The boys were asked whether there were musical instruments or magazines in the home qr not, how often they went to church, how many rooms there were in their apartment, whether they found it easy to be obedient, etc. Assuming that the examinees had considerable insight and were telling the truth, our results might count for something, although even then the bearing of the responses on character is not always evident, but delinquent children cannot be credited with the very qualities which are yet to be proven of them, especially as " no effort was made to check the correctness of the answers to any of the questions ". Hence the differentiation of the groups is not significant.

The daily contribution test is more satisfactory as a measure of a trait, although we cannot be quite certain as to what

---

[1] T. F. Lentz, " An Experimental Method for the Discovery and Development of Tests of Character " : *Teachers' College, Columbia Univ., Cont's. to Educ.*, 1925, No. 180.

the trait is ; and furthermore, the frequency of negative responses interferes with the interpretation of the results. The procedure required every boy to bring every morning for five mornings some interesting bit of material in an envelope provided for the purpose—a news item, a joke, a poem, an advertisement, or even something describing a scene or a conversation in the street. The results indicated that 69 per cent of the unselected group turned in at least one contribution while only 21 per cent of the probation group satisfied the requirement.

The conclusion drawn would appear to be then that the consistent divergence between the two sets of scores proved that the test was a true character test. Naturally one would expect more indifference to a task, laziness, disobedience, and less willingness to accommodate in the delinquent or anti-social than in the social group. There is, however, not sufficient evidence to warrant our holding that the lack of coöperation under such conditions denoted lack of character.

A Surprising Result.   The test is an interesting one, nevertheless, and, in a more elaborate form, might be followed up over a long period of time and with larger groups. The experiment on the whole was valuable in its negative aspects, that is to say, in showing that the other 38 tests, among which are to be found a number of frequently mentioned batteries, did not differentiate the two contrasted groups. In fact— and this is astonishing—the probation group scored higher in the honesty tests which were supposed to represent a miniature life situation. Lentz offers four possible explanations to account for the fact.

First, the government and discipline at the probation school is such that the pupils are especially encouraged to be frank and honest. Second, the Probation Group may be more circumspect and suspicious and thus have evaded the purport of the test. It must be remembered that the validity of any honesty test has not been established to date. Third, it may be possible that honesty is not a factor in school success or, if at all, a negative factor in some schools. Fourth, the motivation may have been different ; the Unselected Group may have been more interested and more anxious to make a high score.[1]

THEORETICAL BACKGROUND OF AMERICAN APPROACH

It is difficult to say whether the conception of the American character testers precedes their empirical work or issues from it as a corollary. The following passage seems to be representative of the American point of view :

> Under the name of character are being ranged for study principally those traits which are of non-moral nature. . . The emphasis is upon the force of activity rather than upon its direction, upon the quality of behaviour in terms of strength, persistence, readiness, rapidity, etc., rather than upon its value as right or wrong, good or bad, wise or foolish, etc.[2]

This seems to be in accord with, or perhaps is based on, Downey's view of the will-temperament which she believes " determines the form assumed by character although it does not determine its content ". Her definition of character involves the organization of native and acquired traits effected through inner subjective factors and outer objective ones.

The behaviouristic leaning of many American psychologists in the general field is also noticeable in the approach to the study of character. Typical of this tendency is the definition that a " person's character make-up would be his exhibition of responses and reactions to inner stimuli and to objective perceivable situations ".[3] It must be repeated here, however, that Watson links character with the demands of social

[1] Loc. cit., p. 31.
[2] R. O. Filter, " A Practical Definition of Character " : *Psychol. Rev.*, 1922, vol. xxix.
[3] J. E. Downey, *The Will Temperament and its Testing*, p. 60 ff.

convention, hence is taking a narrower view than behaviourism would seem to call for, and is practically accepting the popular conception in the most uncritical sense.

Characteristics, Not Character, Tested. Needless to add, I regard the treatment of character by most of the American character testers as altogether too broad in scope, taking in as it does all the non-intellectual elements, and in this way not setting off that phase of personality which properly corresponds with character. The researches referred to in this chapter nevertheless overlap at points with the more delimited territory, and the technique employed and the results obtained often suggest a new tackling point or at least warn against futile methods.

American Testers Reveal Weakness of Phrenologists. On the whole, the American approach smacks of the method of Gall and his co-workers in their attempt to correlate a given protuberance on the head with a definite trait, propensity or capacity. The method in inductive logic, invoked to sanction this type of procedure, would be called that of agreement. It is true that the phrenological doctrine revolved around structures, while the contemporary tests and experiments are centred about the functional side of the individual, i.e. about the question What does he do ? But so long as the connection is not linked up with causal factors, we can never take it for granted that the correspondence which, to the investigator seems preponderant, is anything but incidental. Just as the phrenologist possesses no absolutely reliable information about the alleged amative or philoprogenitive individual as compared with others—for these traits have no significance except in relation to similar ones in other people—so the character tester of to-day must depend on ratings for the most part ; and although our present filing system of characteristics and traits is infinitely superior to the promiscuous miscellany of Gall and Spurzheim, we still have far to go before a classification can be agreed on which would be serviceable even for practical purposes.

Dynamic Note Missing. Such a classification would involve the subsumption of smaller units under large units, but more than that, we should have to gain insight into the cross relationship of traits, compensations, displacements, etc., not necessarily in the narrower Freudian sense, but from the point of view of personality integration. Lastly, the evaluation of traits is of supreme importance ; and for this reason alone a purely mechanistic interpretation of character will yield us no appreciable results. What is more, writers who lack the socio-historical perspective and who are ignorant of the rôle of the cultural sciences in the fabric of modern thought, even if in various German circles this part has been grossly exaggerated, cannot with any competency evolve an applicable system which would stand the onslaught of time.

Cyril Burt, who has had a good deal of experience with these American tests in his professional work as psychologist to the London County Council, finds that they " are too poor for practical work " in spite of the fact that the figures which he hopes to publish in a forthcoming statistical study are encouraging ; and he even holds out the warning that " in this country, teachers and research students should apply such tests very gingerly ". . . [1] For his own work, in order to acquaint himself with the character and temperament traits of his charges, he had adopted the standardized personal interview supplemented by the use of tabular schedules and rating scales.

Chief Value in the Technique. In conclusion, it would be safe to say, however, that the valuable technique of the American character experiments and tests should not be underestimated ; for it opens up at least new possibilities in the matter of checking up impressions and ratings, and holds forth hopes of expansion.

[1] C. Burt, *The Young Delinquent*, 1925, p. 393, footnote.

EXPERIMENTAL RESEARCHES ABROAD

The American technique has not had the same extensive application elsewhere, but beginnings have been made in England and in Germany.   In fact as early as 1885 a study was undertaken by Sophie Bryant at the suggestion of Galton, and afterwards reported on under the heading of *Experiments in Testing the Character of School Children*,[1] which, however, turns out to be a foreshadowing of the Binet method of testing intelligence, and at any rate really bears more on the subject of individual differences in the manner of perception and description on the part of children than on character or even personality traits. Galton's use of the word " character " in this indiscriminate sense, which has already been commented on in Chapter VI, could not be conducive to the development of characterology in England.   Bryant's method was experimental and her main conclusion, viz. that " false perceivers were nearly always ready apprehenders " is important enough, but the only information which even remotely suggests some relation to the characters of her subjects centres about the differentiation between the " reckless " and the " cautious " thinker, who employs in his interpretations such phrases as " I suppose ", or " it is likely " and also about the reference to the " hyper-emotionalism " of some children as revealed by the excessive use of affectively coloured adjectives.

It is gratifying to note that Galton's influence in this direction has not survived and Webb's recent investigation on the character factor in intelligence serves by its very title to accentuate the lack of discrimination in this respect some fifty years ago.

Psycho-Galvanic Reflex and Will Qualities.   Much has been written on the psycho-galvanic reflex in various con-

---

[1] This paper, read in 1885, was published in *The Journal of the Anthropol. Institute of Gt. Britain and Ireland*, 1886, vol. xv.

nections, but the employment of the galvanometer to measure character qualities is a recent development, though not a novel idea. Brown studied the galvanometric reactions (extent and frequency of deflection) of subjects in response to stimuli like a loud unexpected noise, a threat to prick the subject with a pin or to burn him with a match, a pleasant odour, or the offering of candy. Each of the subjects received two independent ratings on various character qualities, and the judges were allowed to revise their markings after three months if they saw fit. The results, after being checked up by several formulæ, show a high correlation between the psycho-galvanic reflex and " those qualities which have an element of ' will ', in the sense of consciously directed activities " ; and it is suggested by the experimenter " that the psycho-galvanic reflex, if it has a real psychological significance, may be closely connected with these ' will-qualities ' or distinctly conative tendencies, rather than with emotions, as has in general previously been asserted ".[1]

Neat Classification of Questionnaire Reactions. In Germany Baumgarten [2] has manipulated the test-experiment successfully with school children from 8 to 14 years of age, among whom she found six or seven different types of reactions. In answer to the question, " What would you do if someone called you a stupid," some children would reply almost mechanically, " I should say, ' You are just as stupid.' " (*Primärreaktion*, " Boomerang " reaction would be a good designation in English.) Others would resort to a more " tangible " response (*handgreiflich*). " I should beat him ", is the reply of this group. The intellectual would demand proof, while the passive would say nothing at all.

---

[1] W. S. Brown, " A Note on the Psycho-Galvanic Reflex Considered in Conjunction with Estimates of Character Quality " : *Brit. Jour. of Psychol.* (Gen. Sec.), 1925, vol. xvi.

[2] F. Baumgarten, " Die Reaktionstypen im sozialen Verhalten " : *Proceed. of 8th* (1923) *Congress for Exper. Psychol. in Leipzig*, 1924.

Then there is a group that would ignore the insult altogether ("I should act as if I heard nothing"). Only five of the types are named and illustrated. Baumgarten does not tell us in her report whether the age of the child has something to do with the type of the reaction, as one might surmise. Her classificatory scheme, however, is adequate because of the clear-cut reactions.

Social Understanding Tested. Another phase of her investigation was to test the level of empathy (*Einfühlung*) manifested by the children, showing how well the subject could appreciate or realize other people's conditions and situations. A number of incidents taken from child life were related to the subjects, who were asked afterwards to anticipate the thoughts and feelings of the individuals figuring in the story. The results of five different tests given to 1,300 children showed six types. There are, of course, the two extremes—those who have no sense whatever for other people and those again who can enter into the situations of their fellow-beings with great aptitude. Between these limits, the writer recognizes four other groups : the children who are inhibited from entering into another person's situation, because of some social injunction, those who are prevented through reflection, deliberation or for some other intellectual reason, the group that can grasp other people's sorrow but not their joy, and, in the class next to the extreme—the cold and correct "empathizers".

CHAPTER XXIV

I

Whether we accept as the pioneer of personality testing Jung, who as early as 1905 devised a series of association tests by which individuals were to be placed in a typological schema, or Fernald, the projector in 1912 of the first set of character tests in the form of questions designed to measure moral consciousness, we find that in the fourth decade of the present century, the psychological atmosphere is precipitate with the measurement of personality elements. I say " personality elements " advisedly, for not even the most sanguine investigator, to my knowledge, will, in the present stage of testing at least, go so far as to claim that he is actually measuring personality as a whole.

An Era of Measurement. This is the era of measurement. In view of the principle that everything which exists, exists in some quantity, *ergo* can be measured, and furthermore, in view of the premise that the more closely a study approaches the scientific ideal, the more frequently its results can be put into quantitative terms, the mathematical movement in psychology is natural enough. It was at first most conspicuous in the numerous reaction investigations of several decades ago, when the Chronoscope was looked up to as a sort of oracle, and perhaps also in the superabundance of psychophysical experiments and discussions which were so zealously conducted in the laboratories and aired in the periodicals.

The intelligence test movement diverted the attention of the average psychologist from the experiment to the test, from the general law to the individual difference ; at the same time

449

it retained the quantitative interest and emphasis on formulae, which Binet himself, the innovator of the intelligence test, could not have foreseen. Nor, would he have relished it, if he had foreseen this aspect. That personality tests, which cropped up first of all in the form of association correlations, ethical questions, emotional tappings, and subsequently will and temperament researches, and motivation analyses, all with a quantitative slant, would follow close upon the heels of the intelligence tests was after all to be expected ; but could anyone have predicted, even as late as a decade ago, the avalanche which bids fair to sweep away from the foreground nearly all interests in American psychology, to the exclusion of personality measurement ?

In 1927, when my *Psychology of Character* first appeared, the chapter entitled " The American Experimental Contribution " with its close to thirty pages seemed quite lengthy as a survey of the field ; at present nothing short of a book would do the subject justice. If our modest ideal at one time was to test traits, one finds that this goal has long been reached or, perhaps better, over-reached. Most personality testers, for reasons which will be examined presently, have sidetracked the trait in order to measure attitudes and interests, opinions and prejudices, complexes and tendencies of all descriptions. In my *Bibliography of Character and Personality*, containing 3,341 titles, there are over 250 references under the quantitative rubric. Since this bibliography was published, the material has been at least quadrupled, and the measuring activity is becoming more intensified from month to month.

On general principles, this approach to the study of character and personality is gratifying. All scientifically-minded people recognize that the subjective treatment of such an important field could not advance our knowledge. It is obvious we must have an objective mode of procedure, if for no other reason than to gain a modicum of uniformity, as for example in the experimental psychology of sensation and perception.

The Purpose of Personality Tests. In surveying the results of the personality tests, our first step is to *ascertain the purpose of the tests*. What do we expect the harvest to yield ? This question has never been asked before, probably because the answer is invariably taken for granted ; and it is taken for granted because the field of testing is scarcely ever viewed in perspective.

As to the question posed, since there seem to be four chief benefits accruing to society from personality measurement, we may say that testing the non-cognitive functions of man has been undertaken, although perhaps not deliberately, for a fourfold reason :

(1) To throw light on the general nature of personality and its mechanism.

(2) To place an individual in relation to others.

(3) To offer a body of sociological data with regard to the behavior of an individual in a group.

(4) To ascertain the best methods for training the young along moral and social lines.

It is evident that the first reason concerns theoretical psychology ; the second bears on psychotechnics, or even applied psychology in the broader sense. To know something about the individual, whether he is emotional or prejudiced, dishonest or generous, is an invaluable guide not only for the employer, but also for the testee. Vocational guidance should be the first beneficiary of personality research, but psychiatry is no less beholden to it ; even medicine and law can acknowledge a certain amount of indebtedness to personality testing, and educators theoretically may gain insight in understanding their charges through the revelations of such measurement. The third purpose is essentially a sociological one, while the fourth is decidedly to promote a pedagogical end, with an ethical (or religious) coloring.

Our next query is : Have the hundreds of quantitative personality investigations borne out their promises ? Can the results of such investigations be placed on a par with the results in the intelligence-testing field ? Do we in consequence of such tests know more about the human psyche both individually and in its social milieu ?

This issue can be dealt with more satisfactorily by reverting to our above-mentioned reasons for administering personality tests (tests to be understood in the widest usage, so as to include questionnaires, interviews, ratings, etc.).

To begin with the first aim : it is questionable, in my eyes, whether the theoretical status of personality has been at all grasped because of the quasi-experimental activity in this field ; and small wonder. We can hardly expect to understand the architecture of a magnificent structure by examining the bricks, mortar, stones, and pillars of the façade. If consensus of opinion, uniformity and objectivity alone were our desiderata, then certainly personality testers have run afoul both of each other and of the mark. The greatest agreement is in the negative direction, e.g., in a tendency to discredit the existence of traits and to break up personality into so many habits and acts.

Results must be referred to a Standard. Has the personality tester succeeded in rating a given individual with reference to others ? This question may be answered " yes and no ". *Every rating presupposes a standard*, but testers are often so busy with correlation coefficients, standard deviations, tetrad difference criteria, probable errors, corrections of formulae, that the standard is lost sight of. It cannot be gainsaid, nevertheless, that the test, if properly conceived and scientifically devised, is of considerable use in diagnosis or even in prognosis. The typologist, pure and simple, unless he possesses an unusually intuitive mind, can scarcely hope to reach the same definiteness and decisiveness as the personality tester achieves by the use of several different batteries of tests. On the other hand, the latter must reckon with different schemes of types or traits, or else his figures will be meaningless. Even in such a rectilinear scale as the intelligence quotient, the mere graduation of the line into 120, 100, 90, 70, etc., *would possess no significance if the figures did not correspond to definite mental levels*, recognized as such in practical life.

An Unexpected Caché. Probably the greatest comparative service rendered by personality measurement has been in the furnishing of interesting data of a sociological nature. This is the unexpected ore discovered in the mines of personality. In the opinions, beliefs, attitudes, and interests of students, to take one group only, we find so many oddities and paradoxes that some of the accepted views in sociological circles will bear revision. It is here that we strike a meeting ground between psychologist and sociologist, and possibly the latter's growing interest in the psychology of personality is largely due to such findings.

Finally, the pedagogical *motif* in the quantitative investigation of personality, it is to be feared, does not fare so well as the sociological groping. Curiously enough, the sociologists received a windfall when they were least anticipating it, while the efforts made by religious bodies to develop the morals and morale of the youth of the country have thus far yielded fruit only in a *methodological* way, which, in itself, is of course no mean asset. Incidentally, the fact that religious organizations have financed quantitative investigations of personality conducted from a behaviouristic angle, as the stimulus-response terminology often shows, is a sign of the times.

II

It is needless to dwell on the shortcomings of most of the scales, batteries, ratings, questionnaires, and personal data sheets ; for by this time the criticisms are fairly well known in characterological circles : the unreliability of ratings, the subjectivity of self-ratings, the inadequacy of information tests as guides of behavior, the inconsequentiality of some of the habits (traits) tested, the inconsistency between what a testee says he would do under the circumstances and what he actually does do, the incomparableness of artificial settings to life situations, and several other such vitiating factors. I have come across tests which incorporate at once three or four of the objectionable features just referred to. One test purporting to give us a clue to tactlessness through the question-answer method lists apparently among tactless acts assault and battery and even murder. This is symptomatic of the omnibus mind bred largely in the United States and intent upon bringing out statistical figures regardless of the incongruity between the correlates.

A Colossal Venture. Instead of examining the minor pieces of research, it would be more to the purpose to take as our instance the most representative of all such investigation, the Character Education Inquiry which was conducted on a gigantic scale by Hugh Hartshorne and Mark A. May, with their centre of operation at Teachers College, Columbia University. The staff of workers engaged in this undertaking, I understand, numbered forty besides the principals and teachers of schools who coöperated with the investigators.

The inquiry lasted five years and was financed by the Institute of Social and Religious Research. Eleven thousand children were tested in various situations for honesty alone. The results of the whole inquiry have been incorporated in three volumes of over 1,700 pages. The enterprise which was carried out with all the technique and efficiency which makes American machinery sought after in every nook and corner of the civilized world, is reminiscent to a certain extent of the organization in the production of a major cinema. We are dazed by the hundreds of tables and figures, scatterplots and histograms, correlation formulae and appendices. If Hartshorne and May had done nothing else than to develop a methodology of character testing, they already would be entitled to a place in the annals of American characterology. Among the subsidiary problems which they probed are the relation of deceit to age ; the relation of deception to intelligence ; the socio-economic background, as well as the cultural background, as a factor in honesty ; differences of nationality and religion ; the honesty reactions of siblings, etc.

It was with some gratification that I noticed that the second volume, *Studies in Service and Self Control*, dealt with the implication of my own doctrine of inhibition as the core of character ; and it is in this phase of the inquiry that the most important and most clear-cut results seem to have been obtained.

In his very comprehensive survey of personality and character-tests, G. B. Watson tells us that

" The considerable attention given to inhibition is probably an outgrowth of Roback's convincing argumentation in favor of ' inhibition of impulses in accord with a rational principle.' as the essence of character. It is to be noted that relatively few of the tests of inhibition follow that definition all the way through." [1] Perhaps that is one of the chief reasons why the consistency or generality of traits has been missed in this project.

The Case for Specificity. The nubbin of this whole prodigious labor appears to be that conduct is specific, and that there are no traits. This *motif* is repeated many times in each of the volumes. Since the children who cheated did not cheat in every test, e.g., some copied, while others would use a key, still others would fake a solution to a puzzle, while not a few would doctor up their answers, or since some would cheat in arithmetic tests and not in completion or information tests,

[1] G. B. Watson : " Tests of Personality and Character." *Review of Educational Research*, 1932, vol. ii, p. 214.

while with others the converse would be true, or since some would steal when the temptation was supplied them, while the majority of cheaters refrained from taking money not belonging to them, it was concluded that neither honesty nor dishonesty was a trait, but that in every case, we are dealing with specific attitudes and habits.

" Our conclusion, then, is that an individual's honesty or dishonesty consists of a series of acts and attitudes to which these descriptive terms apply. The consistency with which he is honest or dishonest is a function of the situations in which he is placed in so far as

(1) these situations have common elements;

(2) he has learned to be honest or dishonest in them, and

(3) he has become aware of their honest or dishonest implications or consequences." [1]

Before we go any further, let us note how the authors stress what they designate as consistency (and what should properly be called uniformity or constancy) and the community of elements in the situation. The attitude or act is, in other words, a function of the situation. Due cognizance of the motive of the child has not been taken except in a separate sheet on one occasion when it was asked what it was that induced cheating in the dishonest. Naturally the answers of the comparatively few " honest " cheaters, i.e., those who admitted copying—answers such as " test too hard ", " Others cheated ", " Lazy ", " Felt like it ', " Test Unfair ", " Too many chances ", " So class would win "—do not give us an insight into the working of the child's mind.

One may go a bit further and express misgivings as to whether a child in grammar school is a fit subject for a character test, the whole weight of which rests on the problem of motivation. For a *genetic* study of character, the school is undoubtedly the best field of operation. It will also be

---

[1] H. Hartshorne and M. A. May : *Studies in the Nature of Character*, 1928, vol. i, p. 380.

recognized that the purpose of the inquiry was largely pedagogical and religious. Moreover, the facilities offered by the
schools and the docility of the children are conditions not
obtainable in factories, plants, and offices.

Rôle of Motives and Viewpoints. At the same time we
cannot shut our eyes to the fact that children of eight or ten
certainly have not yet had the chance to find themselves.
Many of them do not understand the significance of honesty ;
and their inconstancy is, in a great many cases, due to the
fact that they are groping. Situations count, but motives—
and by motives I do not mean merely reasons but the *whole
mental state preceding the act*—count for a good deal more.
Children will cheat in one test and not in another, because

(1) they like one subject more than another
(2) they are more backward in some studies
(3) they have more opportunity to " make a better job
of it "
(4) they feel arbitrarily disposed, or " the spirit moves "
them.

The lack of constancy does not necessarily have to be
explained by the doctrine of specificity. In fact none of the
results, if adequately analyzed and interpreted, militates
against the common sense notion that there are traits governing a multitude of acts, which, though very unlike one another,
are called forth by a similar motive and attitude.

If, as Hartshorne and May contend, the habit and the
situation are the only factors to be considered in honesty and
other traits, then surely since the neural mechanism involved
in copying and in doctoring up answers cannot be the same,
the habit cannot be a common one, and if so, the whole
project of character education is futile, because *training would
have to be applied to every individual set of neuro-muscular
processes involved in every single type of act.* And if the reply
to this objection is that the common elements in all the

specific acts are to be educated in the desirable direction, the concession is obviously made that *there is something which is not specific*, and that that something will have to be discovered before the training could begin. Furthermore, it is more likely that this common element will be a central factor rather than a mere common path leading to an effector. In other words it will be a trait, in which the motive and the viewpoint of the individual are the dominant features.

When a boy in school who is guilty of some mischief in the absence of the teacher rises at the time the culprit is asked to make himself known, he is actuated not so much by honesty as by a sense of bravado and fear of the consequences, particularly by the opinion of his classmates. This is a matter of honor rather than honesty. There is a different congenital tendency affecting the act, just as when a dying gangster in refusing to divulge the name of his assailant acts in accordance with his " code of honor ", although almost every other day he may be guilty of breaking all the commandments of the Decalogue.

Conventional Concepts Without Psychological Foundation. How we can evaluate a certain act and call it cheating or honesty without knowing something about the point of view of the individual in question is a little difficult to understand for one who is not a legalist. *The analysis of a concept must precede the investigation making use of the particular concept.* Honesty is a virtue which exists but rarely, and what is worse, very frequently the term is applied superficially under a conventional purview.

Does the workingman who takes out his family of six for a trolley ride and pays only five fares think that he is cheating the officials of the transportation company who receive individually more in one week than he does for a whole year's hard work ? We say he is dishonest, because in the eyes of the law, his act is culpable, but it is possible that there is a law of equity which judges him differently. Similarly the banker who floods the exchange with bonds for a country which he knows to be on the verge of bankruptcy does not consider himself dishonest, although in reality he is more than dishonest ; nor are senators, in inflating their disbursement sheets at the expense of the tax payers, any different from common thieves, though the neuro-muscular acts are entirely different. The common mental element which connects the two types of behaviour is the knowledge in both cases that the *deed is depriving others of necessities or comforts which are theirs rightfully*, that they are benefiting unwarrantedly by other people's energy. That is what makes the act dishonest—the fact that someone is using another for his personal greed or pleasure without the other's knowledge, consent, or sanction, and without due compensation. Not an act but a principle is fundamental here.

Regulative Principles Produce the Acts more than the Situation or Habit. We must come, in the last analysis, to the conclusion that not a myriad of acts, not a thousand and one independent habits and attitudes constitute character but a few regulative principles curbing the instinctive tendencies through the function of inhibition. In the characterial hierarchy, the acts, it is true, are integrated into habits, but then the habits range themselves into traits, and the traits into principles. The greater the number of elements on a lower level which can be integrated into a higher complex and the more rapidly this organization takes place, the firmer and the sooner has a child's character begun to establish itself. Every intelligent child will learn more from the formulation of a principle as to what type of behaviour is to be avoided than from a whole manual of individual and apparently unrelated rules. Whether these rules, taught in childhood, can be applied to adult situations is another question which cannot be so easily settled, and which adds to the complication of the specificity doctrine. Principles, on the other hand, broaden of their own accord in the course of maturity so as to subsume a variety of situations. The authors make a point of saying that to those who understand the rule of addition, the rule of subtraction must still be taught. That this is actually so may well be questioned. At any rate, it is here that we can perceive a fundamental difference between a rule and a principle.

Far from accepting it as a " fair conclusion " from the experimental data " that honest and deceptive tendencies represent not general traits nor action guided by general ideals, but specific habits learned in relation to specific situations which have made the one or the other mode of response successful ".[1] I should rather consider the results as favoring the view that acts emanate from traits, and traits are a function of constitutional make-up (instinctive urges) and regulative principles.

In his attempt to steer a middle course between the omnibus and hierarchical points of view, G. Murphy asks rather provocatively " If the generalists were entirely right, it is hard to see why one shall need such a very large sampling of specific evidence in order to make a respectable predication in the future. They ought in fact, if completely logical, to admit that an individual having had full opportunity to manifest his honesty in a certain situation could be depended upon to show the same degree of honesty in some new situation ".[2]

Rules and Exceptions. As a matter of fact that is exactly what happens to be the case in everyday life. The convicted forger will not be employed as a cashier or even salesman ; the slovenly matron will not find it easy to secure a position as a cook or maid in a well-conducted institution ; a deserter

---

[1] H. Hartshorne and M. A. May : *Studies in the Organization of Character*, 1928, volume iii of *Studies in the Nature of Character*, p. 372.

[2] G. Murphy and F. Jensen [with a supplement by J. Levy] ; *Approaches to Personality*, 1932, pp. 385–386.

from the army will scarcely be intrusted with a commission of importance even after he has returned voluntarily and become reinstated. It is true, however, that we cannot always predict an individual's behaviour from his previous conduct. An oppressive foreman may be a devoted and kind-hearted husband or father ; a model boy in high school may turn out to be a " wildcat " stock salesman when he gets out of college, etc.

This puzzling feature about character is only natural.

In the first place, our expectations may exceed our rights, considering the scantiness of our knowledge and the chaos of our conceptions, e.g., cheating is a term applied to stealing, copying in school, doctoring experimental results, and extra-marital sex activities. In reality there is very little which is physiologically and psychologically common to all these types of conduct ; and a knowledge of these instinctive urges is most essential. Acquisitiveness and greed are not in the same line as glory-seeking, and both are a bit distant from the pleasure principle manifesting itself in sexuality. The whole mosaic of motivation, as well as the point of view and regulative principles of the individual, must be considered in the predicting of behaviour. Political grafters will not bother with a too small amount, or where the risk is too great, but one can always depend upon their rising to the occasion when a tidy sum is to be pocketed. If there are exceptions, then the exception can be explained. We must surely make allowance for mental conflicts, compensations, fears, physical conditions, and moods in understanding the apparent inconstancy of an individual. After all, that is where psychology is different from physics. Matter cannot determine itself ; man exercises a self-regulative influence. Even inert matter will present difficulties at times. The static of the radio, the problems in television will occur to one immediately, not to mention the indeterminacy of subatomic particles. But the reason why we can predict the behaviour of physical and chemical phenomena is that we *control* the conditions. If we could control in equal measure the mental conditions of the individual we are " sizing up ", the prediction would be just as infallible as in the case of physical entities. We must remember that even biology has its freaks and sports that baffle all efforts at explanation.

A penetrating criticism of the procedure and conclusions of the Character Education Inquiry is contained in P. Lecky's stimulating little book *Self-consistency : A Theory of Personality*, which happens to be the closest approximation to the views expressed in the *Psychology of Character*. We see, incidentally, how the tables are turned on the specificists, in the following cogent argument

> The main objective of the Hartshorne and May investigation was an attack upon personality traits as psychological entities or faculties, an idea which the authors have shown experimentally to be untenable. Yet it seems to us that on the positive side they have swung to the other extreme. The doctrine of specificity appears to be as false and as unpsychological as the notion of faculties. If every act is the function of a specific situation, then, since transfer is virtually negligible, and since the same situation admittedly occurs but once, it follows that behaviour is not predictable at all. For if the situation is unique, then the behaviour which is dependent upon it is also unique, and attempts at training would merely multiply the number of unique acts performed. If this were true, the hope of a science of psychology would have to be abandoned, for a science which can make no predictions is worthless.[1]

A Doctrine which Defeats its Own End. To be sure, the study of character and personality has not reached the high level of reliability enjoyed by physics and chemistry, but we

[1] P. Lecky : *Self-Consistency, a Theory of Personality*, 1945 (Island Press), pp. 12–13.

cannot force the issue by assuming a mechanical attitude toward the whole subject. The didactic object of character research is especially jeopardized by a doctrine which, *ab initio*, spells defeat.

It is well that G. B. Watson, who by virtue of his training showed some leaning to the omnibus school, has come to see the footlessness of a testing which deals with separate acts and habits. In his quite comprehensive survey of character and personality tests he writes :

1. Character testing may be improved by better characterology. We can test almost any conceivable trait, to-day, but are far from testing character.

2. Better characterology will give us better units for study. The inadequacy of the ethical " trait " has been demonstrated too often to need further study. The improvement of character testing will mean testing in units which are the same in their dynamics, their inner structure, in laboratory, home, school, office, or senate.

3. Better character tests will not be content with the measurement of behavior in a few situations, but will present experimental evidence that the pattern really is identical in a wide variety of social and material environments. This is validation.

4. The reliability of tests will be improved, not so much by mere increase in length, as by more accurate insight into the behavior involved, so that errors of misinterpretation and mistaken expectations of consistency are removed.[1]

Reputation as a Guide to Character. What may be considered a sequel to the Character Education Inquiry is the investigation carried on over a fairly long period by Havighurst and Taba with adolescents, principally by means of the

---

[1] G. B. Watson : " Tests of Personality and Character," *Review of Educational Research*, 1932, vol. ii, p. 257.

interview, which, in a sense, affords a more analytic approach than tests.

On the strength of their results the authors believe that " the measures of reputation yield as adequate a picture of character as do several measures of conduct in actual test situations " [1] justifying this finding by the larger coverage which reputation scores involve as compared with discrete test results.

One of the more consequential results happens to be the relatedness of beliefs about honesty, responsibility, friendliness, moral courage, and loyalty in adolescents, which gives evidence of consistency in moral beliefs. On the other hand, the correlation between value rankings and reputation, though positive, has not proved high. Of course, we should realize that ideals, especially professed ideals, do not always go together with practice, but the tests may have been vitiated by the halo effect influencing the opinions of the rating adolescents especially if the ratees were not of the genial type.

An observation which might precipitate a good deal of discussion is " that moral character could be understood only in relation to the over-all personality of the individual. Good character means one thing in one type of personality and something quite different in another. Character is formed differently in different personalities ".[2]

When institutions will realize that in order to neutralize the particular laboratory bias or methodological prepossession of a certain investigator, it is advisable to see to it that the directors of a given piece of research are not like-minded, to begin with, and have not come under the same training influences so that in interpreting and analyzing the results one point of view receives as much consideration as the other —then, and not before, shall we begin to see light in the complicated maze of character and personality tests. Until then we shall still be obliged to ask " Personality Tests— Whither ? "

[1] F. J. Havighurst and H. Taba : *Adolescent Character and Personality*, 1949, p. 309. [2] Op. cit., pp. 87–88.

CHAPTER XXV

There have been many surveys of personality, temperament, and character tests. The two most outstanding of these are by G. B. Watson [1] and by P. E. Vernon,[2] while the whole field of personality has been covered by G. W. Allport and P. E. Vernon [3] who devoted, in their thorough report, a lengthy section to experimental methods. The last-mentioned appeared in 1930. Watson's followed shortly after, in 1932, while Vernon's, which is the most extensive thus far, was published in 1938.

Echoes of the Past. When my own objections to the easy-going presuppositions and sanguine hopes of the American testers appeared in print, they were thought to be cavils showing the bias of the theoretician. So much was then expected of the laboratory activities and conclusions intrenched in statistical computations ; and no doubt much good has come of the testing. New techniques have been devised, fresh angles have presented themselves, and the results had some value *per se*, i.e., where they had not been shown to be invalid by other investigators, but so far as affording us a key to some of the complicated personality and character problems is concerned, we shall see that the criticism brought forth by the present author 25 years ago had been sustained by authorities in their respective fields at different stages until as recently as 1950.

---

[1] G. B. Watson : "Tests of Personality and Character." *Rev. of Educ. Research*, 1932, vol. ii. G. B. Watson is not to be confused with J. B. Watson, the behaviorist.

[2] P. E. Vernon : *The Assessment of Psychological Qualities by Verbal Methods*, 1938, London.

[3] G. W. Allport and P. E. Vernon : "The Field of Personality." *Psychological Bulletin*, 1930, vol. xxvii, pp. 667–730.

We have had occasion to note what G. B. Watson thought of the test procedures in connection with character and personality, in the previous chapter. A more emphatic negative declaration comes from England in P. E. Vernon's 132-page analysis of personality tests, ratings, scales, questionnaires, etc. Here we find the expression " although there is certainly need for objective, and scientific methods in the study of personality, it is difficult to believe that this blind empiricism which takes no account whatever of the psychological significance of the test situation and the test response can yield fruitful results ".

Vernon has himself specialized in psychometry, and he speaks, therefore, not as a " layman " in this instance. If we may regard the year 1940 as another convenient *étape* in the search for trends, we shall find a similar view, in a modified form, stated by a social psychologist who has had considerable experience in testing.

O. Klineberg, in 1940, quoting my statement " it is doubtful whether the combined efforts of all the experimental investigators have established half a dozen new facts or have placed the subject in a new light " added the following comment, " Although considerable time has elapsed since this was written, many psychologists would subscribe to this opinion at the present time." [1]

And in 1943 Stanley Cobb, one of America's representative neurologists and psychiatrists has come out boldly for intuition as playing " a great part even with the most careful psychological investigator of human relationships ".[2]

It is well, nevertheless, that the steady stream of testing still goes on, provided we are not bulldozed into accepting the conclusions, either positive or negative, as final ; and an attempt is made to understand the underlying concepts before resorting to measurement. To some extent the issues

[1] O. Klineberg : *Social Psychology*, 1940.
[2] S. Cobb : *Borderlands of Psychiatry*, 1943, p. 122.

have been threshed out by the present writer as early as 1921.[1]

During the past quarter of a century scores of traits have been nibbled at by means of various empirical methods. Aggressiveness, neurotic traits, and prejudice have been the most frequently probed, but this is not the place to describe or offer specific evaluations of these tests. As a rule, the technique was far in advance of the method,[2] and the theoretical basis or premises were of questionable soundness. Many of the testers are inoculated with special theories, in which often psychoanalysis is merged with sociology or cultural anthropology. This eclecticism can, of course, be turned to advantage in that it is calculated to explain everything, and meet all sorts of objections.

In the course of the last decade or so, the so-called projection tests, factorial analysis, and perception experiments have been in the fore as catalyzers of our characterological insights.

PROJECTION TESTS

Rorschach. The Rorschach ink-blot test which consists of showing to the subject ten cards with symmetrical ink-blots, five of which are in color, and asking for interpretations, is probably the most extensively used and assiduously cultivated of the type subsumed under this heading. Naturally such descriptions are entirely subjective and will show up vast individual differences. What do the different testees stress—form, movement, color, shading, details, white space, etc. ? Many are the conclusions drawn from these perceptions, aside from the discovery of talent or cognitive qualities (intelligence, originality). Impulsiveness, spontaneity, self-discipline, hypercriticism, negativism are only a few of the traits said to be revealed by the responses.

Since Rorschach devised the test, in 1921, it has undergone

[1] A. A. Roback : " Subjective Tests *vs.* Objective Tests." *Jour. of Educational Psychology*, 1921, vol. xii.

[2] A. A. Roback : *Personality in Theory and Practice*, 1950, chap. ix.

considerable change as to the meaning and interpretation of some of the data ; and the norms or standards are by no means uniform for the various Rorschach groups at large, but the reading of the originator's *Psychodiagnostics* alone will be enough to convince anyone of its merit as a sort of personality plummet.

Games and Play. Some of the play techniques developed by Melanie Klein in connection with child analysis, and by David Levy in studying aggressive traits in children may come under the head of projective methods. Klein would let the children play and observe each move while pretending to be preoccupied with her own tasks. The moment, however, the child gave evidence of frustration, blockage, or over-excitability, she would guide and enlighten the child, and in turn gain desired information. Levy had the child interviewed, with several rubber or clay dolls forming a *ménage*. The child would be confronted with various situations and asked how this or that doll would react, it being understood that the child is at the same time projecting his or her attitudes, wishes, aversions, etc. The following quotation may serve as an illustration of the technique.

> In the control situation two rubber dolls of the same type are used. A soft clay penis is placed on one. The girl is told : " This girl sees a boy naked the first time in her life. She sees he has a penis (or wee-wee). She never saw it before. What does she do ? " If a boy, the words are : " This boy sees a girl naked, etc. What does he do ? " [1]

The experimenter seems to have obtained confirmation of Freudian theories positing castration complexes in the boy and penis envy in the girl, whereas J. H. Conn, employing a similar technique, obtained other results, viz.,

---

[1] D. M. Levy : " ' Control-Situation ' Studies of Children's Responses to the Difference in Genitalia." *Amer. Jour. of Orthopsychiatry*, vol. x, p. 757.

There exist varying degrees of acceptance, each to be understood in its own individual setting. Healthy children are not as easily upset as some theorists would lead us to believe. The viewing of the genitals of other children or a glimpse of the parent undressed does not disturb the average child.[1]

Thematic Apperception. A widely known test in the projective category is the Thematic Apperception Test devised by C. T. Morgan and H. A. Murray. The subjects are handed series of indefinite pictures about which they are to weave a story interpreting each pictorial card. Imagination, of course, counts here, but at the same time, the unconscious discloses itself through the longings, aversions, wishes, and complexes which well up in the descriptions. The difficulty is with the interpretation of these themata. There is a tendency on the part of the various workers to read into the accounts different things ; and that, of course, plays havoc with the slightest attempt at standardization. At any rate, the thematic apperception contribution to characterology is thus far still in the exploratory stage.

Completion Tests. A test which involves the choice of one conclusion out of several possibilities in order to complete a series of statements may also be regarded as a projection test. The selection gives us a clue as to the world outlook or attitude of the individual : cynical, buoyant, skeptical, pessimistic, self-indulgent, etc. Like all tests of this type, we are not certain whether the choice made is in terms of permanent or only momentary feelings or ideals, or even masks of sentiment.

The Szondi Diagnostic Drive Test. The Swiss psychiatrist L. Szondi[2] has devised an ingenious projection test employing

---

[1] J. H. Conn : " Reaction to Genital Differences." *Amer. Journal of Orthopsychiatry*, vol. x, p. 754.

[2] S. Deri : *Introduction to the Szondi Test*, 1949.

photographs (six) of each of the following : a paranoiac, a hysteric, an epileptic, a criminal sadist, a catatonic, a manic, a homosexual and a depressive. Subjects are requested to pick out the two individuals in each set they prefer and the two they dislike most. After the forty-eight photographs have been viewed, and the twelve best liked and twelve most disliked have been exposed so that the process could be repeated with these, the selection yields four least and four most disliked. In order to rule out chance, whim, or physiological influences (fatigue, drugs, aches) it is recommended to repeat the test at least six times with a day intervening between successive trials for the series. A supplementary experiment may be introduced by asking the subjects to tell what they can muster about the characters. Hence, in a sense, restricted of course, thematic apperception has its place here.

It is assumed, in the interpretation, that each of the photographs touches off, in some degree, slight or extreme, a different need-system in the organism. Each diagnostic category represents a factor ; and the reactions are said to be *loaded* when four or more choices are involved in any one category (regardless of whether it is a selection or rejection), thus indicating a strong need-tension ; or *open* if the choices are reduced to one, or two, showing either a weakness for that particular need-system or that the tension had been previously relieved or drained.

The positive reactions to a photograph point to unconscious or conscious identification, with the motivational process represented by the particular stimulus-picture, whereas in the negative reaction, there is evidence of a counter-identification although not necessarily a repression of the motivational dynamics in the personality rejected. Szondi operates with Freudian concepts like *id, superego, identification,* but the interpretations do not equate with psychoanalytic mechanisms. On the other hand, there is a good deal of convergence toward field psychology with its vectorial analysis. While the test may seem to be simple, there is an elaborate system evolved in the assessment of the reactions, e.g., choice at one time and rejection at another would suggest *ambivalence*, which again would imply *conflict*. One wonders how the Szondi test would fare in a contest in which graphology, the Rorschach diagnostic, and the thematic apperception tests participated.

The Szondi test has only very recently been put to the touchstone on the part of American experimentalists, and it is too soon to form an opinion of the various aspects. The thesis that after some need had been relieved, the selection of photographs would show a reduced score (because of the " open " reaction in consequence of the absence of, or lowered, tension) is not borne out in at least one investigation reported.[1] The procedure involved a control group and an experimental group of normals and a control group and an experimental group of neuropsychiatric patients. Tests were administered to the patients, both before and after they received electro-shock therapy, and to the normal couples at different intervals after sex relations. No significant differences were found according to the experimenter, which would go to prove that at least in the paroxysmal and sex vectors, the loaded and open reactions have no diagnostic value. Naturally, the test need not be discredited on the strength of some specific bit of contrary evidence, even if conditions were adequately controlled.

Graphology. Among the expressive methods of assessing personality, graphology, despite the traditional strictures on the part of American psychologists who have " inherited " their aversion to it from their experimental mentors, is gradually gaining its status as an empirical approach, thanks

[1] I. A. Fosberg : " A Study of the Sensitivity of the Szondi Test in the Sexual and Paroxysmal vectors." *The American Psychologist*, 1950, vol. v, pp. 326–7.

to clinical progress and interest in psychosomatic circles.[1] Not only are graphologists consulted in large personnel departments, but a number of hospitals both in England and in the United States have not ignored the service of graphology in large-scale investigations. The Harvard University Grant Study which has been conducted for years and will continue to follow up hundreds of students long after they have settled in their career has engaged a graphologist, for some time at least, to delineate the traits of the participants. Certainly graphology affords more clear-cut results than the Rorschach test, which in its present form, does not lend itself as readily to validation.

Field Dynamics. Although, as has already been stated, in the chapter on *Struktur* psychology, the *Gestalt* movement has not, curiously enough, dealt with personality as a whole, it is true nevertheless that it has had some influence in shaping subsequent experimental and clinical procedures. Furthermore since the chapter first appeared, one of the original *Gestalt* group, Kurt Lewin, became the initiator of a sub-school, viz., the topological, and is chiefly associated with the field theory which he has elaborated, supporting it by a series of brilliant experiments.[2] Borrowing his concepts from mathematics and physics, in keeping with the bent of the founders of Gestalt psychology, he adopts the view that in order to understand personality dynamics, we must place the individual and the environment within a field, which we might call *life-space*. Within this field, there are vectors, or forces directed in a given magnitude from organism to some object in the environment, or again from the object to the individual. What starts this force is the *tension* in the organism (hunger, thirst, sex urge), while in the environment are the

[1] A. A. Roback : *Psychology of Common Sense*, 1939, also in his introduction to H. A. Rand's *Graphology*, 1947, and *Personality in Theory and Practice*, 1950.

[2] K. Lewin : *A Dynamic Theory of Personality* (Eng. trans.), 1935.

objects which might relieve the tensions or which may have the opposite effect. These provocative properties, either attracting or repelling, of an object in the field are called *valences*. To a young man in a dance hall, a girl he had not beheld before may have a positive valence, and he would fain make advances to her, but the policeman standing at the door and eyeing him becomes a barrier and, although the valence, i.e., the provocative quality may become enhanced for a while, the realistic barrier will most likely cause a change, and the valence will take on either an indifferent or even a negative quality (change from " the other fellow's grapes are more luscious " to " Oh, the grapes are sour anyway "). The vector is now different both in magnitude and direction, because of the new relationship in the field in regard to the tension of the individual, the barrier and the different sign of the valence (plus to minus). Otherwise, the conflict might lead to frustration and neurosis.

Lewin always considers the present situation. He is concerned neither with its genesis, nor with its goal. Therein lies the strength but also the weakness of the system, for it allows of no predictive cues ; and after all, the objective of all characterology is to be able to foresee future behavior.

In other experiments which have been carried out under his guidance, we do receive some enlightenment as to expectations, e.g., we have been given to understand that interrupted tasks will weigh on our mind and cause tension more than tasks which have been completed, although other non-topological experimenters have found no confirmation of this result. Again, some valuable work on the level of aspiration has come from Lewin's laboratory. What an individual will do when his task becomes too difficult for him, or on finding that he has done better than expected of him, is of course relevant to the problem of traits,[1] but it is still only tangential

[1] A. A. Roback : *The Interference of Will-Impulses*, 1918 (Psychological Monographs, 111). This may have been the first experimental study on the *level of aspiration*. The results obtained therein have been later independently arrived at by other experimenters.

rather than of direct consequence to our subject.

Lewin's investigations of group dynamics have also brought out a number of data useful in tracing the genesis of personality in a social milieu. The artificial creation of " social climates " for a child so as to see how he will develop in an autocracy as compared with a democracy or a libertarian (anarchist) atmosphere is a distinct contribution to experimental social psychology and has some bearing on the study of personality ; but again, the " social climate ", although here the predictive note is not lacking, seems to involve the sidetracking of the very questions which are pivotal to the whole topic, thus shifting the emphasis to interpersonal relations which have, thanks to the sociologists and their allies, occluded from view the very centre of the relations, namely, personality itself, with the result that the individual is lost in a grove or forest of social acceptances and rejections forming a " social atom ".[1]

Factorial Analysis. Of late, factor analysis has been an active form of research in personality. In England, C. Spearman has brought up a whole generation of statistically-minded psychologists at the University of London. L. L. Thurstone, and, to a less extent, T. L. Kelley, have been almost equally influential in the United States first in dealing with mental measurement and then transferring their methodological presuppositions to correlations of personality traits. Perhaps the most articulate of Spearman's students is R. B. Cattell who has had the facilities for engaging in and directing numerous investigations leading to the discovery of all sorts of factors which govern various traits or constellations. Spearman began with a general factor (g) for intelligence and specific ability in a given direction (s) but now the full alphabet would not suffice to label conveniently, with a

[1] Helen H. Jennings : *Leadership and Isolation—A Study of Personality in Interpersonal Relations*, 1947 (Longmans Green). H. S. Sullivan (*Conceptions of Modern Psychiatry*, 1946) was the leader of the interpersonal school of psychiatry.

single letter, each of the large number of factors which investigator after investigator claims to have found. In many cases the factor is simply an X to designate some simple or, for that matter, complex trait.

Cattell is at odds with current experimental methods in tackling the problems of personality, berating the procedure in which the existence of a unitary trait is assumed, without any supporting evidence, a criticism which the present writer has made on several occasions. Cattell, however, goes further. He would not validate tests by life situations, which he regards as peripheral but by the correlations among the test variables —internal validation. Success in life, according to him, is not the real criterion of intelligence. We may grant that, but would internal consistency in correlation of honesty tests be a better criterion of character than actual conduct in life situations ? Perhaps it is again a question of training or predilection as to what one thinks is paramount, and again we are reminded of M. Poirier's dancing master in Molière's *Le Bourgeois Gentilhomme*. Cattell's censure of experimental psychologists as a class goes so far as to say that " the investigator becomes an experimentalist only by ceasing to be a psychologist " [1] simply because the most significant dynamic phenomena dealing with man cannot be brought into the laboratory.

At any rate the primary personality factors as deduced from internal correlation are as follows :—

A. Cyclothymia-Schizothymia.
B. General Ability.
C. Stable Character—General Emotionality.
D. Sthenic Emotionality—Frustration Tolerance.
E. Dominance—Submissiveness.
F. Surgency—Melancholy.

[1] R. B. Cattell : *Description and Measurement of Personality*, 1946 (World Book).

G.　Character Integration—Dependent Character.

H.　Adventurous Rhathymia—Withdrawn Schizothymia.

I.　Anxious Emotionality—Rigid Poise.

J.　Neurasthenia—Vigorous Character.

K.　Cultured Mind—Boorishness.

L.　Surgent Cyclothymia—Paranoia.[1]

These are the twelve first-order factors in rank of importance. Tentatively four second-order factors have been extracted, viz., (a) social status, (b) tenacity tension vs. adjustment, (c) excessive or easy reactivity vs. general inhibition, (d) security—good heredity vs. anti-social qualities.

To be sure, the list provides food for thought ; but, say what you will, there appears to be considerable overlap, and for the life of me I cannot understand, internal validation or not, why surgency-melancholy should be more important in personality assessment than the character-integration—dependent-character correlates, and why the cyclothymia-schizothymia pair stands first and the surgent cyclothymia-paranoia factor is last on the scale. It only goes to show once more that statistics cannot take the place of fundamental valuations. Mathematics might be of great assistance in guiding us to a certain purpose but not in discovering or establishing the value of the purpose in the first placé. However, even if we cannot agree as to the final and long awaited outcome, the lively discussion in the book and some unusual caves are, in themselves, of considerable advantage.

The factorial school is methodologically aligned with operationalism, which aims to achieve a set of mathematical formulations, in the first place, no matter what else may be the outcome of a particular probing. The relationship between

[1] In his later *Personality : A Systematic, Theoretical and Factual Study*, 1950 (McGraw-Hill), he omits J, and adds *M* : Bohemian Unconcern vs. Conventionalized Practicality and *N* : Sophistication vs. Simplicity. Some of the labels are altered too. Thus in H, Rhathymia is replaced by Cyclothymia.

any two measurable qualities or trait will constitute a dimension. Hence, the title of Eysenck's *Dimensions of Personality*,[1] which purports to reveal the correlations among physical and mental characteristics, expressive movements, etc., in the last analysis suggesting a hierarchical structure, in which the most salient factors are (a) intelligence, (b) introversion-extraversion, (c) neuroticism, which, as has been shown above, rank high in the 12-factor schema of Cattell, although the last of the triad, in his case, is broken down into different factors, and assigned a polar position in his table !

Self and Perception. Considerable impetus in obtaining a new angle on personality has been derived from perception experiments. Partly due to the *Gestalt* movement, but partly the consequence of experimental expansion, thanks to the increase of workers and situations, the relation of the self to the perceptual processes which was hitherto neglected, because of the need of isolating the objects, has come in for special study. Since this happens to be a period of merging in the physical sciences (biophysics, physical chemistry, biochemistry, astrophysics) as well as in the mental and social sciences, the least to expect is the rapprochement between topics in the same science. Hence small wonder that the subject for a symposium announced for the 1949–1950 academic year at the University of Texas reads : *Perception : A Focus for Personality Analysis*, and the 1950 Meeting of the American Psychological Association has devoted two full sessions to the discussion of experimental results in this territory, which combines personality with perception.

PERCEPTION AND PERSONALITY

It would seem as if the rôle of organic wants and tensions in perception has only recently been discovered, although psychologists several decades ago made explicit references to

[1] H. J. Eysenck : *Dimensions of Personality*, 1947 (Kegan Paul).

it. Two types of determinants are now recognized in yielding a particular perception (a) the structural which are the external, objective, or factual configurations, whether lines, dots, figures, objects, or organisms ; (b) the functional which stem from our past experience, or are affected by our present moods, needs, and tensions, in other words, what is derived from our own personality. If we have just finished a satisfying meal we are not likely to interpret vague pictures as articles of food, but if we are very hungry, we may well do so. Repression causes us to overlook, to fail to perceive certain items, or to take more time or requires greater illumination. Our friendly attitude toward someone will prevent us from recognizing some of the weaknesses, while attributing flaws in an exaggerated form to those who have slighted us. It has been found that frustration does something to our perception, and that distortion is a function of our state of mind.

It is needless to cite references to the increasing number of investigations in this sphere. Some are of consequence ; others are trivial, e.g., whether or not rich children exaggerate the size of coins, and poor children underestimate it, the result has little significance, even if the experiments should have been conducted under ideal conditions, except perhaps as a lead to something more enlightening.

An Irony. What, however, does strike one as curious is that although William McDougall, more than four decades ago, insisted on the motivational factor in all perception as a postulate of his doctrine of instincts, he was practically jeered at by the generation that had grown up on behavioristic pabulum, but as with the general theory of instinct which had been wholly rejected by most of his colleagues for over a quarter of a century and is now being approached somewhat remorsefully, so the perceptual potentialities inherent in the instinctive components are being discovered anew through neat techniques, and amidst a host and variety of situations devised by a small army of experimentalists. Maybe within a few years it will be discovered who the originator was of the felicitous hypothesis. This very occurrence is in itself, a forceful, if ironic, illustration of the truth inherent in the proposition that our perceptions are influenced by our biases. . . .

The bearing of the whole matter on personality is, however, more marked now than has been the case years ago, for one thing, because once the relationship between perception and personality status is established in quantitative terms, and our objective is not to explore the field of perception so much as personality, then by studying the results gained from perception under certain controlled conditions, we could deduce, in reverse, definite facts as to personality status—a process we might perhaps call " retrojection ". Thus far the experiments and tests throw no light on character in the proper sense, but conceivably such as will apply to it are in the making.

CHAPTER XXVI

THE CHEMISTRY OF PERSONALITY AND CHARACTER

That the chemical constitution of the tissues is something more basic than the build or physique almost goes without saying. Morphological patterns are only cues to personality. There is no apparent causal relationship between mesomorphy and aggressive personality except in the sense that well-developed muscles will be more useful in combat, and will perhaps be more likely to precipitate action, whereas the presence or absence of certain hormones, calcium, phosphorus, or iron may actually be instrumental in inducing a particular state of mind or initiating a mode of behavior. To a certain extent this was assumed in the ancient doctrine of temperament as a function of the humors.

Since the doctrine has no physiological basis it naturally could not thrive ; and although latterly the hormones were thought to be the mainsprings of our temperaments, the chemique of personality did not begin until the researches of Charles Richet and Claude Bernard paved the way for a broader perspective. Léon Mac-Auliffe [1] might, in a sense, be regarded as their successor, and in his lectures at the Sorbonne he dealt with human morphology in terms of differences between animate and inanimate matter in respect to colloids and ions (e.g., the effect of the ions on acidity and alkalinity) and osmotic pressure, leading to the subject of varied hydrophily and its effect on the bodily tissues, which, in turn, produce the flat type in some cases, and the round type in others. (See below, pages 91–93, for the fuller discussion.)

---

[1] L. Mac-Auliffe : *Les Mécanismes intimes de la Vie* (third separately published part of *La Vie Humaine*), 1925.

Acidity and Temperament. About the same time G. J. Rich [1] in a series of experiments found that excitability and irritability depended in large measure on the incidence of acidity; and that creatinine was a like precipitate. D. Laird similarly obtained results which align calmness with a condition of alkalinity; and thus the suggestion was put forth that milk acts as a relaxing agent. Investigations on blood groups tend to show that those belonging to type IV are much less susceptible to mental disorders than those of type I and III. [2]

H. W. Sheldon, too, after setting up his somatotypes is now turning to a consideration of the chemistry that might be involved, and the hunches scattered in so many publications may soon receive experimental validation.

Popular Chemo-Analysis. It may not be amiss even to look into the popular fancies of writers who, without sufficient scientific training, may have nevertheless observed shrewdly over years, and found something which may turn out worth while. Victor Rocine wrote a number of books advocating a new branch of science to deal with an analysis of basic chemical types. He tabulated 19 types. [3] His follower, B. G. Hauser, reduces the number to 11, viz. (a) calcium, (b) potassium, (c) phosphorus, (d) sodium, (e) chlorine, (f) silicon, (g) oxygen, (h) nitrogen, (i) carbon, (j) hydrogen, and (k) sulphur. Of course, the approach is such as would not appeal to serious students of psychology or chemistry; for it appears to take much for granted, but I contend that we should not discard the matter entirely, for amidst the chaff there will still lie a grain of wheat.

According to this theory, calcium and silicon develop the bone temperament and give us the angular face, while the

---

[1] G. J. Rich : " Body Acidity as Related to Emotional Excitability." *Arch. of Neurol. and Psychiatry*, 1928, vol. xx.

[2] F. Proescher and A. S. Arkush : " Blood Groups in Mental Disease." *Jour. of Nervous and Mental Disease*, 1927, vol. lxv.

[3] V. G. Rocine, *Foods and Chemicals*, etc., 1923.

ligaments are built out of sodium, in conjunction with potassium and chlorine. The ligamentous temperament goes with the triangular-shaped face. Sulphur and phosphorus are the basis of the nervous system (brain), hence the mental temperament (what Sheldon calls the cerebrotonic) will be recognized in the pyriform-oval shape of the face. The circular face belongs to the vital types (carbon, nitrogen, hydrogen, and oxygen).

The Phosphorus Type. How these writers settle everything in a jiffy and tell you what to eat, whom to marry, and what diseases to be especially on guard against may be gleaned from the following passage :

The phosphorus type weighs 85 to 125 pounds. She is four feet to five feet two or three inches. She eats like a bird. She is dreamy and abstract. She has large soulful eyes and a gentle, timid bearing. She lacks vim, vigor, fire and animation, because she lacks red blood.

This type has weakened, through non-exercise, the vital and motor consciousness, the systems and organs of work, digestion, and locomotion. Hence, she is inert ; a dreamer but not a doer. She is beautiful, artistic, ambitious for angelic perfection. She has a very broad and high forehead, but a very small and pointed chin, a small neck and drooping shoulders. She may inspire others to work and accomplish things, but she must learn that it is necessary to keep *balance* between blood, brawn, and brain, before she can make her dreams come true without depending upon others. If all people developed as this type has, the race would soon die out.

Affinity Type : The phosphorus type instinctively shrinks from marriage, but she is conventional in traditions and training, and she is dependent ; which are, perhaps, two good reasons for marriage. Her tastes run to elegancies, to artistic environments, to excitement and to society life ;

all of which require much money. Therefore, she should choose a refined and educated potassium type, who is able to make plenty of money, or else a gentleman of any type who has inherited a fortune.

Disease Tendencies : She is too fond of sweets and delicacies in foods, and will run short of the blood and heart salts ; consequently she is disposed to suffer from anemia, heart ailments, and nervousness.

Specific Foods for the Phosphorus Type : Nice, yellow olive oil, as well as chlorine, sodium, sulphur, magnesium, manganese, iodine, potassium.[1]

True, it is difficult to swallow all this whole, but it will do no harm to give the system a moment's thought and consider each turn separately, checking it against what has been proposed by established methods.   Some parts of the farrago may make sense after all when related to what is known of the properties of these substances and bodily tissues. [2]

Calcium and Personality. With regard to calcium alone, J. J. Michaels has reviewed the literature citing 176 references. He pertinently asks :

> Where are the points of contact between calcium (in itself a most inert substance) and the personality as a whole (a dynamic energy system), and where do they become unrelated and disparate phenomena ? When the functions of the nervous system are regarded as integrative activities, where can one fractionate events and decide which events are more important than others ?

Quite reasonable is his tentative reply :

> With scientific progress, facts (constants) are valued not so much in their isolation as in their relationship to each other and in the meaning that they bring to the total situation (irreducible variables). The more complex the problem, the less likely is a single factor to be found as the

[1] B. G. Hauser : *Types and Temperaments*, 1930, pp. 70–71.
[2] See note on page 486.

dominating causal one. Usually there are a number of subtle interreacting forces, a plurality of causes, that seriously complicate the analysis. This finds its most complete expression in the human personality.[1]

As we scan the conflicting findings of the numerous investigators, we can be certain only of one thing, and that is that there are too many variables, and perhaps what may be called " chain reactions ", to warrant the supposition that one substance would be directly responsible for personality changes on a large scale, although nervous irritability has, in many instances, been traced to calcium metabolism factors.

Drugs and Personality Changes. Scores of experiments have been conducted in order to study the effects of drugs like caffeine, benzedrine, or strychnine, in comparison with the barbiturates, on learning and efficiency. We know too that during the Nazi War, courage, or perhaps foolhardiness, was artificially induced in the German flyers by means of drugs like heroin. It is only recently that the investigations have been slanted in the direction of personality exploration. What certain hormone- or vitamin-deficiency does to the emotional tone of an individual has been known for some years. That some drugs are stimulants, others depressants, has been recognized as an everyday fact, but the potency of thyroxin, testoterone, pituitrin, or adrenalin had to be established.

It is via the clinics and psychopathic wards that results come to us, for the most part, showing changes in personality, but our own experiences, e.g. when we " cave in " from hunger (the condition of hypoglycemia in many of us) and become so irritable as to be unpleasant company should have taught us that chemical changes in our body are determinants of special mental states. In some cases of exophthalmic

[1] J. J. Michaels : " Neuropsychiatric Aspects of Calcium as Viewed from the Different Levels of the Personality." *Archives of Neurol. and Psychiatry*, 1935, vol. xxxiv, p. 362.

goitre where it is not wise to resort to surgery, radioactive iodine (popularly referred to as an " atomic cocktail ") is administered to the patient. The change in personality is fairly marked to the naked eye, but one wonders to what extent the change is permanent, any more than it is in the intoxicated. Then again, privations and deficiencies, or else excesses, may raise or lower the inhibitions, and yet in times of mental crises or stress, there is no telling what an individual will do, no matter what his physical condition happens to be, in consequence of his exhausted supply of vital chemicals. Apparently, then, there is something in many of us which can countervail the physical conditions when the goal before us is vivid or strong enough.

Character and Colloids. Perhaps man is, as Jacques Loeb taught, nothing but a mass of colloids, perhaps we may yet discover that nuclear fission and the release of energy have their analogue, on a miniature scale, in the nervous system of humans. Perhaps the physico-chemical constitution of the blood is not without its effect in shaping the course of personality, in some way affecting our character, but that is just the difference between man and the lower animals, not to speak of inert matter. The former *can* rise above the welter of impulses and tendencies. With all the pangs of hunger, he can carry out a firm resolution to starve to death in order to call attention to his grievances. In other words, an idea (whether an idle fancy or an ideal) through its physiological or chemical vehicle, in the last analysis can stir up and rearrange the original electro-colloidal composition of the individual ; and thus it is character which supervenes.

Behavior Analysis. Let us, by all means, study chemical processes as applied to human behavior. Let us expand this new combination which is sometimes called psycho-pharmacology, i.e. the field which is dedicated to the investigation of psychophysical reactions induced by certain drugs, but let us not imagine that because of the causal relation there is no possible self-determination, or that the bond cannot be weakened or even severed through a firm decision.

As K. Goldstein writes, " a chemical description will never adequately explain a biological process. It can never do more than disclose factors—essential ones, we grant you— necessary to the course of the performances, and can only show how they appear under isolated conditions. To understand the phenomena and by means of these to understand the organism, requires above all *behavior analysis.*" [1] Goldstein cites an authority like H. J. Jordan in comparative physiology as sponsor of the view that the explanation of life through causal analysis must be abandoned for all time. Perhaps that is a bit too emphatic, but thus far one might very well agree, chemique or chemism has not fulfilled its promise to account for all our temperamental or characterial differences, or what is more to justify them in face of interpersonal exigencies, i.e. moral and ethical adjustments.

NOTE.—In a far more reliable work, L. Berman brings together a great deal of information on the relation of food to temperament and behavior. As in his book on the glands, more suggestive but less scientific, he now speaks of water-centered and salt-needy types, of sugar, alkaline and acid types, making it all a matter of chemistry and metabolism. " To-day it is known," Berman sums up the story, " that bodymind chemistry is the link between the two sets of effects [climate and culture] establishing a law of relationship between climate, culture, and character." [2]

He stresses the rôle of food and hormone control as against concentration on the genes, since we can do nothing about the latter ; and his conclusion may be stated in the dictum " Stability of character, then, depends upon stability of metabolism ". An interesting dichotomy is introduced between the homeostatic individuals (those whose blood, tissue, and nerve chemistry tends to balance over a long period— perhaps even a life-time) and the heterostatic type, marked by fluctuations. " The true conservative may be said to have a fairly rigid bodymind chemistry . . . the heterostatic, on the other hand, is constitutionally a revolutionary. A rebel, a revolter, a progressive, he must be, because change is the essence of his own dynamics." [3]

Earlier in the same volume, we were told that " character then, is a function of the individual's ability to oxidize energy-providing foods quickly and in sufficient amount ", qualifying this by the reservation that this applies, at any rate, to what goes under the name of endurance. But endurance in a race is hardly of a piece with the fasting, say, of Gandhi.

[1] K. Goldstein : *The Organism* (Eng. trans.), 1939 (World Book), p. 208.
[2] L. Berman : *Food and Character*, p. 342, 1932 (Houghton Mifflin).
[3] Loc. cit., p. 191.

CHAPTER XXVII

If this chapter is circumscribed in its treatment, the fault is not in the paucity of the material but rather in its too extensive scope. We should remember that the philosophy of character is not in any sense a part of the psychology of character, but since it does offer some points of contact with our subject, it is desirable that we should take a glimpse into its claims, at least after disregarding *en bloc* the countless books and articles dealing with the problems of individuality and individuation, the self, and the purely metaphysical discussions of personality in which personality is contrasted with object, world, externality, society, etc.

Character Implies Human Differentiation.—Certainly we are not concerned with contrasts or *a* contrast rather, but with *human differentiation, its essence and application.* Hence the whole philosophical literature on character and personality is only incidental to our task. The locus of our study is not philosophy but psychology, and, indeed, it is possible to maintain that there can be no metaphysics of character, except in a metaphorical sense, similar to that in which Schopenhauer's Cosmic Will is employed.

THE METAPHYSICS OF CHARACTER

Nevertheless, votaries of an idealistic philosophy have always found a way open for conversion of the term " character " into a metaphysical principle, so that it might serve as the *fons et origo* of diversification in man. We are reminded here of Leibniz's doctrine of monads, according to which each monad is different from every other and reflects the Supreme Monad in its own peculiar way.

Objective idealism, together with its recent offshoots, has also assigned a somewhat precarious place to character in its system. It is thought that character emanates from the Absolute, and unfolds itself in society. The particularity of character—that which gives the concept its *quale*— seems to be entirely lost sight of by philosophers of this stamp,[1] with the result that the empirical fund of knowledge about character, its psycho-biological basis, becomes subservient to the preconceived all too general scheme of things Under the circumstances, nothing but an empty formalism can be looked for.

To entangle the subject with philosophy is fatal from the very start in that we are committed *ab initio* to a point of view which is apt to determine the selection of our facts and to colour them afterwards, so that the divergence of views will become more marked with every step of the procedure.

Necessity of Consulting Philosophical Movements. Can we

[1] That this view is not defunct yet may be gathered from E. Pierce's recent *Philosophy of Character* which deals with the subject-matter expected from the title of the book in a few pages, while taking up all the problems of metaphysics in the bulk of the book. The reason given for this apparent divagation is that it is necessary to recognize " the mysterious activity of the individual " which must be free in the sense that it results from inward, not outward determination and " to furnish a complete theory of character would then involve all branches of knowledge " (p. 19).

The subjectivistic note of this philosophy is struck in turns such as these :

" Character as an active force in the world assumes real spiritual individuals . . . Character . . . can be stated only in terms of an idealistic philosophy, a philosophy which holds that reality is mental ".

" The study of character is the study of the activity that produces our universe . . . Thus human history becomes an account of the unfolding of human character."

I admit that there is some truth in these statements, but cannot see any scientific value in them ; for even if they are granted, we cannot do anything more with them, except perhaps to inculcate them into the minds of the uncritical for the purpose of providing an inhibitory stimulus. Otherwise before going to history and philosophy for our guidance, it behoves us to *study the individual human beings* who, after all, are our sole guarantees that there is such a thing as character.

then steer clear of philosophy altogether and confine ourselves to the so-called scientific and literary aspects of character ? Perhaps it would be expedient to do this, but the treatment would suffer from a certain narrowness, inasmuch especially as fundamental issues in psychology have lately become bound up with philosophical attitudes. In Germany the growing prestige of the *verstehende* (interpretative) *Psychologie,* as contrasted with analytic psychology ; the widening rift between the sciences of nature and the mental or cultural sciences which has now come to a head ; above all, the question of valuation which is basic for the conception of character— these and like circumstances make it incumbent on us to view at least the philosophical environs of character.

But there is this difference between such a compromise and an out-and-out philosophical approach : in our present inquiry, we adhere as much as possible to generally accepted facts in the sciences until compelled to resort to theory or called upon to apply our information, in this way staving off the controversy as long as possible.

Philosophical influences have permeated all the sciences ; and this holds true especially of Germany. Even psycho-analysis has been harnessed with philosophy, at least in one of its contemporary expressions, viz., the phenomenological school of Husserl. William Stern, who was practically the founder of differential psychology, has now abandoned his original work in the interest of what he calls *critical personalism,*[1] which gives the upper hand to philosophy in the determination of character.

AXIOLOGY OF CHARACTER

A still greater force has been exerted by the phenomeno-logical school, which has enjoyed the coöperation of the brilliant M. Scheler[2] on the axiological side and has enlisted

---

[1] W. Stern : *Die menschliche Persönlichkeit.*

[2] M. Scheler : *Der Formalismus in der Ethik und die materiale Wertethik* and *Wesen und Formen der Sympathie* (1923).

in its ranks psychiatrists like Jaspers,[1] and, to a less extent, Kronfeld,[2] who bring to bear upon their psychiatric experience a philosophical grasp of unusual scope. The last-mentioned really draws his nurture from Fries through his apostle Leonard Nelson.

Purposive Note in Philosophy of Character. To be sure, there is a great deal of psychological material in the works of the writers cited, and for that reason their contributions are valuable from our standpoint, but because of the extreme systematization which characterizes these and other works of a similar sort, it would be impossible to do justice to them in brief compass. The numerous distinctions drawn, while not without reason, require a rather detailed exposition which, however, would take us too far afield. Another drawback is the somewhat cumbersome terminology with which each of the systems referred to is saddled. What seems a common factor in these treatments is their *purposive approach to the subject.*

To take one instance, Stern speaks of self-ends (" autotelia ") and other-regarding ends (" heterotelia ")—a distinction commonly used in British psychology and ethics. He further introduces such phrases as the " convergence " of heredity and environment, the " introception " of the other-regarding ends into the self-regarding ends, abstract ends (" ideotelia ") and co-ordinate ends.

Stern's Personalism. Conation, as with the British psychologists, holds a foremost place in the dispositions of man. These he divides into (*a*) directive and (*b*) auxiliary tendencies which are always in readiness to serve the former. Character, according to Stern, is the unit of all the directive dispositions of a person, including the two self-regarding tendencies, viz. self-preservation and reproduction, and the three sets of other-regarding ends, viz. (*a*) those which govern

---

[1] K. Jaspers : *Psychologie der Weltanschauungen* (1922).
[2] A. Kronfeld, *Das Wesen der psychiatrischen Erkenntnis*, vol. i (1920).

social or superindividual interests (family, nation, society), (b) those connected with fellow-beings, i.e. the sympathetic tendencies, and (c) those dealing with abstract ends.

The auxiliary dispositions as an organization of abilities and aptitudes (skill) also constitutes a unit which goes by the name of the psychophysical health status. This organization is in the service of the unit of directive dispositions or character.

It is clear then that Stern subordinates the intellect, represented by the dispositions of ability, to the will, which realizes the purpose of the totality of dispositions. It is also evident that we are moving here in a sphere of values, especially as the conflict between the directive and the instrumental dispositions is brought on the scene. It is Stern's view that every physical or mental disorder is the result of such friction between the two orders of dispositions.

Perhaps the central feature of Stern's system is the firm stand against the " mathematization " of personality. A curious concept of " teleomathematics " is developed which strikes a compromise between quantitative measurement and qualitative interpretation. Many of his observations on the various measuring values (*Masswerth*) of personality (" personal zero ", " personal constants ", " personal thresholds ", " personal scope "), his treatment of equation as a purposive function,[1] and his discussion of the transfer (*Überlagerung*) of thresholds (for instance, the change of fine discrimination in certain spheres and under certain conditions as the person's circumstances change) are certainly of considerable importance, but unfortunately it is not possible to condense Stern's presentation, unless we resort to tabulation which would scarcely be of service.

Delving into Hidden Fundamentals. Scheler's point of contact with our territory is not so direct and his exposition

---

[1] W. Stern, *Person und Sache*, p. 349 ff., and *Die menschliche Persön-lichkeit*, p. 20 ff.

is encumbered with a scholastic method which reveals an unusual hankering for the drawing of distinctions. At times it appears that he is juggling ideas, always showing three or four different ones in the air and asking us to note their difference in other respects than those anticipated or established heretofore.

Character to him is the constant of dispositions in a person, whether volitional alone or mental in the general sense, but *person* is a concept which underlies character, which permits of no change and cannot be affected by illness, as is the case with character. The *person* is equipped by Scheler with transcendental qualities, while character takes its source in causal relations.[1]

In a book of less compass,[2] Scheler touches upon another phase of our problem, viz. the manner of comprehending other persons. It is here that he develops his concepts of *Mitgefühl*, which he defines more narrowly than Darwin and Spencer and *Einsfühlung*, a term that is reminiscent of Lipps's *Einfühlung*, but approaches rather the notion of *identification*. This process, according to Scheler, takes place in all situations where the " I " has been absorbed by the " other-I " (hetero-pathic) or where the " other-I " has been momentarily swallowed up by the self (idiopathic). The situations cited are those occurring among primitive peoples, in mystical ecstasy or religious orgies, in hypnotism, in infantile life, in cases of obsession, in love and masochistic or sadistic relations.

Impersonal Intuition—the Instrument of Understanding. It does not take much imagination to realize that Scheler borders on the mystical in his conception of *Einsfühlung* as well as in his view of transpersonalism which denies that we have a more intimate knowledge of ourselves than of others. His impersonal psychic totality, which is akin to James's stream of consciousness, seems to make no distinction

---

[1] M. Scheler, *Der Formalismus in der Ethik*, etc., p. 501 ff.

[2] M. Scheler, *Wesen und Formen der Sympathie.*

between mind and mind. At the bottom of this view is probably the transmission theory in James's later development. In any case, the cognition of human beings becomes from this angle a simple affair which, however, in practice turns out to be well-nigh impossible.

While discussing various types of sympathy, Scheler has occasion to add a grain to the study of character, especially as his psychological insight and keen analysis compel us to reconsider ordinarily received views without, however, necessarily accepting his conclusions even in the rare cases where these are clearly stated.

THE EPISTEMOLOGY OF CHARACTER

Although the title of Jaspers' recent work is *Psychologie der Weltanschauungen*, it, too, is mostly of a philosophical nature. In this comprehensive volume are passed in review the numerous types of philosophical attitudes in systematic order, with special reference to the psychological motives at their root.   Fichte long since declared that the kind of philosopher a man is will depend on the kind of man he is ; and apparently Jaspers has given application to this dictum. It seems as if the author had removed the whole problem of types from the heterogeneous level, where the man in the street dominates the situation, to the cultural stadium where fine shades of difference are readily discriminated. Here a conflict becomes an antinomy, yet the consequences in reaction are analogous, although in the one case they consist in action ; in the other, in thought. Jaspers was not the first to perceive the possibilities of explaining the history of philosophy psychologically.

Importance of Human Types for Philosophical Insight. Dilthey, in a number of brilliant essays, but principally in *Die Typen der Weltanschauung*, maintains that a philosophical system is but the outgrowth of a particular constitution and its experiences, which create certain *Lebensstimmungen*.

" These life-moods," he says, in one place, " the countless shades of world attitudes constitute the lower stratum for the elaborations of world conceptions."   " All world conceptions," he writes further, " regularly contain the same structure. This structure is always a relation in which the questions of the sense and significance of the world are decided on the basis of a world picture, and out of it are derived the ideal, the highest good and the loftiest principles for the conduct of life." [1]

We can perceive, therefore, that with Dilthey the problem of human types antedates that of metaphysics, for it contains the key which would unlock the mystery of its polyphasic cult. "The individual stages and the special aspects of a type are refuted, but its root in life persists and continues to function and to bring forth ever new patterns." [2] Spranger was now able to begin where Dilthey left off ; and in his *Lebensformen*, as we have seen in a previous chapter, he has worked out a " typology " in this spirit.

Phenomenological Influence. Finally, we ought not to overlook Kronfeld's *Das Wesen der psychiatrischen Erkenntnis* which purports to examine the philosophical and psychological foundations of psychiatry on methodological lines. In the promised second volume, the problem of types is to receive much more attention, but even the material in the first volume serves to indicate the influence of the normative and purposive in spheres which only a decade ago were entirely governed by descriptive aims and laws, and were permeated with the empirical bias.

Kronfeld harks back to the school of Fries whose philosophy had been revived by Nelson ; yet the phenomenological terminology in which the volume is steeped gives evidence that

---

[1] W. Dilthey, " Die Typen der Weltanschauung " in *Weltanschauung-Philosophie und Religion in Darstellungen* (edited by M. Frischeisen-Kohler, 1911), p. 11.
[2] Loc. cit., p. 16.

in spite of his disagreements with Brentano and Husserl on individual points, both important and otherwise, Kronfeld lustily wields the instrument of the latter.

As for the organization of types, he repeatedly emphasizes the normative point of view, the rôle of evaluation as basic because of its significance for society. " The social moment, he declares, " is a criterion of psychological type-forms " (*Typik*),[1] and in the individual's reactivity he finds the index of the social attitude, which again has a teleological flavour.

THE ONTOLOGY OF CHARACTER

We have seen that it is possible to point out metaphysical discussions of character, much as the subject does not appear to lend itself to such treatment. The linking of character with the theory of value, as done by Scheler and Stern, and with the theory of knowledge, traces of which may be found in Jaspers' and Kronfeld's works, need not surprise us.   The problem here is not to account for differences in character, but in one of its phases to show the connection between an outlook on life or a philosophical system and character, taken in the broadest sense, while in another phase the task is to settle the question as to the validity of our concepts in the sphere of character and their relative significance. The problem in this aspect has not been formulated by any of the writers mentioned, but the subject-matter touched on by Kronfeld suggests it.

To complete the traditional division of philosophy, we have yet the field of ontology to cover ; and this territory is amply covered by Pfänder and Häberlin, both of whom, although belonging to different philosophical schools and living in different countries, have set out to discover the *essence* of character. They may well be dealt with together, as they are

---

[1] A. Kronfeld, *Das Wesen der psychiatrischen Erkenntnis* (1920), vol. i, p. 466.

both inspired by an animistic bias and guided by a scholastic method.

Fundamental Character. Pfänder's starting point is the sharp discrimination between what he calls the *empirical* character and the *fundamental* (" Grund ") Character. This distinction is not to be confused with the dichotomy of *empirical* and *intelligible* character in Kant's and Schopenhauer's philosophy, for Pfänder's " *Grundcharakter* " is not a thing-in-itself, a mere limiting concept underlying the empirical character. It is rather something real existing at least in time, although it manifests itself only through the empirical character of the individual.

What are the earmarks of this fundamental character ? For we must not take it for granted that it is the sum-total of a person's characteristics.

First of all it is necessary to exclude everything which is perverted, abnormal, or warped from the character. These are deviations which may belong to the empirical character, but are not a part of the fundamental character. In this procedure, we begin to get an inkling of Pfänder's objective. Since " the fundamental character of an individual is the original individuality of a human soul ", we can perceive why all imperfections must be removed before the ground can be so much as examined.

The Typical as the Perfect. The *idealization*—for such it is, and this suggestive thought may be regarded as the core of the whole essay—is justified through an analogy in botanical method. When the botanist is about to describe a plant, he does not consider the leaf that is crumpled or decayed. It is only with the healthy leaves in their normal condition that he is concerned. Now much of the empirical character is in an unhealthy condition, due to circumstances, but our goal is to discover the *quale* of the constant, the genuine, of which the

---

[1] A. Pfänder, " Grundprobleme der Charakterologie ": *Jahrb. d. Charakterol.*, 1924, vol. i.

empirical character is only a symbol, or, to put it differently, which can become manifest only through the working of the empirical character.

After taking us tantalizingly through many *culs de sac* only to lead us out again with the caution not to make such mistakes in the future, Pfänder lets a hint drop now and then, until it dawns upon us that his doctrine is steeped in transcendental idealism. This fundamental character of his is a personal free-acting agency. Then there are general characters and individual characters for both the fundamental and the empirical forms ; the most general type, the genus of character, represents the " character of the human soul in general (*überhaupt*), that peculiar mode of being through which every single individual is a human psychic person, differing from other, non-personal, beings ".

Universals in Character. It would tax the patience of most readers to have to follow much more of this abstruse dialectic. The point which Pfänder is at pains to make appears to be this : we must guard ourselves against mistaking the spurious for the genuine, the transient for the permanent, the warped for the healthy growth in character. There are undeveloped characters (childhood) and also those in their devolutive stages (old age), there are temporarily misdirected characters, or those called "*ressentiment* characters"—a phrase to which, I believe, Max Scheler [1] was the first to give currency as applying to the disgruntled who annihilate theoretically all the values from which they happen to be excluded. These forms, Pfänder maintains, are not basic. They are like the dead petal in the flower which the morphologist would not think of describing in his classification. We are enjoined then

---

[1] M. Scheler, " Über Ressentiment und moralisches Werturteil "' *Zt. f. Pathopsychol.*, 1912, vol. i.

The analysis of this type originated with Nietzsche, who in his *Genealogy of Morals* censures Christianity rather severely for encouraging this resentfulness against the worldly values—a view which Scheler does not share.

to replace the imperfect by the perfect, to reconstruct ; and such reconstruction necessitates idealization. Pfänder is not dissuaded from his conviction by such considerations as the fact that in life his *characterial universals*—for as such we must recognize them, even if he does not employ this term— are not to be experienced. Worst of all, his criteria or marks of the fundamental character are simply based on analogies and prove wholly inapplicable.

Deluge of Qualities. What are these kinds of characters according to their qualities ? Size or range of the soul, the nature of the substance constituting the soul (hard or soft, heavy or light, coarse-grained or fine-grained, compact or rare, flexible or rigid, elastic or inelastic, tough or tender, dry or juicy, luminous, transparent, lustrous ; also qualities according to clang, odor, and taste qualities), the nature of the psychic life stream (volume of the flow, rhythm, rapidity, swiftness, warmth), as well as the qualitative composition of the current (e.g. in one there flows a psychic cod liver oil, in another milk, in a third the stream resembles limpid water, in a fourth—lemonade, in a fifth there gushes a tropic wine or a sparkling champagne), then the psychic forces of tension, and finally the psychic light (aura ?) all enter into Pfänder's estimate of true character. With such a burden on the shoulders of the characterologist, it is dubious whether he can muster the courage to advance the first step ; and certainly the shrewd man in the street with the task reduced to a minimum has the advantage over him. But, as already implied, Pfänder moves in a sphere of ontology, and may regard it as his business to discover the essence of character, regardless of the question whether or not his findings are practicable.

Character as Essence Individualized. Häberlin [1] writes in the same vein in his book on character which forms a companion volume to his elementary psychology (to which he provokingly

---

[1] P. Häberlin, *Der Charakter* (1925).

refers us on almost every page, and sometimes more than once).
Just as Pfänder made a search for the essence of character,
so Häberlin seeks the *Wesenheit* which is never actually
experienced as such, but in its " projection " upon us. Essence
in itself forever remains a mystery. We obtain, however, a
glimpse of it through our personality which is a component
of the universal essence. This elusive concept carries with
it the notion of absoluteness, spontaneity, autonomy, self-
activity, creative production. In individuality, it shows
itself as a mode of the general (*überhaupt*) and takes on a
crystallized form. In that case we secure a relative essence
and it is the nearest approach we have to the mystery.

Personality is the human in general ; character is
personality as it reveals itself in differentiated human beings.
Naturally, then, everyone would appear as a character in some
form or other. Characterless people are non-existent.

What has happened is this : Häberlin started in the clouds
and, without delay, made a dash to the earth, and with such
force that he failed to keep on his feet so as to see man, not
too much from above, but also not too much from below.
Soaring in the heights of essence, he was confronted with a
mystery ; grovelling in the data of empirical psychology he
identifies character with characteristic, and his characterology,
as becomes plain from his book, is another name for
differentiated psychology in its scholastic phase.

Häberlin deals with the relational aspects of character, e.g. :
Is character constant or variable ? Is it a unity or a
composite ? and answers the questions much as would be
expected offhand. It is constant in one sense, and variable
in another. It is not wholly constant, therefore it must be
somewhat variable. But in addition he treats of qualities
which are far more directly connected with personality in its
widest usage than with character. Affectivity, religiosity,
æstheticism, cultural range, genius, energy, constancy,
originality, direction and mobility of drives, periodicity,

reflection, intelligence, memory, imagination and interest, all find a place here. At the same time more complex structures are passed in review; ideals, life-attitude, adjustment, direction of life, outlook, life-problems, etc.

Just as Pfänder prizes the distinction between fundamental and empirical, so Häberlin sets great store by the difference between what he calls *Einstellung* and *Stellung*. It is a difference, I take it, between the bodily adjustment and the conscious attitude.

The " set " (*Stellung*) and the Life-Attitude (*Einstellung*) together go to make up what is called character. It is the attitude which determines the " set ", for when the attitude changes, the adjustment naturally undergoes a change too. The one is complementary to the other.

Interaction of Attitude and Outlook. Häberlin is not content to rest with this dichotomy. He brings in many other factors which bear on both the *Stellung* and the *Einstellung*, dialectically conceived, and so subtly demarcated from each other that one must be in sympathy with the hair-splitting game to subscribe to the formal distinctions. Everything is to be considered in this account from both the qualitative and the quantitative points of view, from both the subjective and the objective angle, and also as regards form and content. The individual is not only differentiated, not only a mode of the total essence (objective relation), but, furthermore, he has a right to his individuation in and for itself. as if it were not merely a mode of the universal. In this way Häberlin obtains the " conduct of life " (*Lebensführung*), the substance of it being the " ' I '-ness (*Ichheit*), the fact of being subject, or as one would ordinarily say, the fact of personal life, i.e. the fact that the individual is not a mere part or something which is made the plaything of life, but is himself the bearer of life, who advances actively and reacts in his own peculiar way, the fact of the separated personality of the individual who voluntarily shares the collective will ". This sentence is a good illustration of the author's presentation both as to form and content and should serve as an indication of the difficulty of expounding briefly such a laboured and obscure position.

The *Lebensführung* is to be set in juxtaposition yet with the *Lebensauffassung*, or outlook on life which colours the *Einstellung*. There is the outlook on life as well as the conscious experience of this outlook. There is the direction of interests as well as the direction of drive (*Triebrichtung*). Altogether we get a formidable array of prolegomena to the actual study of character, which reminds us of the house-that-Jack-built jingle. Even if Häberlin can successfully defend every one of his many nuances in the ontology of character, the question still remains : *Cui bono* ?

Inconsequential Differences. In building a house, we might divide the materials in many different ways, according to colour, shape, roughness, weight, etc., but these qualities are of no consequence as compared with the *practical use* of the materials.

That Häberlin's prolegomena are inapplicable is almost a foregone conclusion. Nevertheless, his mode of approach, because it resembles so much the phenomenological method, is interesting and representative.

Texture of Hegel. As for the philosophical background of Häberlin's characterology, it is easy to perceive that he derives his nourishment from objective idealism, and although he does not mention Hegel in his book, it would seem that this formal analysis is of a piece with the master's *Phänomenologie des Geistes*.

Characterology as a " Science of Essence ". Among the philosophical conceptions of character must be counted Th. Lessing's characterology.[1] Dissatisfied with all the existing views on the subject, he boldly announced his plan to lay the foundations of a new science, which he might

[1] Th. Lessing: "Prinzipien der Charakterologie," *Deutsche Psychol.*, 1926, vol. iv.

have called symbolistics, typology, eidology, or phenomenology, did not others anticipate him in these designations.

Character, maintains Lessing, is not confined to man alone.
Each drop of water, each micro-organism in a cubic centi-
metre of air, each crystal in the depths of the earth reveals
a character of its own, not only in its configuration, but in
essence.

The science of character thus becomes fundamental to
everything else, and must be shorn of sophisticated accretions like subjective and objective phases, or conscious properties. Characterology is the science of essence, and the
lore of essence has three spheres, the knowledge of organisms
(" *Gestaltenkunde* "), knowledge of forms (arrangement, order,
and uses in objects) and the knowledge of ideas. It is curious
that Lessing did not adopt the term "essentiology" with which
to christen his new science or scientific approach. Without
going into the depths of this monograph, which bristles with
paradoxes, it will be sufficient to say that after limiting himself,
for obvious reasons, to the consideration of human character
after all, he takes occasion to expatiate on the psychology of
Ahmung, which he emphatically denies to be the same as
empathy or inner mimicry.

" It is not true that I empathise my sorrow in the meadow,
my pride in the rock, my joy in the cloud, but meadow, rock,
and cloud are (insofar as they are not given me as objects of
consciousness) altogether self-animated : dæmons and spirits
like myself. They are no more dependent on my being alive
than I am anchored to their life."

The word " *Ahmung* " is used instead of " *Nachahmung* "
because the latter would suggest a priority in time of the
object or person toward whom the attitude in character-
grasping is taken. In reality, Lessing thinks, no such priority
is possible. The process of " *Ahmung* " is simultaneous,
complementary, and takes place before the observer's attitude
has had time to become diluted in a sophisticated analysis.

SUMMING UP

Certainly it is not to be supposed that the whole ground has been covered as regards the bearing of present-day German philosophy on the study of character. Typical instances only have been referred to, especially as much has already been written on this head in the chapter dealing with the relation between *Struktur* psychology and characterology. Meanwhile, it has become clear, I hope, that the trend in German philosophical circles to-day is to attach greater significance to the *intuitive*, the purposive, and to elevate the valuative method above its erstwhile status. To this end, several schools have converged their efforts in the same direction, so that no matter in what else they differ, their agreement in this respect is striking.

Aside from the detailed systematization and orientation, the direct contribution to the study of character in the cited works has not been fruitful. These German writers have treated many indifferent points as if they were vital issues, and are prone to spend much time arguing against a minor observation of a colleague, thus losing themselves in an unprofitable controversy, especially as the opponent as a rule can always defend his position through the same verbosity as has been employed against him. Scheler and Kronfeld are particularly guilty of this side burrowing.

Since no two experiences are alike, distinctions may be drawn *ad infinitum*, but the question is first—and this addresses itself to phenomenology in general—how a distinction, a nuance, which occurs to us as valid can be proven to the satisfaction of our adversary, and secondly, after the distinction has been accepted by others: how can we gauge its value ? We are confronted here with the problem whether the distinction is a general one or merely an incidental variation ; and interminable discussions might be started to ascertain this very point.

We might perhaps crudely liken the situation of the German philosophical writers who bring out these ponderous dialectic works to a partnership in, let us say, a huge hardware store where one of the firm takes great pains to arrange the various articles in systematic order, labelling every item and listing it for sale, but no sooner is this executed than another of the partners would enter and re-arrange nearly every article in the store, making out different labels and different prices. Of course, no practical results could come from such a procedure.

One gains the impression on reading these systematic works that the planning is done on a tremendous scale, and the phrase " we must " is, I believe, the most frequently used stereotype, but the executing is never begun, let alone the working out of the applications.

To be sure, it may be retorted that the philosophical grasp of the problem does not entail the practical elaboration of the suggestions, which is the task of the psychologists and perhaps also the psychiatrists, but it so happens that these various disciplines—philosophy, psychology, psychiatry, and logic—are not divorced from one another in Germany. In fact they often appear to be identified with the same person ; and it is rare to find a philosopher in Germany who is not conversant with the problems in psychology or a psychologist who does not dabble in philosophy, whence our complaint about the footlessness of the philosophical approach to the study of character or the problem of types.

CHAPTER XXVIII

BIOGRAPHICAL AND HISTORICAL MATERIAL AS SOURCES OF CHARACTER STUDY

Relation between Biography and History. Without going into the broad issues of historical foundations, I think it is allowable to conceive of history as events carried out by the promptings of individuals, allowable, because I am aware of other conceptions of history, but this is no place for arguing such a portentous issue. It all depends on what we choose to include as history, and on how much weight we are willing to attach to circumstances and conditions. The eruption of a volcano in Italy, the flooding of a river in Portugal, an earthquake in Japan, or a famine in China are surely not to be associated with the doings of an individual. But an uprising, war, and other political or economic upheavals can be traced usually to the operations of some one individual; and the hands of individuals can be detected even in the shaping of events which follow natural disasters or arise in the face of national perils. This view is not altogether incompatible with either historical materialism which ascribes historical events to the economic needs of the people or with objective idealism which regards progress as an unfolding of the Absolute Idea throughout the ages.

The former will have to admit that the masses must always be prompted by a leader (whose biography throws a good deal of light on the historical developments with which he was connected), and, furthermore, the economic storms and stresses are considerably modified by the advent of a great organizer or inventor or even a religious leader or moralist who can pacify the most unruly multitudes.

Hegelians, on the other hand, cannot deny the claim that the Universal idea may be working itself out through individuals on the lines suggested by Malebranche's Occasionalism. It is not for us to take sides in the eternal historiosophical issue ; and, in fact, only by steering a middle course can we rest assured that we are safe from the wrangles of the schools. But it is necessary to reduce biography and history to one denominator for the purpose of character study, not that the biographies of all outstanding men of a certain period will give us the history of that period, nor that the historical method is essentially the same as that of biography, but for the *reason that whatever in history is relevant to characterology* in reality comes under the head of biography. And it matters little whether we accept the position that Napoleon's brow-beating the world can be explained in terms of physico-chemical processes or can be understood only in the light of motives and purposes. This decision will rather hinge on whether we are inclined toward the causal, nomothetic sciences, as Windelband called them, the *Naturwissenschaften*, or lean in the direction of the purposive, appreciative, ideographic sciences, the *Geisteswissenschaften*.

Advance of Modern Biography. Biography as an important department of literature has been cultivated as far back as antiquity, becoming an art in the hands of Plutarch, whose comparisons of famous Greeks and Romans were replete with discerning contrasts. The best examples of this delicacy of shading may be seen in his delineations of the two Gracchi brothers, Tiberius and Caius, in the touching picture of Marcellus the conqueror of Syracuse and, metaphorically speaking, the steel engraving of Cato, the censor. Plutarch's *Lives*, however, is no more than a collection of *memoirs* pieced together without regard to reliability. Legend and fact are here mixed without concern. It is only in modern times that the biographer has taken his task seriously, and has turned historian for an individual, as in the case of Hazlitt's *Napoleon*, Irving's *Columbus* and also his *George Washington*, Masson's detailed account of Milton and his atmosphere, or, better still, the monumental biography of Disraeli by Monypenny and Buckle, and Thayer's devoted labour on Beethoven. The sifting of facts, the examination of documents, the rummaging into archives, the questioning of contemporaries, the scrutiny of letters, the ferreting out of all sorts of information and references, cited with reservations— all this does not seem to have been known of until about a century ago.

Different Types of Biography. Both biography and autobiography may be divided according to the intention of the writer. Biographies are seldom mere catalogues of facts. Nearly all of them reveal the attitude of the writer, and some of them, like tendentious literature, point to a moral or were undertaken in defence of the biographee. Biographies may thus be subjective or objective. Boswell's famous life of Johnson is valuable largely because it is so all-inclusive as to show little prejudice in choosing the details, since the author was so overawed and inspired by the subject of his sketch that he could not consider anything in connection with his hero as deserving to be excluded. For this reason Boswell's *Life* gives a true picture of the great Englishman's character. Macaulay's *Warren Hastings* and *Lord Clive* are pleas in which the subjects of the sketches are to be constructed out of the events and the circumstances which Macaulay marshalls. Such biographies have, of course, their use in offsetting the political libels which an intriguing band had fastened on the men, but a championed character cannot serve the purpose of characterology, except where no other data about the individual are forthcoming.

Value of Voluminous Biographies. It is not always the bulky biography which offers most information about the biographee's character; but other things equal, the more

detailed the biography the greater its reliability.   Political
men of note will of necessity require more space because of the
historical events connected with their lives.   Carlyle toiled
twelve years on his " unutterable " *Frederick the Great*, which
he brought out in several volumes.   Yet Glasenapp's *Richard
Wagner* and Kalbeck's *Johannes Brahms* exceed its bulk,
indicating in part that the artist's life may be fuller than that
of such a renowned sovereign as the versatile Prussian.
Similarly, it took Lockhart about 3,500 pages to tell the story
of Walter Scott, while the life of that human volcano,
Napoleon I, with all his campaigns and political conflagrations,
seems to have been exhausted in the seven-volume German
translation and completed edition of Pierre Lanfrey's *Histoire
de Napoléon I*.   Many of these voluminous biographies will
permit of considerable sifting, but it is safer to have too much
to discard than too little, as instanced in the ten-volume
biography of Abraham Lincoln by Nicolay and Hay.

The Composite Biography.   The *individual* biography is of
value because of its conveying a total impression of the
subject; and also because it enables us to judge for ourselves
instead of offering us a cross section or selection of an
individual's life-history.   But the individual biography, after
all, purports to tell us nothing more than the character of that
individual ;   and if we wish to inform ourselves about other
individuals of the same type so as to draw generalizations, we
must resort to the *composite* or *class biography*, an excellent
example of which is Isaac Disraeli's *Literary Character in
Men of Genius* and to a less extent his *Curiosities of Literature*.

The drawback of such biographies is, of course, their
necessarily fragmentary character, but a greater danger is
often the preconceived theory of the writer, the truth of which
the assembled facts are to establish.   Isaac Disraeli had no
hypothesis to substantiate.   He regarded the particulars
which he was able to unearth as mere curiosities.   Some
literary men had one set of habits, while others were addicted

to others, but there was no scientific conclusion which this delightfully unassuming writer was willing to sponsor.

Lombroso, on the other hand, in publishing his *Man of Genius*, gave us a composite picture which was highly coloured not only in the selection of his subjects, but in the reporting of the incidents and traits. Lombroso's composite biographical draft was highly impressionistic and marked by a tendency—the tendency to prove his well-known thesis about the degeneracy of genius.

The Psychological Biography. The type of biography which may turn out most fruitful for the purpose of characterology is exemplified by Ostwald's *Grosse Maenner*, where we find the oft-cited distinction of classical and romantic types in science. The book, which is the forerunner of a number of biographies of eminent scientists,[1] under the supervision of Ostwald, does not exactly deal with the problem of character, since it was inspired by a question which a Japanese student had once put to the distinguished chemist, viz., How can we discern genius in young children so as to pick them out and give them a special training for the benefit of their country *?* Yet no one can read Ostwald's book without gaining a clear characterial impression of men like Faraday, Davy, or Helmholtz.

Limitations of the Memoir. The memoir which is a condensed biography and usually written by way of introduction to the work of a deceased author is not nearly so satisfactory as its more extensive *genre*, particularly because it is as a rule the product of an admiring friend or worshipful relative. Much, for instance, must be discounted in the description of Sir William Hamilton by his American editor, O. W. Wight, as "A philosopher, who thinks like Aristotle; whose logic is as stern as that of St. Thomas, ' the lawgiver of the Church '; who rivals Muretus as a critic, whose erudition finds a parallel only in that of the younger Scaliger; whose

[1] The latest book of the series is a large volume on Johannes Müller.

subtlety of thought and polemical power remind us of the dauntless prince of Verona ; whose penetrating analysis reaches deeper than that of Kant . . . who, in a style severely elegant, with accuracy of statement, with precision of definition, in sequence and admirable order, will explain a system in many respects new—a system that will provoke thought that, consequently, carries in itself the germs of beneficial revolutions in literature and education, in all those things that are produced and regulated by mind in action." [1]

AUTOBIOGRAPHY

Its Unreliability. One might think that a great advantage is to be had over biography in the accounts which writers give of their own life. Surely here, if anywhere, reliable data are to be expected, for the writer knows all that has happened to himself. Nevertheless, it is one of the curios of human nature that the autobiography does not always yield so adequate a reproduction of one's inner life as do some biographies.

Does not St. Augustine's *Confessions* give the impression that the author has exaggerated his youthful profligacy as if by way of penance for his early sins ? And must it be brought to mind that while the artist-devil Benvenuto Cellini succeeded in exposing his boundless selfishness and ferocious egotism with the same consummate craftmanship he was able to bestow on his handwrought masterpieces, we can never be certain to what extent his spirit of bravado led him to exaggerate his villainy ?

Aside from this, however, Cellini was merely a narrator. He did not apply the reflective torchlight to his traits and conduct.

The weird autobiography *De Propria Vita Liber* of his equally famous contemporary Girolamo Cardano, a most analytic document of a marvellous personality, must also be

---

[1] O. W. Wight, *Philosophy of Sir William Hamilton, Bart.*, p 7.

discounted for the reason that its author at times seems to lack the insight proper to sanity of mind ; and although Cardano is reputed to be the first scientific autobiographer, his superstition, his constitutional defects and his paranoid sallies make it difficult to assign to his pathetic life-history the place it possibly deserves.

Inexplicable Aberrations. What better instance need we of the unreliability of autobiography as a correct impression of the writer's achievement and worth, his motives and ambitions than the *Autobiography* of Lord Herbert of Cherbury, who wrote in Latin a remarkably subtle treatise on Truth, and yet appears to have lamentably concealed the truth about his intellectual attainments in order to magnify his prowess as a courtier, gallant, and swordsman ? There is a good deal of food for reflection in the observation of Sidney Lee in the introduction to a recent edition of this work, that the " contrast between the grounds on which he professed a desire to be remembered and those on which he deserved to be remembered by posterity, gives his book almost all its value."

Certainly this aberration on the part of the English philosopher, poet, historian, and courtier is in itself a character puzzle which requires unravelling and which readily lends itself to the divagations of all-embracing psychoanalysis.

The voluminous *Memoirs* of the celebrated criminal and spy Vidocq has been questioned not only as to its reliability but even as to its authenticity. Rousseau's *Confessions* is notorious for its inaccuracies, many of them deliberately indulged in, and even Goethe's *Dichtung und Wahrheit*, has often been discussed by editors and critics with a view to determining how much of it is fiction and how much of it truth. Goethe, the seeker of truth, in actual life was not meticulous as to the truth of details about his own life ; and Renan, referring to the title which Goethe had chosen for his autobiography, rather approves of it by pointing out " *qu'on ne saurait faire sa propre biographie de la même manière qu'on fait celle des autres* ".[1] With regard to his own episodes which he collected under the suitable name " *Souvenirs d'enfance et de jeunesse* ", he writes with characteristic good grace : " Bien des choses ont été mises afin qu'on sourie ; si l'usage l'eut permis, j'aurais dû écrire plus d'une fois à la marge : *cum grano salis.*" And if Renan, the great apostle of truth, he for whom a contradiction in the Bible meant the shattering of his whole career's dream, if Renan could bring himself to include incidents merely for the purpose of evoking smiles and not to be taken except with a grain of salt, then how much more justified are we in expecting men and women whose passion for truth was less patent to permit themselves to vivify their memories with a rosier tint ?

The Drawback of Reserve. To be sure, Renan was an artist as well as a scientist and philosopher ; and we might perhaps look to the autobiographies of men who are primarily philosophers, e.g. J. S. Mill, Bain, and Herbert Spencer, whose accounts of their own lives are admirable documents, and in the case of the latter, a fairly complete record of his work and personality, but even in these two or three remarkable pieces of self-portraiture we are not certain that the authors have done themselves justice in some things or that they did not overlook others. It is just the philosopher who would be most affected by the virtue of modesty, and try as he would to shake off the personal reserve so prevalent among men of thought, he could not do so altogether without Bacon's injunction *de nobis ipsis silemus* constantly ringing in his ears.

Biography and Autobiography Compared. Gruhle aptly remarks that the autobiographer usually is concerned with his aims and intentions, but it is the motive which the investigator of character is seeking. Why did the man choose such means ?

---

[1] E. Renan, *Souvenirs d'enfance et de jeunesse.* Preface : " It is impossible to write one's own biography in the same way as one would write other people's."

What were the mainsprings of his action?[1] These are slurred by the autobiographer, and where he does make an endeavour to impart the desired information to posterity, he is quite likely to stall before he goes to the very depth of his self-analysis, unconsciously suppressing perhaps the most important items; or else in his quest of motives, he stumbles upon wishes and details them in lieu of the sought facts.

Relevancy and Incident. A rather important point is raised by Gruhle in connection with the genuineness of a given trait, where contradictory evidence pulls in two different directions. The relevancy to and compatibility with the character as a whole are generally regarded as determining the genuine character of the trait in question. But the writer recommends that, in establishing motives for a given personality, we register all tendencies that come to light whether they are compatible with one another or not. The selection of the *essential* will then depend on the frequency with which the various tendencies crop up. Controversies which often break out among historians as to whether a certain trait is characteristic or not, central or peripheral, deep-seated or only superficial, can be settled after some such fashion as this.

This question of the essential in biography has been answered by Stern a decade before somewhat differently. He noticed the need of separating out a certain phase of the total personality " If I wished to describe Moltke as a literary individuality, other characteristics would become ' essential ' than if I were to treat Moltke the strategist."[2]

Theories of Individuality. Nevertheless, he thinks that the direction a biography takes is bound up with the theory of the structure of individuality. He cites three such theories of the past, the historiosophic, of Hegel, which regarded the great man as the mouthpiece of the impersonal objective

---

[1] H. W. Gruhle, " Selbstbiographie und Persönlichkeitsforschung " : *Ber. ü. d. viii Kongress f. experim. Psychol.* 1923.

[2] W. Stern, *Differentielle Psychologie*, p. 322 ff.

spiritual progress of humanity; the psychological theories which will stress either the cognitive or the will aspects of the biographer, according to the general psychological position of the writer (Ostwald is mentioned as a representative of the psychological school) ; and finally he notes the ethical theorists in biography who estimate their heroes from religious or ethical angles.

The natural sciences have yielded other observation points such as the aetiological which views the individual through the *milieu*. Environment, nourishment, bodily attention, and mental influences are components of the formula which Taine employed to explain individuality. On the other hand, there are the racial theories of Gobineau and H. S. Chamberlain, who see in the individual nothing but the product of his race.

As Stern has quite rightly urged, every theory, no matter how useful, already determines the attitude of the biographer, with the result that he is apt to overlook an important detail for the benefit of an unimportant one which may, however, fit into his theory.

Cautions in Interpreting Autobiography.   Several other pertinent suggestions are offered by Gruhle. He warns, for instance, against a well-rounded smoothly written account of oneself, and calls attention on the other hand to those auto-biographers who take a delight in dwelling on their faults and sins, which inclination, as exemplified in the autobiographies of monks and nuns, he takes to be nothing but intentional self-torture. The education of the autobiographer, his age, the circumstances under which the life is written, whether in exile, for instance, or in prison, and finally his fluctuations of mood, should all be taken into account in evaluating its contents.

Gruhle believes that the diary of a young person is more reliable as to the single motives; that the adult is liable to deceive himself about the motives, but is apt to produce a more finished picture of his personality, while the aged individual is the most inefficient of all. If Gruhle is right in his observations, we must regard Hall's *Life and Confessions of a Psychologist* and *Senescence* as exceptions to a tentative rule.

Memoirs. What has been said about autobiography as a whole holds for the various sub-classes of this *genre* of literature. Memoirs [1] and reminiscences seldom give us proper access to the inner self of the writer, who, for the most part, turns out to be the *historian* of a small circle of influential people by whom he was affected. The writer of memoirs or reminiscences is usually more extraverted than the auto-biographer, pure and simple, though he may be more subjective in his interpretations of others and in his attitude towards himself. The autobiographer has a more unified view of his personality and is more reflective than introjective. The memoirs writer is primarily a narrator, relating his own episodes just as he would those of others. We must bear in mind, however, that the label " memoirs " or " auto-biography " is not sufficient to serve as a finger-post to the contents. The choice of the title is sometimes arbitrary. It is the character of the writing' that reveals the nature of the account. (Cf. the *Memoirs of John Quincy Adams*, in twelve volumes.)

FUNCTION OF THE PERSONAL JOURNAL

The Diary. Diaries present the same difficulties as reminiscences. Here, too, there are great variations. The diary of Amiel is not to be put into the same class as that of Samuel Pepys. In the one we have a record of inner experiences ; in the other a storehouse of trivial happenings. True, the latter may be far more important for an understanding of English life in the seventeenth century. The character of a Pepys can easily be reconstructed out of the multitude of bagatelles, just as an individual can be known by every

---

[1] *Memoirs*, in the plural, should not be confused with *Memoir*, in the singular, which is usually an appreciative biographical sketch.

expression of his ; but then, if so, we are evaluating *behaviour*. It is not the author's conscious *meaning* that we are endeavouring to appreciate, but his *work* that we are studying. The autobiographical cast of the diary gives way to a biographical form, and the information is now gleaned second hand.

Limitations of the Diary. The huge diary of Madame D'Arblay in six volumes, as it is edited by her niece and Dobson, actually answers this description ; for although the editors' supplement and explanations constitute but a fraction of the work, they supply the biographical foreground upon a vast autobiographical background.

As to the almost universal weakness inherent in the diarist, there is a pertinent passage in that brimming and ominous journal of Barbellion, *A Last Diary* [1]:—

> James Joyce is my man (in the *Portrait of the Artist as a young Man*). Here is a writer who tells the truth about himself.   In this journal I have tried, but I have not succeeded.   I have *set down* a good deal, but I cannot *tell* it.   Truth of self has to be left by the psychology-miner at the bottom of his boring.

In another place this gifted naturalist and rare self-analyst, who died at the age of 31, allegorically expatiates on the difficulty of revealing oneself in one's true colours.

> Every man has his own icon.   Secreted in the closet of each man's breast is an icon, the image of himself, concealed from view with elaborate care, treated invariably with great respect by means of which the Ego, being self-conscious, sees itself in relation to the rest of mankind, measures itself therewith, and in accordance with which it acts and moves and subsists.   In the self-righteous man's bosom, it is a molten image of a little potentate who can

[1] W. N. P. Barbellion (pseudonym of B. F. Cummings), *A Last Diary*, 1920, pp. 35–36.

do no wrong. In the egoist's, an idol loved and worshipped by almost all men, addressed with solemnity and reverence, and cast in an immutable brazen form. Only the truth-seeker preserves his image in clay-covered, damp rags—a working hypothesis.

A man towards his icon is like the tenderness and secretiveness of a little bird towards its nest, which does not know you have discovered its heart's treasure. For everyone knows the lineaments of your image and talks about them to everyone else save you, and no one dare refer to his own—it is bad form—so that in spite of the gossip and criticism that swirl around each one's personality, a man remains sound-tight and insulated.

The human comedy begins at the thought of the ludicrous unlikeness, in many cases, of the treasured image to the real person—as much verisimilitude about it as, say, about a bust by Gaudier-Brzeska.[1]

One might think that the twenty post-quarto volumes of manuscript which constituted the bulk out of which *The Journal of a Disappointed Man* and *Enjoying Life* were condensed would have given us a clear picture of the extraordinary man, but his brother tells us in the prefatory memoir to *A Last Diary*, that Barbellion

was forever peering at himself from changing angles, and he was never quite sure that the point of view of the moment was the true one. Incontinently curious about himself, he was never certain about the real Barbellion. One day he was ' so much specialized protoplasm ' ; another day he was Alexander with the world at his feet ; and then he was a lonely boy pining for a few intimate friends.

Diarists are usually given to introspection and are therefore prone to create problems, phases and attitudes in the course of their introspection or as food for its nourishment. That is

[1] *Loc. cit.*, pp. 89–90.

one reason why reviewers are inclined to be suspicious of the veracity of the allegations. This misgiving on the part of the literary public gréeted Marie Bashkirtseff's *Journal* as well as the recent anonymously published *Young Girl's Diary*.

The Controlled Diary. The scientific or controlled diary which is kept about someone else the subject of a study, is not to be confused with the spontaneous diary spoken of above. Investigators of child psychology have been known to record the mental growth of their young subjects from day to day for a certain period of time. Examples of such studies are M. W. Shinn's *Biography of a Baby*, G. v. N. Dearborn's *Moto-Sensory Development*, and Clara Stern's *Aus einer Kinderstube*.

In his *Anfänge der Reifezeit*, W. Stern has edited with psychological observations the diary of a precocious boy written some forty years ago during the age of puberty. It is Stern's opinion that diaries of children can be relied on as spontaneous expressions, and that those written at the instance of grown-up people are detectable as artificial, and the recording impulse is of short duration.

CORRESPONDENCE

Character in Letters. Even more care must be exercised by the student of character in the examination of letters. The letters of the sixteenth and seventeenth centuries were, as is well known, written with deliberation and even ostentation. They are essays with a personal touch. For this reason they must be purged of the artificial before finding a place in the list of first-hand sources.

It is curious that the simple expressions of young children in letters will show a surprising amount of individual variation. There is much to be learnt from the short notes, reproduced here, which were penned by children between the ages of 9 and 11, at the suggestion of a teacher in a public school on the occasion of a pupil's illness. We may note that although the conditions of the writing are of the simplest nature, each letter represents not only a different level or mode of intelligence, but a different touch of personality. Although the letters speak for themselves, they have been characterized by a word or two at the top of the letter in parentheses.

SPECIMENS OF CHILDREN'S NOTES TO A SICK CLASSMATE

Russell School,
Cambridge, Mass.
6th April, 1925.

1. (Flightiness, incredulity)

My dear William,

I am very sorry to head[r] that your are sick. When Eleanor told me that you had the measlel[s] I did not believe her. But when I hear(e)d her telling another. I believed her. I am painting now, I hope you will be back soon. To-day we had 19teen examples they were subtraction and addition of fractions. Your school frei[ie]nd,

Jeanne R.

2. (Personal)

The children said you had the measles. I feel sorry for you. When you come back we will treat you as good as we can. And when I have the measles I hope you will send me a letter. Yours truly,

Harry C.

3. (Untactful, revealing the obligatory nature of the letter-writing)

I am very sorry you are sick. We are having a language lesson. All the children had to write to you. We miss you in school very much. Would you rather be home sick [or] in school. I would rather be in school. I will now close my letter Yours truly,

Gertrude B.

4. (Choppy)

I am sorry you are sick, I hope you will be better by next week. We have next week off. I hope you have a nice Easter. Yours truly,

Henry L.

5. (Expansive and sympathetic)

I hope that you are feeling better now. I am awfully sorry you have the measles. Miss C. told us all to [write] to you. Are you feeling better ?   We all miss you terrible.   Miss C. gave the boys a new ball to play (base-ball).   I think it is a grand one.   Which side are you on.   Did you win last time. We all miss you, we want you to come back as soon as possible. Your truly friend,

Louisa R. B.

6. (Sympathetic)

I am very sorry you are sick with the measles.   How are you getting along ?   When will you be back to school ?   We are all writing you a letter now.   I hope you will be back to school soon.   Yours sincerely,

May D.

7. (Cordial)

I am very sorry that you have the measles but hope you will get better soon and be back to school.   I wish you would soon get better, so you could play ball with us.   My dear fre[ie]nd Goodby[e],

Tony F.

8. (Conventional)

Just a few lines to let you know how [are] you getting alone[g] with the measles ?   When do you think you are coming back. I am very sorry William.   Hope you will be back this week. Yours truly

Lucy R.

9. (Perfunctory)

I am sorry that you have the Measles. When are you going to get over with the measles ? I hope you will be better and come back to School. Your friend,

Benton E.

10. (Crisp)

I am very sorr(e)y that(t) you are sick. I hope that you will be back to school soon. Your loving fria[e]nd,

Dominic T.

11. (Businesslike)

I am sending you a few words saying that I am sorry that you are sick, and that you can [can't] come to school. Your friend,

Henry K.

12. (Irrelevant)

I hope you will be able to come to school next week if you get rid of the measles, we miss you. I am one of your friends, at resesse [recess] we play tag outdoors we have lots of fun, when we come in we are sweating, Your friend,

Lloyd B.

13. (Repetition, poverty of expression)

I am sorry that you are sick. I hope you will be back to school soon. I am sorry that you have the measles, everybody in the room is sorry to[o]. Yours truly,

Jennie D.

14. (" Good time " dominant idea)

I hope you will get over with the measles. We are having a good time. I hope you are having a good time. I am very sorry you are sick.

Please [answer] this letter. Good-by[e],

Elwood H.

15.   (Sensible)

I am sorry that you are sick. I hope you will soon get better. We are starting back to the work that we first learn[n]ed. I just wrote you a few lines for it is all I can think of. Your friend,

Edith W.

Even from such rudimentary correspondence we can see that when the famous French naturalist Buffon wrote " *Le style est l'homme même*," he was giving expression to a profound truth.

Qualities in Letter Writing which Count Most. Many letter writers, while charming in their style and information, offer little to the investigator who is eager to read the character of the writer through the letters. The most fruitful type of letter is that which is written in time of a crisis pending a grave danger. Spontaneity is then bound to break through convention, and the inner nature of the writer will be revealed partly in the style, tempo, and phraseology but mainly in the content, in the attitude, and in the course of action laid out. That is why the correspondence between Héloise and Abelard, if wholly authentic, is such a gripping human document ; that is why it belongs to the inspirational literature of the world.

Most intimate letters—Swift's Journal to Stella, for instance—are lyric effusions. The Héloise—Abelard epistles, too, are, of course, lyric in tone but epic in circumstance, in spirit, really in essence. It is as if the authors were so possessed by their common lot that they became entirely oblivious of their own " I " while writing. How differently must be treated in this respect Chesterfield's or Horace Walpole's elegant letters, the epistolary nature of which was a matter of form only.

It is time now to consider a type of biography which has come into vogue only recently in a certain department of science, I am referring to the clinical case.

CLINICAL CASES

The case method which has become so popular of late has been making its way into a number of arts and sciences. Psychiatry and subnormal psychology are especially susceptible to this form of didactic presentation, and as with everything else, from non-existence or complete absence, the method has been put on a pedestal so that the description of the case frequently takes the place of systematic presentation ; and let us not forget, too, that the case is particular and often made typical to fit the theory of the exponent.

A certain amount of citation will always have to be resorted to for the purpose of illustration, but many authors nowadays either cite cases in order to furnish interesting reading and at the same time to give an idea of what peculiar people have come under their scrutiny, or else they select the data with the object in view of bolstering up a particular hypothesis.

Let it be said, then, that nothing is easier than drawing out innumerable forms of behaviour such as would render support to any man's statement ; and when the data are not quite obvious, interpretations and explanations are brought forth to colour the picture.

Pitfalls of the Case Description. The clinical cases offered in textbooks and treatises are, of course, nothing but miniature biographies to prove a certain point and often are presented with a specific bias in mind, this bias determining the selection of the facts and the emphasis on some special points, singled out for interpretation in accordance with the writer's favoured view.

The question which every clinical recorder should ask of himself before setting down his report is : " How typical is this bit of behaviour ? Can it be explained in terms of any other theory than the one I subscribe to ? " Above all, he should see to it that the mode of behaviour is distinct, and not blurred. The safest method of testing this is to ascertain whether it ' runs ' in other individuals too. On the other hand, he must make sure that it does not merely bespeak a common trait with which everybody is familiar, and therefore not worthy of detailed description. The character of a miser is too well known to require further portraying, unless the individual in question possesses something in the way of a remarkable variation. Otherwise the clinical picture reduces to mere gossip. We may be interested in the details just as we are impelled to read day in and day out newspaper accounts of the same happenings in which only the names, places, and minor circumstances are varied.

We are quite aware that no two people are alike, and that every clinical case presents a combination of tendencies peculiar to the person described, but it can readily be seen that there is no end to this process of citation. The inevitable result is the creation of as many types as there are individuals, a result which we have had occasion to deplore in connection with the course of literary characterology in England and in France.

The Raw Case History. More hopeful is the collection of material for the purpose of presenting the *individual* as a whole, and not merely one phase of him. What has been said in the previous section refers to the abridged reports of case histories such as the literature in psychoanalysis and psychiatry abounds in. The same cavils do not apply to the complete case history as set down by social workers in their search of data. Their search must, of course, be somewhat guided by previous knowledge ; but, as a rule, the material is gathered without any interpretations in mind. It is from these records and not from the condensed miniatures that character studies may be made. The field of operation for the case method is naturally restricted, inasmuch as from its very nature it is applicable to those individuals only who require institutional attention, whether they be defective in some one respect, delinquent or psychoneurotic. The normal person, in the conventional sense of the word, can never be subjected to this method.

It must also be borne in mind that the case history is not primarily intended for the student of character. " The nature of a social case history is determined by the kinds of purpose it is intended to subserve," writes A. E. Sheffield, who later goes on to define this purpose as threefold : (1) the immediate purpose of furthering effective treatment of individual clients ; (2) the ultimate purpose of general social betterment ; and (3) the incidental purpose of establishing the case worker herself in critical thinking." [1] The student of character must then treat the case history merely as a mass of material in which he is to do some mining. The competent social worker will, of course, not neglect to indicate various character traits of the individuals dealt with, but the impressions and reports must be checked up.

PATHOGRAPHY

By *pathography* is meant a biographical sketch from the point of view of pathology or psychiatry. It may be thought of as an extended clinical case description of a well-known (usually historical) person who need not have been confined or under observation. The primary impulse behind pathography was the historical interest, and I believe it was Ireland who was the first to follow the mental aberrations of historical and literary characters in his two brilliant works, *The Blot upon the Brain* (1885) and *Through the Ivory Gate* (1889), where he reveals himself the historian as well as the psychiatrist.

Our Debt to Ireland. A generation ago, when Ireland carried on his work of enlightenment, it was not so easy to think of conquerors, of rulers of empires, of leaders in thought and art as tainted with insanity. Lombroso, it is true, had

[1] A. E. Sheffield, *The Social Case History*, 1920, pp. 5-6.

already made his sensational *début*; yet it was just as daring then to stigmatize Swedenborg, Ivan the Terrible, Blake, and other celebrities as to maintain at present that some people are free from neurosis or psychosis.   Moreover, Ireland, unlike his contemporaries who wrote in a similar vein, was concerned with the individual, not with proving an hypothesis.

Ireland's sketches are distinguished for the significance and pertinence of the data. He does not stop while telling his story to show how the facts of the case necessarily substantiate his theory.   He lets the events unfold themselves without added digressions and then proceeds to set forth his conclusions on the view that the strange behaviour of the individuals described was organically caused by adhesions in the brain, mal-formations, abnormal conditions in the *dura mater, pia mater,* or other parts of the brain.   The particulars of each autopsy are given at length in support of the general thesis.

Cultivation of Pathography in Germany. If Ireland was a pioneer in this field, he certainly had a host of successors who may never have heard of him.   Of these, Möbius stands out as the foremost and most thorough investigator who, far more than his older contemporary, was influential in directing attention to the study of pathography through his researches on the idiosyncrasies of eminent literary men and philosophers. Pathography in less than a decade became a useful pastime for both the physician and the psychiatrist.   To what extremes this can be carried will be gathered from a perusal of several of G. M. Gould's volumes [1] in which all the letters and utterances of a number of famous men and women are ransacked for expressions about their ailments, both chronic and temporary, only to conclude, though by what means is not apparent, that all their disorders, both physical and mental, were due to eye-strain, and that an oculist correcting their ametropia could have spared them nearly all their misery.

[1] G. M. Gould, *Biographic Clinics.*

To-day it is not eye-strain but complexes, conflicts, repressions, that are invoked to explain the ills of an age. As is ever the case, we shall always find what we are looking for in these obscure regions, and for that reason it behoves us to be doubly careful.

Nevertheless, it would be captious to find fault with the painstaking researches instituted by the medical writers into the lives of celebrities. Even Gould's work of collecting thousands of references to the ailments of literary men and artists (although some of the quotations have been twisted from the context and misinterpreted) is of no mean service. And certainly the numerous psychiatric studies which have sprung up in the last twenty years, studies on Robespierre, Otto Ludwig, Maupassant, Nietzsche, Tolstoi, Berlioz, L. Sterne, Rousseau, von Kleist, Strindberg, Poe, Weininger,[1] and many others are not to be taken lightly. Perhaps the conclusions drawn are not so valuable as the mass of data gathered which can always be exploited in the light of subsequent knowledge.

Psychoanalytic Participation of Dubious Value. Meanwhile the psychoanalytic camp has brought to bear its arsenal of ammunition in the puzzling out of personality traits of eminent people. Psychoanalysis in this respect is an offshoot of pathography ; and already several interesting studies have appeared from the pen of Freud and his disciples, as the monographs on Leonardo da Vinci by the master himself, on Segantini by Abraham, on Lenau by Sadger, etc. The chief weakness of these " analytograms ", if I may coin the term, is the utter failure to discriminate between the essential and the non-essential on the fundamental assumption of psycho-analysis that *what appears as very inessential or accidental may frequently have a significant bearing on the case.* In this way there is no end to the incidents drawn out and interpreted exegetically and hermeneutically, although considerable

---

[1] Consult the bibliography for the full list of titles and authors.

NN

doubt may be entertained as to whether the incidents alleged form a concatenated series in the life-course of the individual or even whether they require explanation.

PSYCHOGRAPHY

Psychography is a step in advance of pathography in that it records a person's *total* reactions (moral, temperamental, physical and intellectual) under all sorts of conditions. The examination upon which the psychogram is based extends over a period of weeks and sometimes even months ; and specially devised tests are often introduced for the purpose of the examination.

In the practical study of personality one of the desiderata has been the singling out of a number of fundamental traits with a view to individual rating.

Before this branch of psychology had come into its own, the emphasis had been on the study of the self. In 1914 there appeared a sort of introspective *vade mecum* by Yerkes and La Rue, called *Outline of a Study of the Self.* It was intended as a stock-taking memorandum of the individual with a biological bias in its approach. Much of the material was irrelevant, and the whole of it was unwieldy. The most significant phases of the personality were missing, while the sensory and genetic questions were overstressed.

Meanwhile new avenues had been opened to the study. Psychoanalysis led the way in its searching examination, but psychiatry was beginning to realize the value of the personality angle. Amsden and Hoch, in particular, among American psychiatrists, have done yeoman service in calling the attention of practitioners to the personality in probing the make-up of the patient along systematic lines, not that the matter had been overlooked by their predecessors, but there had not been the same emphasis laid on the method.

DEVELOPMENT OF THE PSYCHOGRAPH

From the purely psychological approach, the psychograph

had been developed both in France as early as 1896, by Toulouse, and in Germany, a few years later, by Stern, as an abbreviated description of a given individual's personality. The methods differed both in scope and in point of accentuation. Toulouse, Binet, and in Germany, the chemist Ostwald, adopted a literary approach, somewhat diffuse in treatment. Stern's psychography seemed superior to the French literary form in that it was more concise and systematic, but it was still too comprehensive. Stern was attempting to build up not so much a personality structure as a branch to be known hereafter as differential psychology; and possibly without taking into account Galton's projects in a similar direction, he was following the same procedure. The ratings were to be along the lines of visual or auditory acuity, reaction differences, etc. How else could it be? Psychology was committed in those pioneer days to a sensory and static purview.

The psychographic chart which G. W. Allport introduced was much of an improvement over the older psychography in that it represented in a neat form the profile of a given personality. It permitted of quantitative treatment in that each selected trait could be rated from 1 to 100 on a vertical line, so that in conformity with American research methods, a curve could be drawn which affords at a glance an insight into one's personality.

The chart does not purport to deal with a multitude of separate traits. It consists of a selection of fundamental personality components and represents a neat profile of one's whole make-up, assuming that we approve of the selection and the order of arrangement. Intelligence, we note, is distributed under intelligence proper, under attitudes toward self where it appears as insight, and under sociality as social intelligence. Furthermore, character as we understand it in this book seems to be crowded into the one column headed " Socialization of Behaviour ", even if it might communicate with the neighbouring columns (social participation and social intelligence).

CHART I

PSYCHOGRAPH OF _____ AGE _____

TRAITS OF PERSONALITY

FACTOR OF PHYSIQUE	FACTOR OF INTELLIGENCE	FACTOR OF TEMPERAMENT		SELF EXPRESSION					ATTITUDES TOWARD SELF			SOCIALITY		
GENERAL PHYSICAL SUPERIORITY	HIGH INTELLIGENCE	BROAD EMOTIONS	STRONG EMOTIONS	EXTROVERSION	ASCENDANCE	DRIVE	EXPANSION	MODERATE ATTITUDE	INSIGHT	HIGH SELF-ASSURANCE	SOCIAL PARTICIPATION	SOCIALIZATION OF BEHAVIOR	HIGH SOCIAL INTELLIGENCE
							MEDIAN	LINE					
PHYSICAL INFERIORITY	LOW INTELLIGENCE	NARROW EMOTIONS	WEAK EMOTIONS	INTROVERSION	SUBMISSION	ABSENCE OF DRIVE	SECLUSION	RADICALISM OR REACTIONISM	LACK OF INSIGHT	LOW SELF-ASSURANCE	LACK OF SOCIAL PARTICIPATION	UNSOCIALIZED BEHAVIOR	LOW SOCIAL INTELLIGENCE

RANKS PLOTTED BY { RANK ORDER METHOD (NO. OF CASES _____ MEDIAN _____
SCORING METHOD (AVG OF _____ RATINGS. MEDIAN _____
TEST METHOD _____
INDEX COMPUTATION (FOR ATTITUDES TOWARD SELF)

Offhand one might say that the conative aspect of personality is rather neglected in the chart.

The graphic treatment of personality has both its advantages and disadvantages. The quantitative comparison of individuals is a great gain. That perplexing quantity called the borderline is eliminated. The location is concretely shown, and the direction taken by a given trait is clearly indicated by the ascent or the descent of the curve. In addition, composite ratings are possible by averaging the curves of all the raters ; or an individual's self-rating may be compared with the composite rating of himself by a group.

Shortcomings of the Chart. On the other hand, however, we miss in the plotting method the *qualitative differentiation* of individuals. Can we really compare persons as regards their social participation when their modes of behaviour are disparate ? One individual may never enjoy a theatre performance unless he has a companion by his side ; another attends always alone but is intensely interested in the *social* aspect of the play. How can we measure the social participation of the two men ? Ibsen the individualist served as a powerful medium of social participation not only through his plays but must have been deeply engrossed in the workings of society in order to create the problem play. To take another instance, Chopin was a very poor correspondent. His chief biographer Niecks says somewhere in his life of Chopin that the great composer would rather walk a few miles to answer a friend than to reply by letter. Yet the same Chopin was constantly moving in social circles. Contrariwise, among the scholars and scientists, there is no dearth of men who are in communication with hundreds of people to whom they would rather write than converse with. Tchaikovsky's patroness, who sent him regularly for many years an allowance of 6,000 roubles on condition that they never met personally,[1]

---

[1]Nadejda Filaretovna von Meck feared that a face to face meeting might lower their estimates of each other and tarnish that ideal which had been set up between them.

is an extreme case of this type of person. But even to such a one is sociality not to be denied.

The same cross relationship presents itself with other traits. Aside from the fact that the very one who is extremely ascendent toward subalterns is very submissive in the presence of his superiors, we must bear in mind also that it is quite possible for a man to be ascendent in writing toward the same individuals in whose company he feels submissive ; and, *per contra*, we may find those who are dominating in personal contact while appearing somewhat shy when it is necessary for them to take a definite stand in writing.

Perhaps the psychographic chart would have to make room for more traits in order to allow for a more natural schematization of personality types, for the progressive integration of psychological events or knowledge is such that a viewpoint must be corrected in the light of a new crystallization, even if new data are not available. Allport's schema has obviously been born under the conjuncture of social psychology, behaviorism, and experimental psychology. It is, therefore, not sufficiently dynamic and is particularly lacking in the conative and affective components.

REQUIREMENTS OF A PERSONALITY CHART

But before we proceed further, we ought to look into the methodological requirements of a chart of this sort. The difficulties are not to be denied or overlooked. The problem before us is how to condense the one thousand and one traits of an individual, so that the most significant of them (perhaps only a dozen in number) will stand out and, so to speak, spell the individual. Allport selected the following qualities :

Physique and Intelligence
1. Factor of physique.
2. Factor of intelligence.

Temperament

3. Breadth of emotions.
4. Strength of emotions.

Self-Expression

5. Extraversion and introversion.
6. Ascendance and submission.
7. Drive.
8. Expansion and reclusion.
9. Moderateness and extremism.

Attitude Toward Self

10. Insight.
11. Self-assurance.

Sociality

12. Social participation.
13. Socialization of behavior.
14. Social intelligence.

With the median line forming the boundary between the positive and negative values in each of these traits, we have the means of rating each trait either as a plus or minus.

In applying to the chart the touchstone of methodology, we must ask ourselves (1) whether the most fundamental traits have been singled out, (2) whether some of these traits can be at all rated either by the individual or his friends, (3) whether there is not some overlapping or indication of intercorrelation, and finally (4) whether the resulting curve presents us with a true profile of an individual's personality.

To answer these questions provisionally, let us start with the factor of physique. The term connotes, I think, generally the external structure of the body, stature, build, and figure but only in a broad sense refers to the facial appearance, both features and expression ; and still less does it include the qualities of the voice, which is no inconsiderable factor in the appraisal of personality. Gait, laughter, and gestures will fit into one or another of the three rubrics mentioned.

Instead of the one column, then, dealing with general physical superiority at the top and physical inferiority at the bottom, we should require three columns for the physical traits, so that the lay friend who rates the individual will not lose sight of either the facial features or the voice.

With regard to the intelligence factor, the intellect component should not be missing on the chart, in the case of the intellectual. At any rate, high and low intelligence may not be comparable with high and low intellect. This point, however, may be ceded without too much controversy. The component of social intelligence should also find a place here instead of in the last column under sociality, which as a general category may be resolved. Vision may be included in the intelligence department but only with outstanding individuals.

A far more serious criticism may be made against the restriction of the temperament factor to the double column of broad emotions and strong emotions. First, we may ask whether the classification means much to us without specification ; e.g., let us say that A has strong emotions, what prognosis can we make of him ? Of if B has broad emotions, in what way is his personality revealed to us, other than that some day a certain occasion will call for the display of a certain emotion and he will not disappoint us in our prediction ? But our second objection is more damaging. It appears that we have no instrument for rating either ourselves or others on that score, for we have no standards or limits of range in that respect. To take my own case, I should not be able to state under oath whether my emotions are strong or broad ; and my friends, who naturally could not have observed me under a great variety of circumstances, would be hard put to it if asked to give their opinion on this personal matter.

The breadth or strength of the emotions is a comparatively insignificant question beside the matter of which emotion is dominant, whether fear, anger, love, etc. For once we may be specificists to concede that an individual may show a violent temper and yet not display any signs of terror under the most trying conditions.

Our temperament factor must thus necessarily resolve itself in the old fourfold scheme of sanguine and phlegmatic (in one column) and choleric and melancholic (in another column). The reason why Galen's table persists in spite of incessant attacks is that it is not only human but serviceable. We can in a very short time take the temperamental measure of our interlocutor, without resorting to tests and questionnaires.

As regards the factors of self-expression, there is scarcely anything to cavil against. Extraversion, ascendance, drive, expansion, and moderate attitude top their respective columns and are important traits. One may ask whether expansion and reclusion are not already covered by extraversion and introversion, but apparently Allport thinks that there is an empirical basis for their independent collation. Similarly moderate attitude and extremism (radicalism or reactionism) may to some extent overlap with the next rubric, viz., insight, since an extremist is apt to be deficient in insight.

Under "attitudes toward self", we have the factors of insight and self-assurance, both very important constituents of personality, even if the general label is not clear. Neither of these traits is any more an attitude toward self than toward others. In fact, to possess insight which, however, Allport defines as self-knowledge, is to understand where one stands in relation to others.

Allport's rubric of sociality comprises social participation, socialization of behavior, and social intelligence. In my opinion, social participation can be deduced from the extraversion factor. There may be a few exceptions for some deep-seated reason, but otherwise we may take it as a rule that the extravert will participate in social activity while the introvert will not.

As for " socialization of behavior ", I should suggest as a substitute " behavior factors " and expand the class by introducing the following columns : (1) constancy of behavior (i.e., reliability or uniformity of action) ; (2) conventionality (i.e., conformity to the *mores* of the group) ; and (3) social or inter-individual consistency (i.e., ethical conduct). It seems clear that the three forms of behavior in our age of enlightenment should not be confused with each other, although the man in the street may identify them.

Having dealt with the Allport psychograph as it stands, it now behooves us to consider what a chart of personality should include that the existing psychographs have omitted.

BASIC TRAITS IN PERSONALYSIS [1]

Among the fundamental traits and personality components which we miss in the psychographic chart are to be found egocentricity (and altrocentricity) cyclothymia (and schizothymia), hyperkinesis (and hypokinesis), and the dynamic aspect of the individual (i.e., is he hyperdynamic, dynamic, hypodynamic, or asthenic ?). Perhaps, too, the constitutional picture should be included, i.e., is the person

---

[1] I make no apologies for adopting the word *personalysis* instead of using the cumbersome phrase " personality analysis ". The coining of a word in psychology is no less permissible than in botany or chemistry ; and surely it is not the term so much as the concept which counts. If the word *Amerindian* has been adopted as a suitable designation for the American Indian, how much more appropriate is the word *personalysis ?*

The coining of the term *personalysis* is not a gesture in the direction of the abbreviated government agencies, like O.P.A., V.A., or proletcult, Amvet, comsomol, etc. These abridgments are conveniences or luxuries ; *personalysis* is a necessity, and certainly as eligible to lexicographic naturalization as the term *psychonalysis*. Technically, I propose the term to be linked with a chart in which a given individual's personality traits are delineated in condensed fashion, yet more fully than in a psychograph, which does not list the defects under the various rubrics. Generally speaking, *personalysis* would denote any discussion with regard to the *analysis* of personality, not coincident with the whole subject of personality, but with one aspect of it.

pyknic or leptosomatic ? But if Kretschmer's doctrine is accepted, then cyclothymia and schizothymia will be sufficient for our purpose, since the cyclothymic will correspond to the pyknic and the schizothymic to the leptosome. Naturally as in the field of intelligence testing, it is superfluous to include two classes which correlate too highly with one another.

Certainly we should reserve a place in our personalysis for the impulse factor, i.e., answering the question whether the subject is hypomanic, impulsive, inhibited, or obstructed. The sense of humor is another basic personality factor which cannot but enter into all social relations and yet is not to be derived from or correlated with either intelligence or gregariousness.[1]

The life-interest factor corresponding to the *Lebensform* of Spranger is another item which we cannot afford to eliminate from our compass. We may not agree with Spranger as to the relative value of the different life interests, but surely to know that a person is money-minded or artistic in his make-up or power-seeking gives us a rather important clue as to his or her behavior in the future.

The habit life of an individual, although *ex vi termini* it cannot be on a par with the fundamental traits, nevertheless, is of paramount importance in our appraisal of a man or woman, not only because the formation of a habit is, as I have contended elsewhere, definitely to be linked up with some native predisposition, but even if this postulate is not to be granted, the fact remains that our attitude changes materially when we discover objectionable habits in our interlocutor. It is not so much smoking or drinking that one has in mind nowadays, as general uncleanliness, habits like picking the nose, drilling the ears, belching with gusto, sucking the teeth

---

[1] According to Allport, the sense of humor has been omitted because it correlated so highly with insight. This is a significant fact, which should be followed up. Cf. *Personality : A Psychological Interpretation* 1937, p. 222.

noisily in order to remove some particles of food, etc.

Finally, or perhaps better ultimately, the integratedness or lability of the personality must be considered, for that constitutes an index of how well the whole personality hangs together.

As we view our newly constructed chart, we perceive that our aim was to achieve comprehensiveness in the bounds of serviceableness. It is for us to ask ourselves whether the *particular trait or component* will be of diagnostic value. It makes no difference whether the subject is of dark complexion or fair, unless it can be shown that the coloring will enable us to predict something about the individual's behavior.

What Determines Inclusion or Exclusion ?   Similarly, we cannot go into the qualities desirable for filling a certain post. The Y.M.C.A. application blank will probably assign a place for leadership. A denominational college will inquire into the religious principles of a candidate for an instructorship ; and probably the matter of a headmaster's sex life is of considerable magnitude to the administration of a boy's boarding school, but these are all specific requirements. Leadership, to take one instance cited, is not a fundamental trait, but a conglomerate ; and besides, it is a variable concept differing with the circle or milieu, in its general usage bearing a politico-religious connotation. We need not discuss the inclusion of the creed ingredient in a personalysis, but the eligibility of the sex factor is a mooted point, the question before us being whether the diagnostic value of the information is sufficient to compensate for the complications arising out of the exploration of such delicate regions.   To state that X is homosexual, a transvesite, or sadistic, to mention only the commoner forms of sexual deviations, would in no way enlighten the subject who is supposedly acquainted with his or her tendencies and it is problematic whether, except in the case of medical treatment or matrimonial contemplation, the revelations are useful. I admit, however, that the point is debatable, and if strongly urged, I could bring myself to introduce this extremely important component of personality, provided, of course, these sex characteristics could form a continuum comparable with our other series.

The endocrine factors have been intentionally glossed over, because they should figure on the clinical chart rather than on a personality chart. To what extent the glands affect the personality is not definitely known, and what we usually do is to reason backwards ; in other words, if the individual is excitable and vivacious, we say that there is hyperthyroidism ; if very energetic and swarthy in appearance, we associate the condition with the adrenals ; and so on. Naturally in this state of affairs, we cannot expect to offer much sound knowledge in our personalysis.

Psychoanalysis in Order but Out of Place. It may seem a bit strange that the Freudian mechanisms do not figure in our present scheme. The primary reason for this apparent neglect is that they are too deep-seated and serve an ætiological purpose, i.e., they help to derive existing conditions, but are not fundamentally diagnostic. Furthermore, they involve too much speculation, if they are to be applied diagnostically or prognostically. Another disadvantage is that many months would need to be consumed before a personalysis could be charted for any individual. We shall see later, however, that at least some of the psychoanalytic mechanisms or dynamisms will be dealt with under the proper rubrics below the trait columns.

Perhaps it must be explained that the phenotypical aspects of personality must in such a practical device as a personalysis take precedence over the genotypical constituents, which of necessity are obscure and fraught with controversy at every turn. To make an issue of every disputable factor in the dynamic substructure of personality would lead us away from psychology, and into the realm of metaphysics. To be sure, the genotypical elements, especially where there is some consensus of opinion regarding them, may throw a great deal of light on the perceptible personality.

To illustrate further, even if we should ascertain that the individual examined is troubled with a mother fixation or anal eroticism, it would be difficult to obtain further results out of this discovery. Rather should we expect the fact, if actually revealed by psychoanalytic treatment, to be liquidated by the very discovery. Most of the other Freudian dynamisms are too general to be applicable to specific individuals significantly ; e.g., sublimation, compensation, rationalization, etc. When, however, we come to such a dynamism as projection, it is a different story. Undoubtedly we have before us a definite trait, which can be established by other than the psycho-analytic method ; and it is a trait which looms large in the contacts of life. Thus we see that *serviceableness, applicability, and the degree of empirical observability determine the inclusion or elimination of psychoanalytic factors in our personalysis.*

Combination of Quality and Quantity. One of the novel features that the personalysis is to introduce centers around the designation of qualitative stages on the graduated column as milestones or as fingerposts, perhaps, to the rater. Not only the layman but even the psychologist is in need of a reminder in common-sense terms, in addition to the graphic division lines. As in the intelligence quotient scale, where 70–80 denotes a state of moronity, and 110–130 superiority, we may find it convenient to set down the trait of quarrelsomeness in the choleric-melancholic column as 90, morose as 80, sensitive as -10 to $+10$, and depressed as -90. The plus values and negative values naturally do not possess for us any more than a referential significance, for 90 may be no more desirable a position to hold than -90 in the various columns.

There is one other avowal which should be made, indicative

of the writer's point of view, and that is the point where the qualitative gradation interferes with the quantitative treatment of a given generic trait. It is the former that has the right of way, for to my mind the qualitative classification is more telling, more definite, and in doubtful cases will permit us to check up on the quantities, especially when the rating is done by lay people. In other words, there is apt to be more agreement as to whether an individual is sensitive or not than on the particular quantity to be marked as an ordinate for our curve.

Finally a word might be said about the clinical observations or conclusions to be noted at the bottom of the chart under the respective rubrics ; e.g., under the explosive-inhibited column, abulic or anancastic tendencies may be checked, or under the physical make-up, definite malformations and defects may be enumerated.

From the psychograph, as it is originally constituted, we cannot tell whether our subject is an eccentric, fanatic, boaster, hypochondriac, or neurasthenic. Our personalysis aims to present a total picture of the individual's personality, particularly helpful to the clinician. It is self-understood that these designations and findings will frequently offer controversial points, but I think it cannot be denied that the proposed chart will be of heuristic value to psychologist, psychiatrist, and social worker, as well as vocational director ; and all the information can be had on one large sheet of paper.

One of the objections which I can anticipate is that our chart will be so cluttered up with traits that for the trees it will be difficult to see the forest ; and perhaps at this juncture my own strictures of Klages', Pfänder's, and Haeberlin's systems will be recalled as taunting spectres. On consulting, however, these authors, it will be perceived that not only is the list of traits in their works many times larger than the total number of components in the personalysis, but that on the basis of classification, their rationale for appearing as fundamental traits is not in evidence. It seems as if the authors under discussion have thought now of this quality and now of that and decided to lump them all in the cauldron of personality or·character, as they each, in spite of their different approaches, may denominate the field.

Moreover, I am quite willing to reduce the categories if some trait which appears in the personalysis is shown to be non-diagnostic or slight, or else perfectly correlated with another already mentioned.

The Source of Our Information. The psychographee should first rate himself by placing a dot in the centre of each column and connecting the points so as to obtain a graph.

Other charts are then passed to each of five associates who know the person well (near relatives are to be avoided). Most of the terms are self-explanatory to intelligent people ; others need a few words of explanation. The average (algebraic summation first) of the five ratings is then obtained for each column as a new graph, which is traced in ink of a different color on the original chart. The difference in the two curves will, to some extent, indicate the amount of insight in the person charted, on the assumption that insight is the quality of seeing ourselves in relation to others objectively.

In order to secure our information, all the methods in vogue must be appealed to. If the individual himself is also harnessed for the task, we have the introspective method in addition to the method of observation, the questionnaire, tests, the interview, and, last but not least, graphology. Psychoanalysis is invaluable but cannot, because of the various restrictions (time, expense, factional exclusiveness), be invoked regularly.

Personalysis—A Species of Human Parsing. The relation-ship of grammar to the classification of psychopathic phe-nomena has been remarked on more than one occasion. Southard, probably deriving his cue from Kraepelin, has been particularly fond of pointing out parallels between certain functions in grammar and human behavior, as is evidenced by the charts that used to hang in the Boston Psychopathic Hospital.

Indeed we need not wonder at such a tendency. Grammar as the logic of speech must be grounded in the same principles as are at the root of all our methodology, but, in addition, it has the advantage which does not attach to philosophy (logistic), viz., that it is not too artificial, having evolved out of the psychological folk-urge. In this way grammar is closer to our subject, to wit, the phenomena of human behavior, than is logic, pure and simple.

As we go back in our recollections to the sometimes irksome task of parsing, we may remember what satisfaction was ours after completing the parsing of a difficult word, or rather a word in a complicated sentence. Now we may view our individual whose personality is to be analyzed as the analogue only a thousandfold more complex—of the word, and the world as the analogue of the sentence, only a million times more complicated. The function of the parsing exercise was to place a given word in relation to all other words in the sentence, so that its position would be clear from all angles. Now is it not just this that we are trying to do when we analyze personality in a specific case—placing the individual with reference to others, by discovering his particular combination of traits, idiosyncrasies, defects, and possibilities ? And in so doing must we not bring to bear the weight of all the different schools, in so far as they tend to explore a new region of personality ?

The benefit accruing from such analysis is not merely of an applied character, i.e., helping the person gauged, but contains a theoretical element, for it is calculated to further our knowledge of the much disputed problem of traits ; and it cannot but serve to bring out the differentiae of certain qualities which are generally treated as if they were identical, e.g., moroseness and sullenness or timidity and cowardice.

That the chart submitted here is not without its flaws goes without saying. G. W. Allport has offered two or three objections which may briefly be dealt with at this point.

His chief objection is to treating the temperaments, and particularly the life interests, Spranger's *Lebensformen*, as if each set formed a continuum, whereas in reality each of the temperaments and each of the value directions are claimed to be a separate category, deserving a rating in itself, especially as there are tests devised by Allport and Vernon for the rating of these value directions in an individual.

Undoubtedly the criticism is not without ground from the point of view of pure quantification of traits, but there is an underlying difference between Dr. Allport's position and mine. While he is committed to a numerical treatment of personality factors, making an exception only where an individual is made the subject of an extensive independent investigation, I should prefer to qualify the quantification whenever possible, even in the primary analysis. Secondly, he is skeptical of the type theory of personality, while I am in favor of accepting the doctrine of at least dominant tendencies ; that is to say, while recognizing the difficulties of pigeonholing an individual under so many rubrics, I am of the opinion that the majority of people exhibit characteristics sufficiently pronounced for typal identification.

With regard to the specific charge that I make a continuum of traits and qualities which are incomparable on a scale, I must appeal to the differentiae upon which the classifications in point are based. I think of choleric and melancholic as opposites, or contradictories rather, on a scale, because the temperaments which they represent differ from one another both as to speed and intensity. Similarly is it the case with the sanguine and phlegmatic traits. The concept of a continuum requires only the condition of linking homogeneous extremes without a break in the series. It is true that a melancholic person may be choleric. In that case he would be sullen or morose, which is a piece of supporting evidence that the two temperamental phases form a continuum, for one quality combines components of both extreme ; and thus is effected, in a sense, a compromise. Sensitiveness, too, is a function of both the choleric and melancholic, but lower down the scale. The sensitive or " touchy " person is a melancholic with a choleric lining.

As to the life-interests (*Lebensformen*), again it is my feeling that the six fundamental value directions are intended to form a continuum, with the economic or money-minded person lowest in Spranger's scale (although assigned positive values in keeping with some of the other traits with which they may be correlated, incidentally showing that the negative values on the chart are not necessarily undesirable any more than the positive values are always socially desirable) and the spiritual life-interest highest in the scale. Now, of course, I realize that it may be simpler to expand the column of life interests into six rubrics, placing each of the life interests at the top of their respective columns and the deficiency of each life-interest at the bottom, but this not only overemphasizes one approach in our personalysis but savors of Porphyry's system of dichotomy—methodical but barren.

May we not assume that there is a value *élan* which expresses itself in a theoretical urge in one individual, in the quest for power in another, in the drive for money in a third, in artistic impulses in a fourth, and so on ? And is it not true that empirically money-mindedness and spirituality are mutually exclusive and that the pure theorist is not an artist, nor is the *Machtmensch* weighed down by considerations of love for his fellow-men ?

When we decide that an individual is money-minded, we

accord him a narrow range to begin with and place him somewhere in that circumscribed sphere. We are not *rating him so much on his money-mindedness, as on his value élan* ; and if found to be money-minded, then his place is more or less established, although in comparison with other money-minded individuals he may be assigned a higher or lower position.

We are not primarily concerned with how much of other interests the same individual may possess, but with ascertaining his dominant interest. If, however, we discover the *rara avis* that actually partakes of two life-interests almost in the same outstanding measure, then for once we mark our notch in two different places in the column of life-interests and obtain a delta-like spot in our curve ; but certainly this would be the exception, and should not invalidate the purpose of our chart. It would scarcely do, because of these rare exceptions, to introduce six rubrics in our already too elaborate chart and supply six artificial opposites at the bottom of the column merely to carry out our dichotomy.

Relation between Biography and Psychography. Psychography is contrasted with biography by Stern as (*a*) dealing in a psychological manner with the manifold of characteristics of an individual instead of treating him as a unit, and (*b*) concerning itself with the average person as well as with the outstanding personality who represents the subject of the biographer.[1] Perhaps in a work on individual differences it is better to keep the biographical method and the psychographic method separate, but it is not necessary to draw an antithesis between them, for not only is psychography in the service of biography, as Stern himself admits, but actually a psychogram overlaps much of the territory that is included in biography ; and Toulouse's and Binet's psychographic sketches of eminent men are psychograms in every sense of the word, even if their technique is found wanting. Nor is there any reason why Ostwald should not be justified in

---

[1] W. Stern, *Differentielle Psychologie*, pp. 327–328.

PERSONALYSIS OF_____

	PHYSICAL MAKE-UP				INTELLIGEN		
	Physique and Dynamique	Facial Appearance (Mimique)	Voice	Constitution	Intelligence	Insight	Soc Intelli
	(Includes: Posture Stature Build Gait Gestures)	(Includes: Smile Regularity of features Expression Glance Charm)	(Includes: Laughter Inflection Modulation)	(Take outstanding examples for models)	(Standard to be found in successful efficiency engineer or other profession)	(Ability to see ourselves objectively in relation to others)	(The j hoste cleve mat stanc here)
+100	Very superior	Splendid	Most pleasing	Pyknic	High intelligence		High intelli
+ 90							
+ 80							
+ 70							
+ 60							
+ 50							
+ 40							
+ 30							
+ 20							
+ 10							
0				Athletic		—MEDIAN LINE	
− 10							
− 20							
− 30							
− 40							
− 50							
− 60							
− 70		Furtive glance	Nasal				
− 80		Scowling Stolid	Gruff Raucous				
− 90	Very inferior	Asymmetrical	Very disagreeable		Low intelligence	Lack of insight	Low intel
−100		Very poor		Leptosome			

Slouch Dwarfishness Obesity ———— Nervous habits Chorea Blinking Tics	Prognathism Strabism	Contravocalism Tonguetiedness Stammering Cleftpalate voice	Dysplasia	Moronity Imbecility	Inappreciativeness Faddism	Boori

ICE FACTOR			AFFECTIVE LIFE				
rial igence	Intellect	Sense of Humor	TEMPERAMENTAL FACTORS			Extraversion	Ego tric
			Sanguine	Choleric	Cyclothy-mic		
fine ss and r diplo-are our lards							
social igence	Profound and cultured	Brilliantly witty	Euphoric	Quarrel-some Sulky Sullen Morose	Capricious Changeable	Socially reactive	Conce Egoti Self-cent
				Sensitive			
social ligence	Lowbrow Shallow	Dull Insipid	Phlegmatic Apathetic Torpid Lethargic	Depressed Melancholic	Schizothy-mic	Introverted Shut-in Autistic	Altroc

OBSERVABLE DEFECTS, ANOM

hness				Litigious-ness ——— Inferiority feeling Extreme self-con-sciousness Anxiety complexes	Extreme moodiness Cycloid behavior ——— Schizoid behavior		Bragg Narci Eccen Projec ——— Fanat Religi

cen- ity	Reactionism	Ascendance	Self-Assurance	Life-Interests	Impulse Life	Drive	For
ited stic ered	Nazi Fascist Chauvinist Tory Conserva-, tive Mildly liberal	Brazen Aggressive Forward	High self-confidence	Economic (money-minded) Political (will to power) Social	Hypomanic Explosive Impulsive	Hyperki-netic Energetic	Hyper-dynar Dynar
				—MEDIAN	LINE—		
centric	Socialist Communist Theoretical Anarchist	Reserved Submissive Timid	Low self-confidence	Theoretical (scientific philo-sophical) Aesthetic Artistic Spiritual	Inhibited Paralyzed	Hypo-kinetic Indolent	Hypo-dynai Asther

ALIES, IDIOSYNCRASIES, ETC.

| ing sism tricity tion icism osity | | Superiority attitude
——
Phobias | | | Compulsive tendencies (anancasis)
Ceremoni-alism
——
Abulia | Quixotism
——
Listlessness | Neurai theni: |

	Set-Goal	Social Habits	Constancy of Behavior	Conformity of Behavior	Social or Inter-individual Consistency (*Character*)	COHESION OF FACTORS Integratedness	
mic	Purposeful	Personable Clean Tidy	Uniform Reliable	Moral Convention-al	Ethical	Well-knit Stable	+100
nic							+ 90
							+ 80
							+ 70
							+ 60
							+ 50
							+ 40
							+ 30
							+ 20
							+ 10
							0
							— 10
							— 20
							— 30
							— 40
							— 50
						Emotionally unstable	— 60
							— 70
			Bohemian Paradoxical		Unethical	Loose	— 80
mic		Untidy Uncouth	Unreliable				— 90
nic	Aimless	Infantile	Spasmodic	Unconven-tional	Unscrupul-ous	Labile	—100

| | *Idée fixe* | Nose picking Belching Ear drilling Teeth sucking | Habit-slavery —— Flightiness | Cowardice Contrariety | Scrupulosity Crimi-nality | Hysteria Psycho-pathic personality Dissociation Dual personality | |

face p. 546

calling some of the sketches [1] which he afterwards incorporated in his *Grosse Männer*—" *Psychographische Studien* ". Psychography in the broadest sense would include biography ; in the narrow sense it forms a part of biography written from the psychological standpoint.

It is through such a method that the French psychologist Toulouse was able to obtain the most astonishing comparison of the novelist Zola and the mathematician Poincaré. The results belied our expectations in most respects ; for the novelist turned out to be the more methodical, the more systematic of the two, while the serious-minded mathematician proved to be more flighty, less stable, and more given to moods. [2]

The scope of psychography was considerably enlarged through the efforts of W. Stern and O. Lipmann. Stern's review of the experimental literature with special reference to individual differences practically ushered in that branch of the science which we now call differential psychology. Latterly, it is true, Stern has abandoned the course he had earlier mapped out so laboriously, yet at the same time enthusiastically, in order to range himself with the other representatives of the *Struktur* movement which would have nothing to do with atomizing a personality, but the foundation which he has laid can still serve as a substratum for a new structure ; and a reconciliation between the analytic method and the intuitive is not unlikely, especially when we reflect that the latter receives most of its support from theoretical quarters pervaded by the individualistic vapours of metaphysics.

So far psychography has not been of much use in the department of character study. The technique has been lacking in this domain of investigation. On the reactive and the cognitive sides, all sorts of types were discovered ; and only within the last few years have the possibilities in character testing begun to open up and gradually take shape in definite suggestions for the separation and classification of types.

[1] W. Ostwald, *Annalen der Naturphilosophie*, 1907, 1908, 1909, vol. vi, vii, viii.

[2] E. Toulouse, *Henri Poincaré* (Enquête médico-psychologique sur la supériorité intellectuelle).

CHAPTER XXIX

SOURCES AND METHODS OF STUDYING CHARACTER TYPES

(RECAPITULATORY)

Equivocal Use of Term "Method". Before going any further it would be advisable to say a word or two about the use of the term "method" which is often employed ambiguously, thereby leading to confusion in classification. Methods are means taken in order to obtain certain results. But these means, may be instruments or vehicles, so to speak, or, again, they may constitute routes traversed. In reality we ought to distinguish between the *vehicle* and the *avenue of approach*. We may go to Japan by way of the Atlantic or the Pacific, but it is possible to use different vehicles in order to reach it.

In the enumeration of methods by which the study of character may be furthered, there is apt to be an overlapping or evidence of cross classification because of the circumstance referred to above. Ordinarily, to take a single instance in exemplification of the dilemma, we may speak of the historical method or the biographical method when our approach is that employed in history or biography, but in the investigation of character, the method is not historical or biographical, except by courtesy or for the sake of expediency. It is the point of view, the material exploited, which is historical or biographical. *The means we adopt of handling the material or applying the point of view* is either experimental, of the questionnaire sort, literary, etc.

Two General Types of Methods. Owing to the development of the subject and its intrinsic nature as well as the moorings to which it is attached, we must make allowance for two

548

METHODS OF STUDYING PERSONALITY

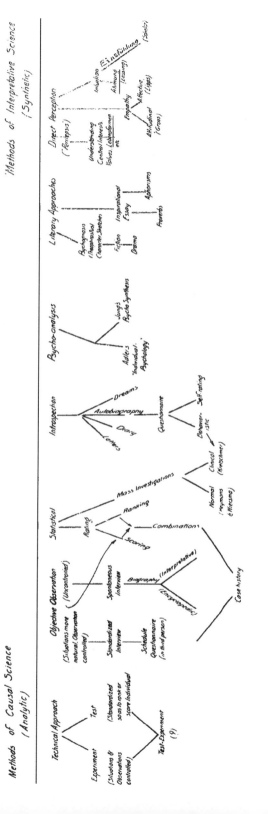

Methods of Causal Science
(Analytic)

Methods of Interpretive Science
(Syntistic)

different types of methods with intermediate combinations. The first must be envisaged as coming under the purview of the causally related sciences (the *Naturwissenschaften*), the second type must look up to the interpretative, intuitive, or understanding sciences (the *Geisteswissenschaften*). Experiments and tests come under the first head ; the exploitation of proverbs, literary sketches, etc., belongs to the second category, while questionnaires or statistical treatments contain the elements of both types, in which interpretative material is usually cast into a *naturwissenschaftliche* mould, so that it might be described and explained after the fashion of the exact sciences.

Observation in Twofold Sense. The method of observation, likewise, may be *introspective*, in which case it is open to question as to whether it comes within the jurisdiction of the natural sciences, or it may refer to objective behaviour, but even here there are different possibilities. A proverb or folk saying is certainly based on objective observation. It has the accumulated experience of the race in its favour ; yet since it was not scientifically arrived at, it belongs rather to the intuitive type of methods.

With these precautions in view we may arrange our methods according to the accompanying chart.

It goes without saying that the scheme is anything but perfect and that it has not escaped the danger of overlapping, since statistics may be applied both to questionnaire material and to the direct observation of other people's behaviour. The questionnaire, again, may deal with introspective facts or data about others. (Schedule.) But since every other arrangement will offer similar difficulties, we may resign ourselves to the present one with the understanding that it is adopted for the sake of convenience and in the hope that, as a given investigation comes up for consideration, the preliminary remarks will help to distinguish which are the primary methods and which the subsidiary.

I am aware that the rubrics fiction, proverbs, character sketches, inspirational essays and aphorisms are not strictly speaking methods but sources, and as such are secondary means of gaining information, making use primarily of observation and intuition, yet for the modern theoretical characterologist they constitute avenues of approach which serve the same purpose as a method in the broad sense of the word. It is well not to clutter up a complex classification with too many divisions, classes and sub-classes, so long as the distinctions are noted and allowed for in the text.

The Strictly Empirical Methods. Most of the methods and sources appearing in the chart have been amply discussed in the text. The experimental method of character investigation has come into vogue only lately and is best illustrated by the work of American psychologists (Chapter XXIII), particularly in the technique of Voelker. Tests, too, for the purpose of collating and identifying human types have been introduced recently, and though cultivated for the most part in the United States, beginnings have been made under favourable auspices in other countries, England and Germany, and to some extent in Russia and in France.

The test-experiment of which the Downey Will-Temperament tests furnish an example combines the control factor of the experiment with the sampling convenience of the test, but is not necessarily on that account the best kind of method, for a good deal of interpretation and assumption is involved, as may be gathered from our earlier discussion.

It may be questioned whether a combination like the test-experiment is possible on the ground that every experiment, if positive and clear-cut results are obtained, eventuates in a test, or in other words, the test is a standardized experiment. Nevertheless the distinction between a test and an experiment being that the former applies a general result to an individual in order to place that individual on a particular scale, while the experiment is undertaken to establish a general principle, we may easily conceive of material which can serve the purpose of both the test and the experiment. Since the experiment is designed to bring out a *qualitative* fact, and the test a *quantitative* fact (rank on scale) a test-experiment could be applied so as to satisfy both demands. An individual may be tested as regards his tendency to contrariness, yet the material might be used in mass experiments so as to obtain light on the dynamics of this trait. The material in a test-experiment then must be standardized and yet allow for variational handling.

Direct observation is what we ordinarily fall back on in judging our fellow men, but the man in the street usually has no rules to guide him in this " sizing up " of character except his own prejudices, and certainly has no idea of the possible human types, nor is he in possession of the training and knowledge required to discriminate between one human being and another.

Methodical Derivation of Biography. Biography is a source of character study which is based on the method of observation, either direct or indirect. As a rule the observation is indirect ; for not only is it impossible for even a veritable Boswell, on intimate terms with his Johnson, to set down all the facts about the hero or subject of the biography, but in most instances the writer is obliged to piece together numerous accounts about a person he has never had the opportunity of seeing.

In any case, whether the biographer is acquainted with the subject of his sketch or not, he must apply the *interpretative* method not only by sifting and selecting the facts reported but in *understanding* the inner unity of the personality written about. All biographers must in a certain measure be sympathetic, but even the most impersonal setting down of pure chronological data entails the process of selection, and selection implies interpretation. Thus biography is a combination of observation and understanding and derives its methods from the natural as well as the interpretative sciences.

Statistics. The statistical method, as instanced in the researches of Heymans and Wiersma, may deal with biographical and autobiographical data as answered in questionnaires. Tests may also be treated statistically for the same purpose. Various handbooks and reference works like *Who's Who* are often consulted when some one point is being investigated, as in Giese's inquiry into the recreations and avocations of prominent individuals so as to determine the compensative value of personality.[1]

Treatment of Introspection. Introspection, from the very nature of the case, cannot be used as a method of studying human types unless in conjunction with the introspection of others, subsequently to be collated and treated statistically. The introspector himself can of course gain some insight into his own motives through this method ; but again, it will be necessary for him to compare his own behaviour and mental states with those of others.   Examples of this type of character study or rather self study are Yerkes and La Rue's *Outline of a Study of the Self*, and F. L. Wells' *The Systematic Observation of the Personality*.

Orientation of Autobiography. Autobiography is an extension of the introspective method just as biography is an extension of the method of observation.   It is a sustained introspective process over a period of long duration and recorded with an eye to unity of treatment.   Like the biography, the autobiography must resort to interpretation or rather, with reference to the self, insight.   Thus it also draws on the interpretative methods ; and the autobiographer in order to be successful will always endeavour to understand himself.

Marks of the Diary. The diary is a species of auto-

---

[1] F. Giese, " Kompensationswerte der Persönlichkeit," *Bericht ü. d. viii Kongress d. exper. Psychol.* in Leipzig, 1923 (1924).

biography lacking the element of unity. To be sure, the diarist will reveal his outlook and his temperament both in the events he chooses to register and in his style, tempo, etc., but while the autobiographer has his savings to take into account, the diarist lives from hand to mouth, so to speak, never knowing what he will regard as important enough to enter a month hence. He moves in the specious present, and his composition consists of nothing but staccato notes. The objective diary, i.e. where the entries refer to a third person, is more satisfactory.

The autobiography and the diary differ in another essential respect, in that as a rule the latter is given to the recording of acts and events, thoughts and feelings being given a secondary place therein. There are of course notable exceptions like Amiel's *Journal Intime* ; but even here the expression of the writer's sentiments takes the form of objective reflections, rather than presentations of his own state of mind. For this reason the diary leans more to the observational side and draws on the behaviour methods rather than on the interpretative attitudes.

Correspondence. Letters are a valuable aid in discovering character cues, and though they express one's personality only in isolated moods or in relation to certain people—relatives, friends, acquaintances, or business associates, they have the advantage of often reproducing the writer's mind unawares. Beethoven's letters speak for the man unmistakably, and his individuality is stamped even in the three-line notes which he would scribble sometimes without regard to orthography. As compared with Kant's gentle tone and carefully guarded language, Beethoven's impetuous phraseology is a revelation of his rugged personality. Similarly is Chopin's choleric temperament evident in most of his letters.

The Rôle of Dreams. As to the source of dreams, it should be explained that the method I have in mind here has little to do with psychoanalysis, which regards the *dream as a symbol only*, pointing to a latent content which, in its turn, is to throw light on the patient's trouble. I think it has been generally overlooked in the dream literature as a whole that the dream often gives us an opportunity of finding ourselves in a situation where we could hardly imagine ourselves being in waking life. We likewise may in our dreams see others in characteristic poses which are nevertheless beyond our waking ken. Probably every one has had the experience of getting up sometimes with a feeling that now he has learnt just what he would do or say under circumstances which he was never in. Our imagination cannot have the same sweep in our normal conscious state as it has in the dream, when our mental processes are not directed *by* us but *for* us through the subconscious operations, and are therefore more *objective* than in waking life. The repartee we never made, the joke we never cracked, the command we never gave in actual life were unborn not because it is not " in us " to express ourselves thus, but for the reason that so far the occasion has not arisen. The dream then, in its *manifest content serves to make us see ourselves and others in a characteristic light under hypothetical conditions*, and as such it constitutes a subconscious form of self-observation and, through the process of mental incubation, sometimes of the observation of friends and acquaintances.

Types of Questionnaires. The questionnaire method, strictly speaking, applies to introspective material, though of course the questions put may and often do refer to others. The point at issue would be to determine whether the answers are not primarily introspective in character, but we need not go into so academic a question. For the most part the questionnaires relate to oneself, and may refer to a future hypothetical situation, as " What would you do if confronted with such and such a problem ? " (Baumgarten in Germany.) F. H. and G. W. Allport in the United States, on the other hand, frame questions relative to past and present experiences of the individual. The most extensive questionnaire of this sort is the *Woodworth Personal Data Sheet*.

Locus of Psychoanalysis. Little need be said about the psychoanalytic method in view of the prominent position which it already occupies in this book, except to point out that it is meant to embrace all that is customarily treated under that head. The questionnaire in a very restricted form beginning and ending with the individual (the data not to be used for statistical purposes) is the foundation of the psychoanalytic method, since even dreams are reported at its behest, and the method of free word association (Jung) may be considered a species of questionnaire. The examination of humour, however, as also of the various types of slips must be included too. The kind of slips one makes in writing certainly throws some light on the personality of the writer. In my own experiments on interference in writing, I have found that there were different reactions to the stimuli-words dictated at a high speed. Furthermore I noted that patients in the psychopathic hospital were more apt to omit r's in their words and to make different lapses from those of normal subjects. But the curious thing is the unwillingness on the part of Freudians to view slips as symptomatic of personal traits. Instead, they interpret these phenomena as the breaking through of unconscious desires, wishes, and complexes, thus taking this important section of human behaviour out of the field of character study.[1] And this affords one more instance of the psychoanalytic tendency to leave the obvious for the sake of the speculative and conjectural.

Psychoanalysis must embrace the doctrines of all those who were at one time associated with the leader of the movement, though afterwards repudiating their master. Jung's

[1] Cf. A. A. Roback, " The Freudian Doctrine of Lapses and its Failings " : *Am. Jour. of Psychol.*, 1919, vol. xxx.

system, sometimes spoken of as psycho-synthesis and Adler's " Individual-Psychologie " as well as Stekel's unlabelled system are all to be comprised under the term of psycho-analysis.

Inspirational Essay.   The distinctive feature of the inspira-tional essay is its inspiration, which may possibly be regarded as an instrument of gaining insight. There is probably a religious keynote at the bottom of the eloquence of Emerson and Smiles, who seem to be filled with a realization of values as the dominant in character. Their fervour has nothing in common with the causal sciences and derives its strength wholly from the world of motives, purposes, and meanings.

Parœmiological Approach.   Proverbs, epigrams, and aphorisms are alike as sources of character-information, the conclusions based on observation of what people do and how they compare with one another, but while proverbs are more direct expressions of the common people, aphorisms and reflections are less spontaneous and issue from the more or less outstanding mind. They are more subtle, often more elaborate, more specific and more artistically expressed, but do not necessarily come nearer the truth than the sayings circulating among the masses.

Psychognosis.   The literary character sketches are a cross between direct observation and imagination, united by the method of interpretation (*Einfühlung*) ; and it will be remarked that the less the sympathy for the subject of the sketch, the poorer and less successful for the purpose of characterology the delineation. The *understanding* of the individual or of the type is of paramount importance here, and the grasping of essentials will determine the nature and the division of the types or classes.

Character in Fiction.   Fiction comes under the same rubric, but the imaginative component is of greater proportion than that of direct observation, and, in addition, the type is particularized or individualized. In fact, the great characters in fiction are not to be found in everyday life. We can hope to discover only approximations to them. There are thousands of sharply drawn characters in fiction, yet they cannot be said all to represent different classes of people.

Intuitive Methods. Finally, we come to the intuitive methods proper which have been made so much of in the latest schools of the *Geisteswissenschaften* in Germany. We have no suitable words to designate that immediate grasp of one's personality which is recognized by most German philosophical and psychological writers of to-day as superior to the experimental and observational methods used to delineate the sum-total of an individual's personality traits under the technical label of a psychogram (Stern).

In search of a Generic Term. A term like *Einfühlung* or empathy in Lipps's sense has an aesthetic connotation and was intended for the person-object relation. Scheler's *Sympathie* or *Einsfühlung* (identification) is more suitable in the connection where we are dealing with one person understanding another, but the stress on the affective side of man, to the exclusion of the cognitive and the volitional, is too patent to warrant accepting either of the two words employed by Scheler for our generic caption. In Scheler's philosophy,[1] the heart takes precedence over the head, and naturally we cannot commit ourselves in an unbiassed classification to some one standpoint in present-day German thought.

For the same reason, the word *Ahmung*, employed by Lessing,[2] which over-emphasizes the *attitudinal* phase of man, or Münsterberg's " will-attitude " is not appropriate as a class name for the intuitive methods. The weight logically would have to be placed largely on the effectors (muscles and glands) in this type of understanding which, I

---

[1] M. Scheler, *Formalismus in der Ethik und die materiale Wertethik.*

[2] Th. Lessing, " Die Psychologie der Ahmung ": *Archiv. f. d. System. Philos.*, 1917, vol. xxiii.

should think, would come close to Karl Groos's "inner mimicry", notwithstanding Lessing's repudiation of the latter.

Certainly the simplest course would be to resort to the plain word *understanding* as a comprehensive class name, but here again the flavour is that of cognition. When we *understand* a person, it is taken for granted that we have studied him, that we have penetrated him through the intellect, and not by means of the feelings or our attitudes. It is true that in order to understand, we must take a sympathetic attitude which would involve both the affective and the will functions, nevertheless a prepossession in favour of the cognitive would arouse the just protests of representatives of the other wings of the *Struktur* movement.

Perilepsis. It would be best if a neutral word were found the equivalent of the Greek περιλαμβάνω, signifying to seize, grasp, encompass, or "*umfassen*" as the German would express it. If a word like *perilepsis* could be coined to do duty for this concept of snapping a person's make-up with one click, as it were, without the cognitive or the affective or the conative function receiving more weight than either of the other two in this neutral process, we should have a suitable class name for these intuitive methods.

Psychiatric Auxiliary Devices. In addition to the methods charted, we ought to take cognizance of the indirect contributory methods devised and extensively used by psychiatrists in their endeavours to clear up the riddle of personality. The hypnotic trance brings to light much that is hidden from view in the waking state, and whether the technique is that advocated by Charcot, Bernheim, Janet, Prince, or Sidis (hypnagogic), the anamnesis, dissociation, automatism, and other phenomena brought about are most revelatory of a patient's inner life.

Again, the grammatical analysis (active and passive voice) introduced into personality descriptions by Southard, the application of psychoanalysis to behaviouristic doctrine by Kempf, the systematic observation guides of Amsden and Wells are to a certain extent covered by some of the headings in our chart, but still each one of these auxiliary suggestions has something additional to offer toward the solution of the problem.

Four Fundamental Points of View. The whole field of character is, on close examination, really dominated by four fundamental points of view, each making use of a method peculiar to its own requirements and range of experiences. The basic concepts, too, which each of these points of view manipulates—or perhaps, better, their products—are different in each case. Let us see what this composite picture looks like.

In the first place, although the ethico-religious or exhortative approach has not been accorded a prominent place in this book for reasons stated in the introduction, we cannot afford to ignore it wholly even in a *psychology* of character. We must remember that the *normative* method, with its *idealization* premises, serves to stabilize, in some degree, the constituents of character. The ethico-religious precepts or maxims form a centre of reference, never quite attained in actual life. The *moral experience* is the phenomenological product of this point of view.

Secondly, there is the historical point of view with the biographical material which is at its foundation. The chief method which it makes use of is the interpretative one of the *Geisteswissenschaften.* Other methods have been introduced but the former still remains the best instrument for understanding personalities of the past. In the historico-biographical rapids, the waters swirl with purposes and intentions. The end-products are creations—not, as in the natural sciences, constructions.

We now come to the biological point of view with its physiological data. The method *par excellence* here is

PP

experimental and the chief aim is to *correlate* facts so as to establish *causes, constructions.* Quantification of results is the *desideratum* in this sphere of activity. To know a character here is to give it a definite place on a scale and to understand the functions of the various traits in terms of their organic substrates.

CHART OF FUNDAMENTAL POINTS OF VIEW

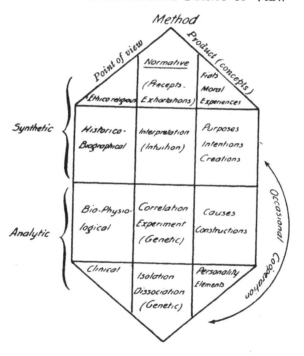

Finally we have the psychiatric point of view, with its clinical data and isolating method. This isolation consists partly in dissociating or disintegrating the personality complex into its components, and partly in magnifying the elements. Just as the ethico-religious point of view idealized the character of man and then imposed this ideal upon the world through precept and exhortation, so the psychiatrist (including the psychopathologist, delinquency investigator and clinician) unfurls the human bale and discovers that the texture underneath is of coarser woof than that on the exterior. Or the figure may be represented differently : We may regard the psychiatrist as bringing to the surface the excretory vapours of the human personality through his searching examination of the data. Like the industrial chemist he may find that a fragrant personality odour sometimes contains at least one repulsive ingredient.

The genetic method is employed on behalf of both the biological and the psychiatric points of view, yet in a different dimension.

The four conceptions of character, with special reference to their methods, might playfully, and for mnemotechnic purposes, be designated as (a) the inspirational point of view (religion, ethics), (b) the " conspirational " (history, biography), (c) the " perspirational " (experiment), (d) the " expirational " or " transpirational " in its original sense (psychopathology, etc.).

It is the business of psychology in its treatment of character to consolidate these four viewpoints so as to form an integrated whole.

PART IV

CONSTRUCTIVE

CHAPTER XXX

INHIBITION AS THE BASIS OF CHARACTER

Having devoted considerable space to the historical development of our subject, I shall set forth my own views as briefly as possible.

In the first place, though the discussion so far has included the concepts of temperament and personality (since it is not always possible to isolate the subject of character from a general treatment of personality,, which in some presentations is identified with it) it is necessary to remind the reader that character is regarded here as one aspect of personality, the others being intelligence, temperament, physique, and other mental and physical qualities.

If character is a psychological entity we must endeavour to examine it by means of psychological methods and place it on a psychological basis.

Delimitation of Term " Character." But there is another condition that must not be lost sight of, and *that is the cumulative meaning of the word through the centuries,* a meaning which psychology cannot supplant without actually talking about a different thing. The concept may, of course, be grasped in a different setting in order to be invested with authority, but its nucleus must remain intact.

The reason why the tripartite division of mind is inadequate to furnish us a classification of characters is primarily the overlapping of the divisions with respect to the two allied subjects—character and temperament—as well as the resulting confusion. I think it is well to keep the temperaments in reserve for the affective side of man. To talk of an affective character is not instructive, and to institute further divisions by hybridization such as " cognitive-affective " or " active-sensitive " reveals the weakness of the position, and serves but to escape the necessity of pointing out definite categories on which we can put our fingers when we come to apply the findings in real life. In the last analysis, instead of psychological types, we see before us verbal categories ; and the core of character in its original denotation is missing to boot.

Nor can we be satisfied with the resort to speed and intensity as the foundations of character. Perhaps these criteria would be suitable for the classification of temperaments, and it is remarkable that, over two thousand years ago, these principles were mentioned in the Talmud to differentiate the four mental types of man, as may be seen in the following passage from *Pir'ke Aboth* :—[1]

" There are four types of mental disposition : (*a*) He who is easily irritated and easily reconciled, thus offsetting his liability by the asset ; (*b*) the one whom it is difficult to anger and difficult to appease, thus counterbalancing his gain by his loss ; (*c*) he whom it is difficult to provoke and easy to pacify—the saint, and (*d*) the one who is easily provoked but reconciled only with difficulty—the villain."

We thus have the speed of the reaction in the time it takes for the anger to develop and the intensity in the time it takes for this emotion to subside under proper conditions.

Speed, energy, intensity, perseverance—these are all significant traits, especially in the matter of engaging employees, but in our relationship with friends, and in the appraisal of historical personages they do not loom so large. Character counts for much more ; and it is the distinguishing mark of this character that we are in quest of.

---

[1] ארבע מדות בדעות: נוח לכעוס ונוח לרצות, יצא הפסדו בשכרו;
קשה לכעוס וקשה לרצות, יצא שכרו בהפסדו; קשה לכעוס
ונוח לרצות, חסיד; נוח לכעוס וקשה לרצות רשע. (Aboth 5 : 14)

Contradictoriness Due to Ignorance. Often we are deceived by the use of such terms in that they have practical application only when coupled with an objective. The indolent scholar may turn out to be an energetic professional baseball player or a hustling politician. The slow eater and awkward manual worker may nevertheless be a quick thinker and writer. *The persons who display most of the article we call character are the ones to offer the most contradiction in their make-up. The contradiction, however, lies not in them, but in those who do the judging and who are not provided with a key to the objectives.*

Instincts Provide Possibility of Character. But to what psychological entities, then, can we hitch character? The answer is: *The Instincts.* We shall soon see that through such a procedure we can meet the requirement of the man in the street, and at the same time move safely on psychological territory without taking recourse to hazy categories combined in sets of two or three. An instinct, after all, notwithstanding the attempts made in certain quarters to evict it from the psychological purview, is a definite mechanism which operates visibly enough to convince us of its existence.[1]

Roughly speaking, one of the major differences between men and infra-human beings is that the latter do not inhibit their instinctive impulses except after a painful training; and that is the chief reason why character cannot be ascribed to animals. If speed, intensity, perseverance, and other such traits were to be the basis of character division, we should expect animals, since they present marked individual differences in regard to such traits, to partake of the classes of characters drawn up for man.

---

[1] A reading of McDougall's two papers, one entitled " The Use and Abuse of Instinct ", in the *Journal of Abnormal Psychology*, 1922, vol. xvi, the other " Can Sociology and Social Psychology Dispense with Instinct ?" in the *American Journal of Sociology*, 1914, vol. xxix, will be sufficient to prove the validity of the older position.

SYNTHETIC CONCEPTION

The view proposed here also makes use of the tripartite division of mind, not, however, in a way to break it up into strips, eventually to be pasted together in various combinations, but in a synthetic manner, so that each character may be said to consist of cognitive (intellectual), affective, and conative elements.

Definition of Character. My definition of character accordingly is as follows : *An enduring psychophysical disposition to inhibit instinctive impulses in accordance with a regulative principle.* Each of these conditions must be fulfilled before character can be attributed to the individual. The possession of instinctive urges is of prime importance. The inhibition of the urge stamps the agent with character, though of varying degrees. Not, however, until we have the regulative principle as a clue, can we determine to what extent the man or woman we are judging possesses character.

Since every instinct is grounded in both conation and affection, and since inhibition is wholly a matter of conation, and finally since the determining factor of this inhibition is or has been reflection of some kind, we perceive that the older categories still have a place in our scheme when properly arranged so as to form a synthesis, the affective part furnishing the condition, the conative supplying the raw content, and the cognitive factor colouring it with significance, giving it status and suggesting a possibility of measurement.

Criticism of Instincts Irrelevant. To the objection that our knowledge about the instincts is limited and that controversy is rife as to their number, one might easily reply that it is not necessary to have detailed information about every instinct before we can work with any of them, any more than we have to give up talking about the elements in chemistry until we shall have discovered their exact number for all time.

It is quite sufficient to base our study of character on the more palpable instincts, such as self-preservation, sex, acquisitiveness, self-aggression, or the will to power. We must remember also that not all instincts are of equal intensity. Many, if not most of them, can be placed on a scale according to their universal intensity. Thus it is quite certain that the instinct of self-preservation is more potent than the mating impulse or the food drive. The inhibition of the latter is therefore not so expressive of character as the inhibition of the former, other things being equal.

Degrees of Character. As regards the logical principle regulating the inhibition, it must be pointed out that inasmuch as different people will be guided by different principles or sanctions, there will be various degrees of character. Little boots it to say that we all rationalize our actions. *It is the type of rationalization which counts.* In our everyday life we can recognize this especially in our dealings with men (and perhaps women, too). Some excuses we accept as reasonable, others we reject as chronic alibis. The Freudian over-emphasis of rationalization, then, is apt to mislead and in fact has misled many educated people. In calling attention to the tendency of the average man and, we may add, the average woman to rationalize their actions, Freud has universalized a truth which was noted in the past by acute observers in their own spheres ; but if, on that account, the barrier must be broken down between Socrates' reason for refusing the opportunity to escape an unnatural death and that of a soldier's wife in attaching herself to a paramour while her husband is at war ; if one reason were no more of a *libido* [1] manifestation than the other, then it would have been better perhaps that the universalized truth should have remained restricted to the unscientific area of individual sages than to have appeared in such a distorted form.

General Operation of Character. Instead of classifying the characters according to affective or intellectual pre-

---

[1] Jung's term is more appropriate here than Freud's.

dominance or traits, such as quickness, firmness, energy, etc., we should on our scheme range them *as to kind* in accordance with what instinctive tendencies are or are not inhibited by the individual. As a rule, the *man of character in the full sense of the word exercises a distributed inhibitory power in keeping with a general principle which subsumes under its authority more specialized maxims.* But we do find irregularities manifesting a weak spot in some specific direction, as in the case of Byron, noble in many ways, but lax in sex relations, or as exemplified by Beethoven, whose character (not his temperamental make-up) seems to have been unimpeachable but for his unreliability in the matter of adhering to contracts, especially in his dealings with publishers. The epigram about the famous actress Adrienne Lecouvreur, who was regarded as Voltaire's mistress, that she " had all the virtues but virtue ", strikingly illustrates the point that the contour of character may be broken at some particular spot.

There is no reason why we should not look for a general character factor and specific sub-factors, such as Spearman contends to be the case in the sphere of intelligence. Perhaps the strength of a single instinct is greater in one individual than in another, but for the most part I should ascribe the cause to the relation between the impulse in question and the guiding principle.

We all like comforts and what are vulgarly called " good times ", and we all know that the acquisition of money is the only road for attaining that object ; but then, if our ruling principle is not to " do " the other man, or, in the more dignified language of Kant, to treat every person as an end and not a means, we shall not indulge in telling lies, a practice which is condoned in business, or what is perhaps even worse, engage in flattery in order to gain advantages with influential people, so as eventually to satisfy our material cravings.

Popular Fallacies. It may be urged that the inhibition

of one instinct is only the furtherance of another, e.g. in shunning society for the sake of accomplishing a cultural piece of work we are swayed by the will to power in downing our gregariousness. That such a reciprocal interplay between the instinctive impulses goes on is perhaps beyond question, but it hardly touches our problem. For what gives the stamp of character to an individual is not the mere fact that some instincts have been subordinated to others, but the nature of the guiding principle, whether, for instance, the man's purpose in life is to add to the sum-total of knowledge, to benefit humanity in some way, or merely to increase his fame, to become, in the slang of the street, an intellectual " go-getter ". The difference between a Spinoza and a Voltaire with respect to inhibiting certain social pleasures for the sake of achievement —and even the latter was obliged to repress at times his gregariousness, or else his output would not have been so vast—is an instance of like inhibitions inspired by different reasons.

Nor are we to infer that character is attached to the operation of the so-called higher, altruistic, or other-regarding instincts as against the baser, egoistic, or self-regarding congenital urges. Whether such a division of instincts is at all useful is questionable in this connection. What I should like to emphasize is that characters are evaluated *from the point of view of such principles as truth and justice rather than on the strength of altruistic tendencies.* The masses who mistake disposition, mood, or what-not for character are often inclined to form wrong opinions in this regard, especially as their judgments are based on the attitude the person takes toward them. A " good " railroad conductor is frequently one who takes but a fraction of the fare from passengers, which he keeps for himself, thus cheating the company out of the full fare. A " good fellow " in politics is one who cherishes no principles in life and whose corruption is shielded from view because of the many individual favours he is willing to grant those who assert themselves. On the other hand, many a criminal thinks of the " hard boiled " judge who sentences him to a long jail period as an objectionable character.

Character Not Bound Up with Sympathy. The truth is, however, that character is not dependent on human emotions. Many persons of touching sympathy are devoid of character, and, conversely, most of the great characters known in history have been ruthless in dealing with evil. The man of high character (and there is just as much reason for talking about high character as about a high intelligence quotient) is exemplified by the Roman father who sentenced his fiendish son to death, thus inhibiting the paternal instinct in deference to the principle of justice. Firmness is the quality which typifies character at its best ; and firmness goes peculiarly well with inhibition, for the greater the inhibition the greater the firmness.

An Arena of Action Necessary. In this light we can readily conceive the insight contained in Goethe's famous couplet—

> *Es bildet ein Talent sich in der Stille ;*
> *Sich ein Charakter in den Strom der Welt.*

The man who leads the life of a hermit has fewer opportunities to inhibit his instinctive urges. His inhibitions cannot compare either in scope or in number with those of the man of affairs in the bivouac of life. It is on this account that only statesmen are potentially able to realize the highest there is in character, though, unfortunately, they nearly all slip before they reach the summit. And that is what marks the greatness of Lincoln, and perhaps also of Wilson— the uncompromising political idealism in the face of a *force majeure.*

An Important Issue Examined. One objection to my conception of character, I fancy, would be the apparent negative definition to begin with. It may be said that the mere inhibition of an instinctive tendency does not lead to action, as is classically illustrated by Hamlet. Were this to constitute a serious objection, it would, of course, undermine the foundation of my whole view, but we must be mindful of the fact that the material to yield an estimate of character consists of both acts and restraints. Now, in many cases, for instance, in the matter of refraining from being dishonest—the inhibition is sufficient to warrant the making of a notch on behalf of the agent. But even the case where the man is called upon to act in the face of death is covered by our definition, since naturally the inhibition there centres around the instinct of self-preservation and unless he does act in a manner to renounce his life if necessary, there is no evidence of such inhibition.

We also know that the inhibition of one tendency will lead to the expression of the opposite tendency, so that absolute inaction as a result of inhibition is restricted almost exclusively to neurotics and characters in fiction. Even the waverer *par excellence*, the much ridiculed Prince of Denmark, was throughout his inhibitive " pandering to thought " waiting for a better opportunity to undo the villain that slew his father. In justice to the scorned Hamlet, it should be mentioned, too, that he was not absolutely certain of the crime.

Inhibition a Positive Force. We are altogether too prone to interpret a concept statically, as if its context did not matter. Inhibition conveys to the mind the picture of inactivity, and therefore is thought to be a negative process. In reality, however, it is a positive force.

It takes students some time before they accustom themselves to think of a synapse, the mere juncture between two neurones, as something worthy of a name. This gap they later discover is perhaps more important than the actual cell itself. In mathematics the practical boy or girl finds it difficult to understand why we should talk about negative quantities and surds. A little training in this direction convinces us that a negative concept may have a very positive part to play. Inhibition involves definite physiological processes and manifests itself in definite positive acts, except where the individual is pathological. Otis is quite correct when she argues that the resistance to suggestibility which she found in the children she experimented on is " the positive trait that is measured by the test as here described ".[1]

Analogy from Physics. We may, however, go a step farther and point out that all energy or force is measured in terms of what may be regarded by analogy as physical inhibition. The weight of a body is ascertained by the amount of resistance it offers against the pull of gravity. Similarly work or heat is measured by the amount of force it takes to overcome the original inertia of a body. For our purpose the effect is positive. The body in question has moved over a certain distance in a given period of time, but we must not forget that the motion is only one phase of the resistance, and is a function of it.

Inhibition Not Necessarily Pathological. In questioning the significance attached to such a quality as inhibition in the estimation of character, some will seek to show the ineffectualness of inhibited persons. They will point out that inhibition is more of a liability than an asset, that it is apt to paralyse one's capacity, and that the great characters in history were all dynamic personalities.

My answer to this criticism is as follows : first of all it is evident that to those whose interest lies in psychiatry, psychoanalysis and therapy in general, the term inhibition bears a connotation savouring of the abnormal. We must remember, however, that the original use of the word was derived from physiology and experimental psychology. It would not be fair then to set up a derived and special

[1] M. Otis, " A Study of Suggestibility of Children " : *Arch. of Psychol.*, 1924-25, vol. xi, p. 95.

sense of the word for our standard of reference. We may as well depreciate the serviceableness of volition because it is in this sphere that impulsions or compulsive ideas develop.

The abnormally inhibited, as a matter of fact, *do not inhibit their instinctive tendencies.* As a rule they, in a large measure, give way to them, whence arise their onsets of senseless immobility. For instance, the man who refuses to budge from his position, in the middle of the room, which he had taken up during a thunderstorm is merely yielding to his fear instinct. He who attends to his business in spite of the terrific bolts, which at least suggest danger, has inhibited the fear tendency. Probably all abnormally inhibited persons are weighed down by an exaggerated fear, either of congenital origin or acquired in the course of events (shell shock, remorse, anxiety, regret, etc.).

When it is urged that there are too many people to-day who are given to inhibition, attention might be drawn to the fact that the steadily growing army of malefactors would argue the opposite, viz., that inhibition is not sufficiently exercised.[1]

Why Character Cannot Be Measured Except Through Inhibition. Suppose we were to measure great historical characters by their so-called positive traits, what would it entail ? Would it not be necessary to draw up a catalogue of virtues that these men and women practised and a list

---

[1] The word " control " which has been suggested to me in place of the term " inhibition " is inadequate not only because of its commercial background and atmosphere, but for the additional reason that it does not even pretend to cover the facts of any physiological or psychological dynamics. Besides it is used too loosely, sometimes to denote suppression ; at other times, merely governance to the point just below excess. But Blake has so cleverly said in his *Proverbs of Hell*, " You never know what is enough, unless you know what is more than enough." Control carries with it an air of sophistication. It serves well the diplomat who controls his impulse of pugnacity in deference to prudence, but does not inhibit his instinctive tendency after he has secured the upper hand and successfully carried out his scheme.

of vices that they refrained from ? At best a number of cardinal virtues like those enjoined by the ancient moralists would have to be selected out of the vast inventory and the character of the individual judged thereon. Now in the first place, virtues are *primarily ethical and not psychological facts. They are as such not bound up with any of the mechanisms treated in general psychology*, and our whole psychology of character would then in consequence be reduced to a loose and popular ethical discourse.

Aside from that, let us for a moment grant that what counts most in character is the positive trait : courage, goodness, honesty, truthfulness, etc. These traits are of course virtues because they further altruistic ends. They subserve a useful purpose, but if courage were not honoured because of the dangers it involved ; if honesty were not extolled because of the temptations it is necessary to resist in order to cultivate the trait, then the singular weight attached to character in our system of values remains a mystery. The man of great courage should not be placed higher in our merit scale than the woman of great beauty, were it not for the fact that the latter requires practically no renunciation in order to retain her beauty, while the hero in the true sense of the word must necessarily overcome tendencies which exert great power over the reactive system, especially where the step is not a momentary one, but is preceded by reflection and the opportunity of deliberation. Genius too derives much of its rating from the amount of labour that it takes to fully realize itself.

Analysis of Virtue Reveals Negative Core. When we stop to analyze all the virtues, we shall find that what stamps them with that attribute of worth or excellence so characteristic of them is that depreciated negative quality which actually characterizes the behaviour. To be just is not to wrong anybody. To be truthful is no more nor less than to refrain from falsification. In fact, we almost always translate conceptually the positive fact into a negative one in order to understand to the full extent its significance. To illustrate : if someone draws our attention to a person walking along the street and says, " There goes an honest man," we immediately, in order to obtain a characterial picture of the individual, imaginatively put him into all sorts of situations where he does *not* play the cheat or blackguard. Similarly to do one's duty is *not* to abandon a certain cause. The positive effect of the duty is of course what accomplishes the end, but whatever it be, whether fighting on the battle-field, staying at one's post under the most trying conditions, or assisting those in distress, the behaviour itself is praise-worthy only because some principle was not violated.

It may be pointed out that such traits as persistence, energy, vigour, and the like are essentially positive in nature, and that the leaders in the history of mankind have all possessed a large share of these characteristics.   Yet is energy not to be considered *per se* as a fundamental in character. Some rodents possess more energy than many human beings, yet they are not qualified on that account to receive character ratings.   As to persistence, what does this trait mean other than that a certain idea will recur again and again in conjunction with the inhibition of that instinctive tendency which otherwise would prevent that particular idea from expressing itself into action ?   I believe it was Goethe who said that whenever a great idea and a great character meet, then is a great event likely to take place.   Cromwell has made history by dint of his great energy and intelligence, but his character stands out because of his tolerance, for-bearance, and integrity.   Milton, although lacking the initiative and vigour of his fiery contemporary, did not fall below him, but if anything surpassed him in the *ensemble* of qualities which go to make up character in the sense understood here.

Essence of Character Illustrated.   In short, we must not be deflected from our path by mere grammatical categories, or by historical fireworks. Achievement is one thing ; character, while not in opposition to it, is yet something apart from brilliant exploits. And the most striking illustration in support of this view may be had in Jesus of Nazareth who, though, from all evidence, wanting in energy and vigour, yet became for most of the civilized world the symbol of perfection. The more persistent and dynamic St. Paul, who was responsible in large measure for the spread of Christianity and, therefore, the remaking of history, is never so much as thought of as comparing with his Master. The unswerving devotion to a cause, the unyielding spirit which adheres to the right in spite of threats and warnings, such is the texture of which character is made. The garment may seem to be turned inside out, when so much stress is laid on what is ordinarily supposed to be a negative quality— inhibition. Let us remember, however, that the inside of the garment is next to the wearer, and that the outside is for show. If we wish to examine how the garment is made, we must turn to the inside. If it is to be mended or repaired, the operation again starts from the inside. From the point of view of the tailor in fashioning the garment, it is futile to ask whether the inside or the outside constitutes the garment. So it is with inhibition, which may be thought of as the warp and woof of character. It may possess a negative implication but it transcends the difference between the positive and the negative in its actual operation. What Goethe said with reference to Nature is applicable to character as regards its positive and negative aspects.

> *Natur ist weder Kern noch Schale ;*
> *Alles ist sie mit einem Male.*

CHAPTER XXXI

THE INDEX OF CHARACTER

Description Plus Evaluation. Turning now to the application of the inhibitory view of character, we shall be able to test its validity through the instances cited. Since the character of an individual is to be *described* in terms of the instinct which offers most trouble to the inhibitory mechanism and further *evaluated* according to the ruling principles through which the inhibition of the other instincts has been effected, we have two distinct tasks before us. Below, there is the criterion of inhibition ; above, there is the analysis or interpretation of the inhibition. The one without the other is practically valueless.

Each particular inhibition of an instinct *derives its significance only from the logical motive* which governs the restraint. The highwayman, especially of the type depicted in the romantic novel, certainly inhibits his instinct of self-preservation, as does the circus dare-devil in his hazardous stunts. They are not, however, governed by a *principle* but are rather led to their eventual destruction by a *less important instinct*, whether it be acquisitiveness, display, or the will to power. Hence, though the most potent instinct has been suppressed by the bandit, the estimate of his character is on the minus side because of the violation of absolute principles. Similarly the North American Indians, although possessing the making of character in their self-control and physical discipline, cannot, because of their deficiency in principle, be credited with character of a high type.

Asceticism not an Element of Character. It is here wherein the present account, though in substance resembling it, differs from the excellent discourse of MacCunn in his *The Making of Character* which merits the wide popularity it has received in the last quarter of a century. MacCunn also flouts asceticism and eloquently points out that the repressive systems fail in that they " build upon a few exceptional motives, love of God, passion for souls, self-sacrifice if not self-immolation, absolute devotion to a Church or a Brotherhood, and in order to accomplish their end, they make wholesale use of Pain as an instrument for repression ".[1]

What really renders asceticism undesirable, to my mind, is rather its being rooted in some instinctive core, such as fear, superstition, pathological love (as in the case of many of the mediaeval saints), eagerness for reward in the next world, etc. Reason does not enter into its counsel-hall and therefore cannot be said to guide it. Hence mere repression does not satisfy the definition of character as set forth in this treatise.

Nietzsche and the Ascetic Ideal. At this point perhaps it would be in order to refer to the vehement attack on asceticism by Nietzsche who, in the vein of present-day psychoanalysis, interprets asceticism as a refuge for the weakling and a source of self-elation for the philosopher. In his well-known essay " Ascetic Ideals " he asks, " What then does the ascetic ideal mean in a philosopher ? " And he answers this question with his characteristic sneer at the professional moralist or for that matter the intellectual in general : " When he sees this ideal, the philosopher smiles because he sees therein an *optimum* of the conditions of the highest and boldest intellectuality ; he does not thereby deny ' existence ', he rather affirms thereby *his* existence and *only* his existence, and this perhaps to the point of not being far off the blasphemous wish, ' *Pereat mundus, fiat philosophia, fiat philosophus, fiam* ! ' . . . "[2]

---

[1] J. MacCunn, *The Making of Character*, pp. 35–6.
[2] F. Nietzsche, *The Genealogy of Morals*.

Nietzsche's reaction is, of course, an *argumentum ad hominem*. Nowhere in the essay does he make any attempt to disprove the value of the ascetic ideal. What he does is merely to impugn the motives of those who preach or practice it. The advocate of asceticism is, according to this precursor of psychoanalysis, one who suffers; he therefore invents this perverted ideal in order to invest his suffering with a meaning. His will, his pride, is saved; for no longer is he a passive toy in the hands of Fate, but an active agent who suffers for a purpose.

Psychological *versus* Moralist Point of View. MacCunn does not inveigh against the ascetic. He merely finds fault with his narrowness, and I can heartily subscribe to MacCunn's conclusion : "We must decisively part company with the ascetics, even while tendering to their self-devotion our tribute of admiration," but my own view will not admit " the more practical policy of repression by developing the desires which, in the light of a more generous ideal, demand development ", or that " passion must be evoked to cast out passion "—at least not until it is mediated by reason. If character involves the repression of all instinctive tendencies, then using one as an antidote for the other is like taking heroin to overcome excessive fear—a method which we should not particularly extol. The position taken in the present work is that instincts are neither good nor bad, but because of their insistent driving force the ability to inhibit them becomes the distinguishing mark of the man of character. MacCunn, like all other moralists, evidently thinks that some instincts are good and some are bad, and the good ones must be used to oust the bad ones.

Levels of Character. Again, he who inhibits the prime instinctive tendency as a result of military or social pressure must be accorded some measure of recognition, but character in the proper sense he has not necessarily on that account.

Higher in the scale is the religious martyr who dies for his belief, yet expecting to reap some benefit in another world. But the only perfect evidence of character in connection with the self-preservation instinct is that to be found in the thinker who gives up his life for a principle which he would not renounce merely in order to satisfy authority.

Let us seek confirmation in another direction. The sex instinct is no doubt a powerful congenital tendency. Yet the inhibition of this instinct does not evoke so much admiration, nor does the expression of this instinct, even in illicit modes, call forth so much condemnation *per se*, i.e. without reference to violations of absolute principles like justice and truth, as in the case of other instincts. Only a philistine would consider Oscar Wilde, in spite of his unfortunate practices, low in character and less of a gentleman than an officially respectable grafter or fraudulent broker. The reason is not far to seek. *The sex instinct is not governed by absolute principles.* The exercise of the sex function in a legal and legitimate manner has no bearing on the estimate of character. Nor is the celibate who completely represses his sex life credited thereby with a superior character, though, of course, the capacity to subdue such a potent force, assuming that there is no psychophysical defect in that regard, is indubitably a mark of character in the rough. When, however, a Roman Catholic priest, vowed to celibacy, indulges in sex relations even with a woman whom he has secretly married, his character is rightly called into question, but not on account of his worldly indulgence, as every clear-sighted person will admit.

Guiding Principle of Paramount Importance. It is possible to apply a similar analytic course to other instinctive impulses. The inhibition of the reactions which attend the emotion of fear comes under the category of character only if effected on logical grounds. But if the tendency to flee has been thwarted by a pugnacious impulse or the self-administration of a drug, the inhibition loses its force.

Fanatics and Don Quixotes, in spite of their frequently self-denying inhibitions, lack the higher type of character because their guiding principle is often stubbornness. We shall see later that the *highest types of characters can be realized only in the highest types of intelligence*, and if, as Webb has tried to prove in his dissertation, there is a character element in intelligence—what corresponds to persistency of motives [1] —the converse of the proposition should not be lost sight of, viz., that there is an intelligence factor in character.

The observation made by so many thinkers about the characterlessness of women also brings out this conclusion. The typical woman in some respects manifests even stronger inhibitions than the average or even superior man, but her inhibitions are imposed upon her not by the dictates of reason but by public opinion, convention, fashion, and instinctive urges.

Character Rating. The rating of character will always remain a troublesome problem, and it is idle to deceive ourselves that any quantitative procedure could ever be devised to approximate the method of testing intelligence. Rugg has in a series of articles [2] shown the magnitude of the task and the drawbacks attached to it even when carried on under conditions which the rigours of a great war have laid at the disposal of the investigators. In one place he observes, " The unordered—yes, the chaotic—character of the judgments appears, irrespective of what traits are considered or of what kinds of scales are compared."

Inadequacy of " discrete " View. Perhaps Rugg has gone too far in underestimating the value of the results. Then, too, he is referring to the estimation of character on the strength of ratings. He does not consider the body of results

---

[1] E. Webb, "Character and Intelligence": *British Journal of Psychol. Monograph Supp.*, 1915, vol. i, part 3, p. 58.

[2] H. Rugg, " Is the Rating of Human Character Practicable ?": *Journal of Educ. Psychol.*, 1921 and 1922, vols. xiii and xiv.

that have grown out of the various tests so ingeniously administered by a number of American workers. Many personality traits have been probed in one way or another with various degrees of success.

Let us note, however, that what may be termed the " discrete " character investigations are fraught with disadvantages that do not apply in the more restricted treatment of character. The " discrete " view assembles a number of traits arbitrarily, or in accordance with practical demands, and proceeds to the rating of individuals as regards some particular trait. But these single traits are often very complex. Leadership includes so many qualities; and besides, the concept of leadership is by no means standardized. The Y.M.C.A. notion of leadership, the revivalist's idea of a leader and the intellectual's requirements of a leader are vastly different things, so that each judge will rate this article according to his own temperamental inclinations.

The interesting scale of tests which Downey has devised for constructing a will-profile, though a valuable contribution to the subject, suffers from the further limitation that the only general criterion to serve as guide is that of motor co-ordination in the form of writing under various conditions, which can hardly cover or correspond to all the important types of situations by which a man would be judged in actual life. Of course, we may hold that as in small things, so in great things; but we must first be certain that there is an actual correspondence and not merely work on that presupposition. If a high correlation is proved by the results, there will be the further question to settle as to whether the most important traits have been included in this profile.[1]

---

[1] Incidentally, the factor of inhibition figures considerably in her tests, and the most important traits are judged on the ability of the examinees to overcome their original impulses, as shown especially in the motor inhibition test. (J. E. Downey, *The Will-Temperament and its Testing*, pp. 132–134).

Judgment and Action Not Parallel. Of a less satisfactory nature is the method of self-questioning, unless checked up by others, and even then we have no reliable ways of establishing the validity of the ratings. *What we think we should do on a given occasion and what we actually do on such an occasion often do not coincide.* Light on such hypothetical situations can be had with greater reliability in dreams. In the questionnaire method there are the following obstacles to guard against : (*a*) the disconnection between a given question and a particular trait which the question purports to test, (*b*) the personal bias, (*c*) the imaginative bent which is unequal in the various examinees.

By omitting the purely affective and temperamental phase of personality from our conception of character, and taking the instinctive tendencies as our field of operation, we not only are in a position to deal with something definite and traditionally continuous, but in addition can treat character as a unitary pattern, in which each of the points considered has its position, and not as a pincushion where the different traits are stuck helter-skelter.

To be sure, our scheme would not be so useful in rating the ordinary man and woman as in judging the outstanding individual who, in the first place, would possess a more typical character in our sense, and, secondly, whose actions would be better known than those of the ordinary mortal. The students of history and biography would be the gainers on such a basis rather than the executive and the administrator, but even the character of the comparative stranger, if he submitted to a series of tests especially devised to tap instinctive tendencies and their inhibition, through the use of the ingenious technique contrived by the American investigators, could come under our scientific scrutiny and receive a definite rating or place on the character scale. We need not therefore underrate the importance of a safe, though somewhat restricted, guide on the ground that it is not immediately practicable in the plant, factory, or department store.

A TENTATIVE SCHEME OF CHARTING CHARACTER

In charting an individual character we might mark off our scale of motivating principles as ordinates, and the instinctive tendencies, *sufficiently differentiated to make allowance for the objectives of the tendencies,* as *abscissae.* The scale of guiding principles would include the well known sanctions, such as the physical, legal, social, religious, aesthetic, and ethico-logical. The highest type of character would be found in that individual whose inhibitions are brought about by motives of the ethico-logical class only. It is questionable whether the legal sanction is sufficient to prove character. Certainly the physical is not ; and it is herein that we discover another feature of character, and one which clearly differentiates it from a characteristic. While a characteristic is *immutable,* character suggests *variability in accordance with a rule or principle.* The wetness of the water or its tendency to run downhill will for ever remain its property in consequence of natural law, but not only is a man of character subject to a lapse, but his conduct will differ according to principle so that, to the outsider, his behaviour may seem at times contradictory.

There is one other observation to be made in this connection. The higher the sanction which regulates the individual's conduct, the more integrated, better-knit, and more pronounced is the character, though, as already stated, there is no reason why we should expect a perfectly unbroken or regular pattern, even in the highest type of life. Conflicts unfortunately cannot be avoided, and their bearing on the appraisal of character should be clear to everyone, but, unlike Holt, who thinks their very occurrence is culpable,[1] or what would amount to the same thing in our discourse, prejudicial in

[1] E. B. Holt, *The Freudian Wish.*

CHART V

SHOWING THE POSSIBILITY OF A CHARACTER INDEX BY APPLYING THE STRATIFICATION OF THE REGULATIVE PRINCIPLES TO THE INHIBITION OF SPECIFIC INSTINCTIVE TENDENCIES

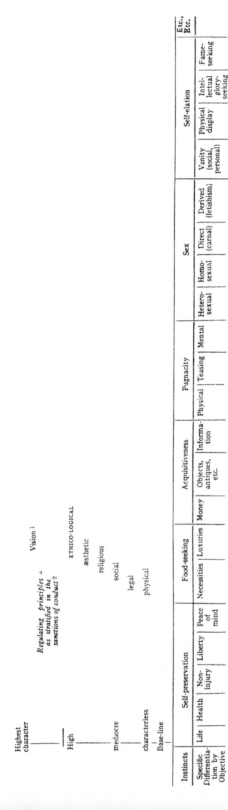

Highest character

High

mediocre

characterless

Base-line

Regulating principles as stratified in the sanctions of conduct[2]

Vision[1]

ETHICO-LOGICAL
aesthetic
religious
social
legal
physical

Instincts	Self-preservation					Food-seeking		Acquisitiveness			Pugnacity			Sex				Self-elation				Etc., Etc.
Specific Differentiation by Objective	Life	Health	Non-injury	Liberty	Peace of mind	Necessities	Luxuries	Money	Objects, antiques, etc.	Information	Physical	Teasing	Mental	Hetero-sexual	Homo-sexual	Direct (carnal)	Derived (fetishism)	Vanity (social, personal)	Physical display	Intellectual glory-seeking	Fame-seeking	

EXPLANATION OF CHART

[1] Since the highest characters cannot realize themselves except through vision, the ethico-logical principles guiding the individual of high character must be joined to vision, on the intellectual side, in order to produce the consummate character.

[2] We may obtain our character curve by fixing points over the proper column and on the level corresponding to the sanction by which the individual is guided. These dots represent inhibitive reactions to specific instinctive tendencies. The usual non-inhibition of an instinctive impulse, except through physical restraint, brings the dot down to about the base-line which corresponds with character-

the appraisal of character, I should hold that the *mental conflict is rather indicative of character*, so long as the stronger instinctive tendency has eventually been overcome in obedience to the higher sanction or maxim of conduct

The Ethico-Logical Sanction. But lest it should appear that this essay is written in the interest of ethics and is a moral exhortation in disguise, I must take the opportunity to emphasize the fact that we are not concerned with ethical acts in the evaluation of character. The mention of ethical sanctions is no more than a reference to *logical principles in relation to behaviour*. The mother who is constantly watching over the welfare of her child will probably be regarded as an ethical being in that respect. But she will not gain an iota from such behaviour so far as the evaluation of her character is concerned. Similarly, the benefactor who in a burst of sympathy for a crippled beggar creates a fund for him so as to maintain the unfortunate in comfort for the rest of his life will be hailed as a moral hero, and will by his deed call forth the approbation of at any rate the vast majority of people ; but his philanthropy has not set him one whit higher as regards his character. If anything, it has lowered him, for, instead of inhibiting a congenital impulse (though sympathy is not, strictly speaking, an instinct) he yielded to it without consulting the principle of justice or fairness, which would dictate a more equitable distribution of his beneficence. In his case, the individual whim has not been overruled by a principle which claims universality. As Scheler has observed, "Sympathy then is in each of its possible forms fundamentally blind as regards values "[1] (*prinzipiell wertblind*).

But then, suppose he discovered a starving refugee and gave him no aid, let it not be inferred that on our view such behaviour would be indicative of character ; for the instinct

---

[1] M. Scheler : *Wesen und Formen der Sympathie*, p. 2.   Spranger in his *Lebensformen* expresses himself to the same effect.

of acquisitiveness is here allowed to *express* itself in the form of miserliness, and this is a more potent inborn tendency than that of sympathy.   Besides, there is no logical principle citable to call forth such conduct, which is in direct contravention of the dictates of justice.

CHAPTER XXXII

THOUGHT AND CHARACTER

There is probably enough implied in our presentation to show that character is not so much linked up with morality as with reason or intelligence, on the one hand, and instinct on the other. Webb,[1] in his interesting study on the relation between intelligence and character, has come to the conclusion that there is a volitional ingredient in intelligence, what he calls an ω factor. Now, we are apt to overlook the truth of the converse proposition, viz., that there is an intelligence factor in character, or, to put it more explicitly, other things being equal, *the highest type of character will be manifested only in those individuals of the highest type of intelligence, or rather intellect* ; for it is doubtful whether the mental alertness conception of intelligence has anything to do with character. But it is not to be gathered that, therefore, a mighty intellect would necessarily give evidence of a high type of character, although from biographical material it would be possible to construct the view that profoundness of mind correlates highly with a well-knit character, and the psychographic results of Heymans and Wiersma tend to show that the predominance of what they call the " secondary function " (comprising such qualities as seriousness, persistence, depth, etc.) is an indication of a solid character.

The Function of Judgment. The reason why character in its highest forms is to a certain extent dependent on intelligence should be almost obvious. Judgment is indispensable in the shaping of a character. The mind which conforms to the rule of the tribe, it is true, partakes of character, but in a lower degree than that mind which sees

[1] Cited earlier.

589

thousands of years ahead and acts in such a way as to set a guiding ideal before humanity.   The Prophets belong in that category in so far as they were the apostles of truth and justice.   In other respects they might have fallen short of the highest standards.

In every great system of ethics, intelligence took its place as a virtue.   Socrates made knowledge the basis of all virtue.   Plato recognized it as a cardinal virtue.   Aristotle included judgment in his ethical system ; and if we turn to the Chinese code we shall again meet with wisdom as a fundamental.

Nevertheless, the positive relationship between character and intellect is by no means to be taken for granted, and it would be a serious omission to ignore the position of Schopenhauer on the subject, who at times is inclined to agree with Goethe's stricture,

> *Er nennt's Vernunft, und braucht's allein,*
> *Nur tierischer als jedes Tier zu sein.*[1]

Schopenhauer's Arbitration.   Schopenhauer's various discussions of the affinity of intellect and character, though teeming with pregnant remarks, are not untainted by his dominant desire to prove the primacy of the will over the intellect.   The passages which are to be cited will presumably reveal at least the somewhat wavering attitude in this respect of the otherwise pertinacious philosopher.

In his essay *On Human Nature* the great pessimist writes : " No one can live among men without feeling drawn again and again to the tempting supposition that moral baseness and intellectual incapacity are closely connected as though they both sprang from one source. . . That it seems to be so is merely due to the fact that both are so often found together and the circumstance is to be explained by the very frequent occurrence of each of them, so that it may easily happen

---

[1] The quotation, as it appears in Schopenhauer's version, is slightly different.

for both to be compelled to live under the one roof. At the same time it is not to be denied that they play into each other's hands to their mutual benefit ; and it is this that produces the very unedifying spectacle which only too many men exhibit, and that makes the world to go as it does. A man who is unintelligent is very likely to show his perfidy, villainy and malice ; whereas a clever man understands better how to conceal these qualities."

Yet in his *Ethical Reflections* the same sage allows himself almost to contradict the above by claiming that " genius and sanctity are akin ". " However simple-minded," we read, " a saint may be, he will nevertheless have a dash of genius in him ; and however many errors of temperament, or of actual character, a genius may possess he will still exhibit a certain nobility of disposition by which he shows his kinship with the saint."

The most explicit statement on the connection between the two chief personality factors is contained in the essay entitled *Character*, wherein Schopenhauer furnishes us the key to the situation and in reality cedes his point, when he discriminates between " two kinds of intellect : between understanding as the apprehension of relation in accordance with the Principle of Sufficient Reason, and cognition, a faculty akin to genius, which acts more directly, is independent of this law, and passes beyond the Principle of Individuation. The latter is the faculty which apprehends Ideas, and it is the faculty which has to do with morality ". The next moment his oscillation again becomes apparent, for he fears that " even this explanation leaves much to be desired. *Fine minds are seldom fine souls* was the correct observation of Jean Paul, although they are never contrary ".

What can account for Schopenhauer's indecision in the matter ? To my mind it is the conflict between his insight and his metaphysical dogma of the omnipotence of the will. It is Schopenhauer, the doctrinal metaphysician, combating

Schopenhauer, the keen psychologist. The two kinds of intelligence mentioned at the beginning of this section tell the whole story, and, recalling what has been said there, we are in a position to secure confirmation of Schopenhauer's point of view as expressed in his essay on character.

Settlement of the Question. The implication is that, while intelligence and character show no correlation, intellect and character are far more closely connected in that the higher types of intellect involve a character factor and *vice versa*.

The attempted sharp dichotomy between the will and the intellect in Schopenhauer's earlier and crowning work need not detain us, except for the quotation of one passage, where the author points out that " it is not the really great minds that make historical characters, because they are [not ?] capable of bridling and ruling the mass of men and carrying out the affairs of the world ; but for this persons of much less capacity of mind are qualified when they have great firmness, decision, and persistence of will, such as is quite inconsistent with very high intelligence. Accordingly, where this very high intelligence exists, we actually have a case in which the intellect directly restricts the will ".[1]

The issue which Schopenhauer has raised here is too ponderous for examination at present. But it is needful to guard against the insidious identification of certain concepts, like character and will ; and it is in illustration of such possible confusion that the argument used by Schopenhauer has been adduced. In reply to Schopenhauer's observation it must be urged that the man of will-power and energy is not necessarily the man of character in the sense described in the present treatment, and, furthermore, it is just because *the man of affairs possesses more will than character that he can get himself so placed as to rule the masses ; and, conversely,*

[1] A. Schopenhauer, *The World as Will and Idea*, Second Book, Chapter xix, Sect. 5.

it is for the reason that the man of character who may at the same time be an intellectual giant is not prone to waste his time and lower his principles on the follies and vices of man that he chooses not to rule the destiny of the masses directly, but indirectly, yet with greater permanence. Let us not be misled by the notion that the ability to forge ahead or, as Münsterberg put it, that power to keep the selected motive dominant is the essence of character.

To come back to the original query as regards the relation between intelligence and character, there can be no denying that the fools do not happen to be the knaves, nor are the knaves known as fools. It has been abundantly proven that some types of criminals are characterized by their sharp-wittedness. And a director of an institution for juvenile delinquents is impressed by the recurring fact that a bright boy, as happens in so many cases, will be devoid of all consideration for others and will take the downward path contrary to his better knowledge, while a moron may show himself obedient, courteous, kind, and trustworthy.

Vision an Essential of High Character. These commonplace discrepancies are simply to be taken for granted. It has never occurred to me to maintain that there is an actual correspondence between level of thought and level of character. All I have contended is that those with restricted intelligence and a narrow field of activity are precluded from entering the class of supernormal characters, which is reserved only for those with vision, those whose very ideas, especially if they possess dynamic force, are bound to provide for them an arena. It is doubtful whether the moron, be he ever so virtuous, is ever guided by principle, spontaneously applied ; whether his placid obedience, tractability, and other such passive traits may not be due in large measure to the forcefulness with which the elementary rules of morality have been inculcated in his very receptive mind. We should not go so far as to deny him a moderately high grade of character, but the issue is, of course, whether the most virtuous moron can be on a characterial par with the conventionally less moral historical figures of great vision who have not only clung to their principles but have fought for them.

What Vision Means. It has not occurred to me that such a conversational word as *vision* requires special elaboration, but one or two reviewers stumbled on it. Particularly was this true of the reviewer of the *London Times*, who curiously or, better perhaps, carelessly enough, referred to vision as one of my " sanctions ", and then again, as if it were a regulative principle, " the highest," as he puts it,[1] although I have made it clear that vision is a phase of intelligence which is essential for the exercise of the highest type of character. It is neither a sanction like the physical, social, religious, esthetic, or ethico-logical clamps on our instinctive tendencies, nor is it a regulative principle, like justice or liberty, to serve as a goal. Vision is like a light-tower which illuminates the dark waters ; the stronger the light, the greater the area it enables us to see—the safer our guidance.

There is no definition of the term in Warren's *Dictionary of Psychology*, except in the literal and technical sense of " retinal vision ". Webster's Dictionary includes, as one sense, " unusual discernment and foresight." The Oxford Dictionary attaches to the term an occult or mystic meaning. Vision is not synonymous with intelligence, or insight, or intuition, since its territory ranges over the future rather than the present. It may be said that what intuition is to the present, vision is to the future. The ancient Talmudic scholar who defined the sage as one *who visualizes what is to happen* [2] (literally, " to be born ") has revealed himself a clear thinker. We may note also that it is not the prophet who is placed in this prized category. In fact, another widely quoted

---

[1] London *Times Literary Supplement*, 16th February, 1928.
[2] Tractate *Tomid*, fol. 32, " *Eyzehu khokhom horōeh es hanolad* ".

Talmudical dictum emphatically states that " the sage is superior to the prophet ".[1]

General and Specific Factors.—Vision, like intelligence, may also be said to embrace a general and specific factors. The sage possesses an all-round vision, but he may be deficient in some restricted field because of inexperience. On the other hand, a man of much less vision may be commercially or politically shrewd, so as to sense a trend many years ahead. Such, however, is the unpredictability of the conjuncture of events that no one can foresee the course of history even within a quarter of century. T. G. Masaryk, a man of the highest character and rare vision, could certainly not have anticipated the vicissitudes of his beloved country, either when he was agitating for its independence, or especially after he gained his objective ; and how can we hold it against him, when the world at large still does not know whether his worthy son took his own life or was hurled to death as a political measure ?

Metternich, in his day, was rated as one of the most astute statesmen in history ; but could he have foreseen the plight of Austria, in 1950, not to mention its annexation in 1937, he would have felt less proud of himself. Similarly the blustering Bismarck, who must have gloated over his successful plan to precipitate the Franco-Prussian War, could hardly have possessed vision, even in the political sense, although political acumen may have been his forte. Disraeli, when he acquired India for Great Britain and Queen Victoria was crowned Empress of India in 1877, could not have anticipated that, in less than a century India would form two independent states with but slim ties to the British Empire, yet Disraeli, like Cavour, will go down in history as a man of great vision ; for

---

[1] *Khokhom ōdef minovi.* (I am not using the Sephardic phonetic system—employed in Israel). Another observation of Talmudic origin is " The ignoramus cannot be pious ", in other words, it requires judgment to know how to serve God.

we cannot be reasonably certain that India, *at the time*, would have been better off if left to her own devices.

Without actually mentioning it by name, Winston Churchill in his War Memoirs, eloquently refers to this endowment without which character, in men of influence, cannot reach a high level, when he writes :

How vain are human calculations of self-interest ! Rarely has there been a more convincing example. Admiral Darlan had but to sail in any one of his ships to any port outside France to become the master of all French interests beyond German control. He would not have come like General de Gaulle with only an unconquerable heart and a few kindred spirits. He would have carried with him outside the German reach the fourth Navy in the world, whose officers and men were personally devoted to him. Acting thus, Darlan would have become the chief of the French Resistance with a mighty weapon in his hand. British and American dockyards and arsenals would have been at his disposal for the maintenance of his fleet. The French gold reserve in the United States would have assured him, once recognized, of ample resources. The whole French Empire would have rallied to him. Nothing could have prevented him from being the Liberator of France. The fame and power which he so ardently desired were in his grasp. Instead, he went forward through two years of worrying and ignominious office to a violent death, a dishonoured grave, and a name long to be execrated by the French Navy and the nation he had hitherto served so well.[1]

Illustrations of vision in laboratory research are so plentiful that the history of science is replete with them. Frequently, too, a physicist or chemist will not foresee the application of his discovery, e.g. Einstein could never have supposed that his early transformation equation would facilitate the making

[1] W. S. Churchill : *Their Finest Hour*, 1949 (Houghton Mifflin), p. 230.

of atom bombs, but there are remarkable cases of foresight in regard to the periphery of a project. Thus when Ernest Rutherford, during the first World War, was asked why he did not abandon the tiny atom and turn to something more impressive, his reply was that the outcome of the work on this bagatelle would prove more important than the War itself.

Gifted Children Show More Character. It is gratifying to draw some support in favour of this view from recent experimental results as well as from biographical material. The data obtained in the investigation of some thousand gifted children by Terman and his associates warrant the conclusion that there is more character evinced by the gifted than by the mediocre. The curves show decidedly that there is a positive correlation between intelligence and character traits. This conclusion is further borne out by the evidence of May and Hartshorne's honesty experiments referred to in Chapter XXIII.

Explanation of a Common Fallacy. The popular notion that the average man is more honest than the one occupying a more prominent place in the social order will probably stand revision. In the first place, it ought to be kept in mind that the popular notion, for obvious reasons, would favour the average man. Secondly, we are apt to judge in such matters by the force of the impression. The lapse of a prominent professional man, e.g. will cause a greater stir than that of an ordinary person, with the result that the one instance is sufficient to create an altogether erroneous belief in the mind of the public which is not likely to take all the circumstances into consideration, but will pass judgment on the strength of what transpires in the light of its expectations. Now, an individual of some intellectual calibre is not supposed to make a moral slip; such an occurrence, therefore, is magnified in extent until it begins to affect the reputation of the whole class to which the individual belongs. There is, of course, no way of telling what

the mediocre man would do if placed in the same position
as his more fortunate brother ; but even in the absence
of an adequate foundation, one would be tempted to gather
that, just as in the case of the gifted children, the more
capable individuals *as a class* possess greater character than
those who are clustered about the median line in intelligence.

The Maligned Genius. It is true that much fault has been
found with the genius. Those writers who have had an axe
to grind have represented him as egotistic, selfish, capricious,
cruel, in short as a degenerate in embryo. To attempt to
minimize the number of personality defects in genius would be
a futile task, although here again, the " expectation fallacy "
vitiates the interpretation. We are so accustomed to look
up to the genius as a paragon of perfection that the discovery
of a flaw in his make-up is enough for some people to relegate
him to a subnormal level, as if, taking one instance, to entertain suicidal ideas were on the whole more characteristic
of the genius than of the common man, or as if that impulse
were symptomatic of degeneration.

As regards character, genius has been sorely maligned.
Lombroso in his *Man of Genius* argues for the moral insanity
of various celebrities on very flimsy grounds. Proverbs
which, as is well known, may be found to satisfy every claim,
rumours, legends, and other questionable sources, provide
him with his ammunition against the man of superior parts.
He quotes George Sand's indictment of great men, of which
she had probably delivered herself in one of her despondent
moods, perhaps after a quarrel with one or another of her
brilliant lovers. He makes out Aristotle to have been a base
flatterer (of Alexander the Great). Schopenhauer's moral
insanity apparently consisted in despising his countrymen.
Tolstoï's sin was to have disapproved of patriotism. (Had
Lombroso lived to read the Journal of Tolstoï's wife, he would
have found a good deal more to complain of in the character
of the famous Russian.) Even Jesus is credited with

emotional anaesthesia because of some of his utterances as reported by the Evangelists. In *L'Uomo Delinquente*, Lombroso takes a more moderate stand. There he says distinctly that "criminals are but rare apparitions in the scientific world ". In the same book [1] he accounts for the negligible amount of criminality among scientists by saying that more than other men they understand that every culpable act is not only unjust and illogical but also without advantage, since it always recoils on the head of its author. In other words, the scientist, according to Lombroso, would be guided by regulating principles as well as by prudence.

Lombroso's Method Faulty. Lombroso's cavils against the *savant* in his *Man of Genius* will not bear examination. His acerbity is too transparent when he describes in uncomplimentary terms the gatherings of academic men or scientists, or when he magnifies some peccadillo of a celebrity. To be sure, genius has its small quota of reprobates ; but on the whole, the leaders in thought (not in the arts and crafts) show a remarkably clear record in matters of conduct. The Bacons and the Rousseaus are rare after all, while the exemplary lives of the beacon lights in the history of thought more than make up for the few serious character defects that may be singled out at century-long intervals. By Lombroso's method of ferreting out some alleged misdemeanour on the part of a notable, it would be possible to make out of a saint the devil incarnate. If men of great intellect reveal at times the common foibles of mankind, it is not because of their genius but in spite of it. Had Lombroso shown that the average man was less jealous, less selfish, less cruel, less treacherous, etc., than the highly capable person, he might have proven his case. As it is, he has only demonstrated that *even* the genius is human, despite the universal expectation that he would have raised himself above the weaknesses of the flesh.

[1] C. Lombroso, *L'Uomo Delinquente*, vol. i, part 3, chap. 9 (4th ed., 1889).

We may, therefore, still maintain with confidence that character in a high degree will be found, on the whole, more among the intellectual than among the average run of people, and that the exceptions are too few to disprove the rule.

CHAPTER XXXIII

PSYCHOLOGICAL SOURCE OF THE REGULATIVE PRINCIPLES

I am aware, of course, that the problem of character is not pre-empted by making it hinge on the instincts on the one hand and rational principles on the other. One might ask whether the possibility of a certain instinct being much stronger in one person than in another might not call for a greater amount of inhibition and, therefore, warrant a higher rating, if such an instinct has been successfully modified.

Weighty Matters Leading to Interminable Discussion. Another question bears on the genesis of the inhibitory force. What explains the different capacities to inhibit instinctive tendencies in different individuals? If a congenital affair, then are we not claiming *ex hypothesi* that character is an instinctive tendency dominating other instinctive tendencies? And if, again, we are born with this disposition, then is not Schopenhauer justified in denying the possibility of modification in a person's character, contending, as he does, that we are but the tools of Fate? And if such is the case, are we not bound to reduce the proportions of the dignity and greatness attached to character?

It would take us too far afield for our present purpose to examine each of these questions at length. Yet a word is necessary to show the psychological origins of character, and particularly that element of it which has been referred to under the heading of regulative principles.

In the first place, as regards the varying strength of the instincts in different individuals, there is reason to believe that even the miser can under certain conditions curb his stinginess. Most prisoners, no matter how refractory and intractable they are in ordinary life, are, as is known, held in check by the jail warders. We have also the testimony of some of the noblest characters in history, such as Moses Mendelssohn, to the strength of their passions, which, however, they were able to rule with perfect ease. Furthermore, the biographies of great men have in a number of cases revealed the subjects to have been given to profligacy in youth, though in later life devoting themselves to the loftiest purposes. (St. Augustine, Tolstoï.) [1] It is well to point out at this juncture that the free will shibboleth does not enter here and should not be introduced to befuddle the issue. So long as the determining factor of a given act, indicative of character, is not brought about by physical pressure or in duress or mainly through social considerations, the causative nature of the evidentiary act does not concern us. So long as the inhibition is from within (regulative principles) we must be satisfied that there is character back of the restraint:

Supreme Distinction Between Character and Intelligence. Any instinct, then, no matter how intense, *can* be overcome ; and it is in this regard that character is so disparate from intelligence, for no amount of effort would turn a 'moron into a superior intelligence, but the most defective character can be changed at least for a short time, provided its possessor makes up his mind to take a firm stand, that is to say, provided sufficient inhibitory force is exerted. But then, what about those whose inhibitions are feeble compared with those of others ?

That some persons are capable of controlling themselves better than others goes without saying, but it is not so generally known that even children at a tender age may be differentiated according to the seriousness with which they take instructions. The influence of the environment, tradition, and customs cannot be invoked to account for the perceptible germs of character displayed by three-year-old

[1] Cf. also H. Begbie's *Twice-Born Men.*

children. *We may reasonably assume that some persons are born with greater nervous plasticity than others, and plasticity in this sense does not mean merely resiliency of the tissues or elasticity, but organization in such a way as to allow the nerve currents to take different paths without serious disturbance.* Naturally the psycho-analytic schools would eagerly point to the many neuroses and psychoses as evidence of the impossibility of such an organization ; and I do not feel it incumbent to dispute their doctrines. All that is set forth in this connection is the fact that with our apparently fixed instinctive mechanisms,[1] we inherit also an element of modifiability, not in the form of a lever or a muscle, like, say, the tensor tympani on the tympanic membrane, but in the actual concatenation of the instinctive steps. Mechanically, the greater inhibitability would call for greater slowness in the instinct to run its course.[2] *Brakes and gears could be put on at more points and with greater effectiveness in the more inhibitive individual than in the less inhibitive.*

The Inhibitory Process. So far, then, we have seen there is no necessity to posit an inhibitory mechanism as such. The variability of the instinct is to be looked for in the instinct itself. But, besides the facility of inhibition, there must be a something to bring about the inhibition. Now, this agency may be another instinctive urge operating in an opposite direction. Anger may be turned aside through

[1] The word " mechanism " as employed here merely represents the physical basis of the disposition and is not meant to indicate that instincts are merely mechanical forces devoid of purposiveness and adaptability. A mechanism is the enduring arrangement which engenders a particular disposition and is invested with the potentiality of modifying the given disposition in accordance with various circumstances. It is clearly not a machine.

[2] The " all-or-none " principle which Rivers has taken over from physiology (Symposium on " Instinct and the Unconscious ", *British Journal of Psychology*, 1919, vol. x), applying it to the course of an instinct, is of little service even if it were proven to hold true of instincts in general.

fear. The threatening finger of the law is sufficient to inhibit the acquisitive impulses of many people within certain limits. Such inhibitions, arising out of purely instinctive sources, cannot be considered as revealing the earmarks of character. It is doubtful whether even social inhibition can be claimed as a criterion, but since in most cases it is scarcely possible to discover the real motives of conduct, we can afford to be charitable and give the benefit of the doubt to all whose actions do not betray evidence of merely seeking social approbation. Similarly, the religious and aesthetic sentiments exercise their inhibitory power over the primitive instincts, but it is only the ethico-logical principles which count in full measure toward according to character its proper value.

Certainly these principles are not implanted upon us by some mysterious force. They may be regarded as sentiments, that is to say, affective complexes, deriving their nourishment out of the individual's social milieu, but I think it is worth while emphasizing the universality and absoluteness of these principles, which are more logical than psychological, inasmuch as they attach to cognition rather than to affection or instinct.

Chief Mark of Regulative Principle. Lest, however, the impression be gained that these principles represent a sort of *deus ex machina* device which has no psychological basis, I should remind the reader that even striving in the cause of truth and the religious exercise of justice are not beyond the possibility of inheritance. As McDougall has observed, " The innate structure of the human mind comprises much more than the instincts alone . . . There are many facts which compel us to go further in the recognition of innate mental structure, such facts as the special facilities shown by individuals in music, in mathematics, in language, and other aesthetic, moral and intellectual endowments." [1] These

---

[1] Wm. McDougall, " Instinct and the Unconscious " : *British Journal of Psychol.*, 1919, vol. x, p. 37.

principles differ from instinctive drives particularly in this respect, that, while an instinctive expression is no more than a *particularization* of an act involving one's own self, the guiding principles which are under discussion represent *universalizations*, involving naturally also the individual who is acting, but directed toward humanity in general, of which this or that person appears as a case. Anger, too, is directed against somebody else, but no universalization takes place in expressing this emotion. It must be remembered that justice has been distinguished from sympathy in another chapter, and the difference holds here, too, and consists in the fact that *sympathy, though, as Adam Smith taught, it may be the root of all our moral sentiments, is primarily a particularized act, immediately generated by an impulse suffused with feeling, while a just act is more impersonal, less immediately generated and mediated through reflection, momentary as it may be.*

In spite of what has been said in the above paragraph, L. P. Thorpe in his *Psychological Foundations of Personality* (1938), p. 10, brings up the objection that " Roback's regulative principle might not be a righteous one. Theoretically, it could be the code of gangsters ". Thorpe might have realized that a regulative principle operates in the direction of progressive humanity. A gangster's code would not be a principle, for one thing, since it could not be consistently carried out because of too many clashes, and then it could not be called " regulative ". What would it regulate ? Not even one man's life.

The Sanctions. It will have been noticed by this time that the use of the words " principles " and " sanctions " is not clearly demarcated, the former being employed sometimes to cover only the purely .ethical determinants, such as truth and justice, while at other times they are intended to designate the standards of action. The reason for this apparent looseness in language is that *all recognized standards* *of action are merely popularized versions of the ethical standards diluted with the appeal to fear and the incentive of reward* so as to gain a hold on the average man and woman. Even though the social sanction often encourages flattery and hypocrisy, it without question originally took rise in the community desire to safeguard the interests of its members ; and this could not be realized without invoking the primary ethical principles as a *sine qua non*. In spirit, then, all approved standards of action are the same, though they sadly differ in application. The purely ethical appeal may, therefore, be looked upon as containing the various other sanctions in their ideal form, while these other standards may be considered as a graded stratification of the ethical principles governing action.

Knowledge and Practice. But even these ethical principles have two sides to them. It is one thing to recognize that fairness should be the mark of all dealings, but quite another to observe this rule in practice ; and character value depends on the observance, not on the mere observation of the maxim, because it is in the practice that the crucial test lies. That all normal people, that is to say *all*, excluding the aments and the demented, possess a sense of justice, can be readily seen from the fact that they seize on every opportunity to set forth their claims when they believe themselves to have been unfairly dealt with. The next to receive such consideration is their kin, then their affiliated groups, etc., but what must appear so puzzling to a logical mind is the disinclination of the vast majority of human beings to apply the same measures to themselves and to others.

Now there are two paths open to us in explanation of the two divergent approaches. One alternative is to assume that the recognition of right and wrong is not sufficiently potent to actuate most people in the cause of others. But then, if the notion is dynamic in one's self-interest, something else must be sought to account for its inertia otherwise. It is within reason, I think, as our other alternative, to postulate a *consistency* urge as the basis of all conduct typifying the person of character. It is this medium which helps to depersonalize our instincts, merging the " mine " and the " thine " into an impersonal cause.

THE CONSISTENCY URGE

Since the word consistency is often understood in the sense of acting uniformly and merely this, it must be explained that in our present connection tne term refers to the relationship between one's expectations from others and behaviour toward others. A person is consistent in our sense not when he merely repeats his acts in the same way under similar conditions, but only when he employs *one standard* of action both for himself and others, it being obvious that where only one course is open, such as in saving either one's own life or another's, one's own interests come first. This surely does not run counter to the principle of consistency, for we expect everybody else to act similarly under the same conditions, although true nobility of character might prompt one to self-sacrifice on certain rare occasions—in accordance with the consistency principle. But the habitual miscreant who performs his acts consistently in the popular sense, would certainly think himself unfairly dealt with if he were treated as he behaves towards others. To be consistent, then, is to act in accordance with what one considers to be right and to refrain from what one considers to be wrong.

By this time some impatient reader will come to the conclusion that the consistency principle is merely another name for the " Golden Rule ", whether in its positive or negative aspect. After all, it will be remarked, is all this not a circuitous way of saying, " Do not unto others what you would not have them do unto you," or, in the positive version,

" Do unto others as you would be done by ? "

Difference Between " Golden Rule " and Principle of Consistency. My answer is as follows : (a) The psychology of character does not deal with maxims or precepts except to explain their connection in a system of mental facts ; (b) underlying the " Golden Rule " is, of course, the consistency principle which has its root in an inborn urge. But that is where the resemblance stops. Every concrete precept is defective in that it lacks a broad perspective to make allowance for unanticipated possibilities. Many acts can be thought of that might come literally under the sanction of the " Golden Rule " which would yet be frowned at. The ladies' man who makes advances to women might contend that he is not averse to receiving similar attentions from them. The ethical maxim, however, based on our psychological view of character would remove this loophole by making the injunction read : *Inhibit your instinctive tendency in accordance with the principle of consistency as you would wish it observed from the angle of an impartial spectator.* There are two features which distinguish the injunction as formulated above. In the first place, it provides a rule which is psychologically applicable and which covers the widest range of cases without the possibility of quibbles entering in as a wedge. Secondly, the relationship is neutralized and therefore made objective. It is no longer a question of what *you* would like done, but what the detached judge in you would have done.

In the conventional moral maxim, on the other hand, the relation is solely between the agent and the individual to be acted upon.

The Use of Maxims. The stress laid on inhibition would act as a logical damper on the ardour of, let us say, an annoying suitor, but it would not with reason curb the heroic impulse of a life-saver from carrying out his praiseworthy act, for in so doing he is actually inhibiting his most potent instinctive complex—self-preservation. Not that many are really governed in conduct by perceiving the superiority of one maxim over another. Actually few stop to reflect at all before making a significant plunge on the spur of the moment. Just as logic is useful to test the validity of our thinking, rather than to determine the results of our thinking, so the establishment of rules of conduct helps us more in estimating the rightness of the act already done than in affecting our course of action in the first place.

We must not digress, however, into a field which has been too greatly cultivated and too little harvested. The consistency urge which, it is here contended, exists in embryo in every person who has attained self-consciousness, and which alas is the earliest connate tendency to become perverted, chiefly through rationalizations, requires, as one might expect, sufficient time for maturation.

Manifestation of Principle in Young Children. Young children seldom give indications of this tendency, yet it is possible to detect significant differences in reactions to others on the part of even five-year-old youngsters, and that in spite of their being brought up in the same environment.

To attribute the differences to education is to put the cart before the horse; for the fact that some children will benefit by the strict injunctions and others will not ought to convince us that there is something in the child which accepts the consequences, rather than that it is the nature of the injunctions which brings results. In some, the argument: How would you like me to take that toy away from you, as you did from that little boy? produces a ready and desirable response, while others, though they seem to understand the injustice of their act, make no effort to mend their conduct, and still others find some either wholly fictitious or else totally irrelevant excuse to justify their budding rapacity. Women, too, are, as many great novelists and essayists have remarked, incapable of acting with consistency, and, unless moved by pity, are prone to commit many unfair acts on various pretexts, chief among which is that, being the weaker sex, or the weaker of two of their own sex, or having " gone through " more than their rival or expecting to enjoy life less than someone else, they ought not to lose at least this opportunity of making up for the hardship either already endured or in store for them.

Consistency Lacking in Women. Such a warm champion of woman's cause as Moll, tries to gloss over this character defect by an explanation which leaves much to be desired. " When women," he writes, " are so frequently denied the sense of justice, it is . . . a matter of the present motive preventing other considerations from presenting themselves." [1] What is this but an admission of the fact that they are not considerate of others, in other words, that they lack the impulse to apply to others the same measure as they apply to themselves ?

We hear it said and repeated almost *ad nauseam* that women are prompted by their feelings rather than by their reason. But such a hollow statement possesses no scientific value. Many women reason well enough at the very time they are supposed to be guided by their feelings. Their reasoning, however, lacks consideration for others. It is the element' of consistency alone which is wanting—a gap which is sometimes filled by the substitute of pity. If the above time-honoured and apparently universal belief about the main-springs of women's conduct is to be invested with any psychological meaning, we should necessarily hold to one or the other of these alternatives : either that women, on the whole, are born with stronger instinctive tendencies, or else the consistency urge is weaker in them than in man. The former alternative does not seem plausible, more especially as the maxim of parsimony would lead us to explain the phenomenon

---

[1] A. Moll, " Sexualität und Charakter " : *Sexual-Probleme : Zt. f. Sexualw'ft. u. Sexualpolitik*, 1914, vol. x.

through some weakness in the one factor rather than in the many.

It is, therefore, not in the relative strength of the instinct that we shall find the reason for the lack of objectivity in female conduct, but in the relative weakness of the fundamental principle of conduct which has its root psychologically in some mechanism making for consistency. In fine, then, consistency in action, which is one of the chief determinants of character, can be traced to original connate tendencies ; and if this smacks too much of Descartes' innate ideas doctrine, I might point out that there are vast differences between the two classes of concepts. If it is true, as is generally conceded, that men differ as to the relative strength of their instinctive tendencies, then may it not be taken for granted that they also differ as to their nervous constitution in respect of inhibitability, and in the application to others of what they consider to be fair for themselves, and above all in the strict adherence to an abstract principle, like liberty, for instance, in the face of great danger to the acting individual ? It is in connection with the recognition of the issues to be championed that intellect is of service, so that it becomes indispensable in the make-up of the most typical specimens of character.

Inborn Basis of Consistency. Let us *per contra* assume that there is nothing in the original make-up of man to determine the disposition to observe consistency both in theory and practice, that sympathy in conjunction with the inculcation of moral precepts is wholly responsible for the part justice plays as an ideal and for what little of it is actually done of one's own accord. Now in the history of the race, as already suggested, the same foundation may underlie sympathy and the consistency urge, but there is abundant evidence for rejecting any such close relationship in the same individual. There are too many sympathetic people in the world who by their very acts, either heedless or intentional, create the occasion for sympathy, and indeed often in a greater measure than those situations which elsewhere move them to compassion. Need we cite James's example of the lady who sheds bitter tears over the fate of the fictitious character in the play, while her coachman is freezing outside the theatre waiting for the performance to end?

Suppose we furthermore accept the view that the principle of consistency has grown out of the perception that consistency in some form must be erected into a tradition—if society is not to revert to its original state of perpetual warfare, *bellum omnium contra omnes*, to quote the words of Hobbes—there is still to account for the co-operation of the individual under conditions which would render him immune from legal responsibility. Is it that one man is more suggestible to the imposition than another? Very well then, this *individual suggestibility which is peculiar to action in relation to others*— since there is no such thing as general suggestibility and, moreover, as the least suggestible of people (in the sense that they rarely accept personal suggestions) are usually the most consistent in conduct and *vice versa—has an inborn source.* That is all I would be pleading for. No matter how much we try to get around this fundamental conclusion, we shall come to it in the end, although in a more roundabout way.

In Flugel's review, cited previously, the cavil appears to the effect that my theory of the consistency urge is novel but not explained as to its derivation. Surely, it would be rather easy to draw a series of diagrams showing the topography of the trait, or, following the psychoanalytic procedure, one could pile up layer upon layer of premises, but neither course would constitute the semblance of a proof. On the other hand, the very fact that people do differ in regard to consistency, even in the logical sphere (Emerson, for example, thought that to strive invariably for consistency is a species of slavery) would argue for an original disposition, perhaps in conjunction with other traits, either positively or negatively linked. I see no greater difficulty in positing genes that are responsible for this urge than, let us say, in accounting for a consuming interest in and talent for music, languages, or mathematics.

CONSISTENCY AND THE CRIMINAL

The essence of punishment consists in forcing upon the criminal's mind the absoluteness of the principle of consistency which he had denied through his action ; and it is significant I think that nearly every culprit who pays the supreme penalty and admits the dastardliness of the crime also thinks that he is receiving his just desert. " If I could undo, or make amends for anything I have done, I would suffer my body as I now stand to be cut in pieces inch by inch," [1] Charles Peace, one of the most notorious criminals of his century, feelingly said when visited a few days before his execution.

Similarly. Webster, the chemist, who murdered his benefactor, in answer to the sheriff's question about his reported contemplation of suicide replied : " Why should I ? All the proceedings in my case have been just. . . it is just that I should die upon the scaffold in accordance with that sentence."

" **Moral Insanity.**" The extreme degenerate who, as in Andreyev's *The Seven that Were Hanged*, keeps repeating, after a revolting murder, " I must not be hanged, I don't want to be hanged," until he brings himself to believe that he will never be executed, is so rare as to make us class him with the low grade imbecile or the insane. What has been called " *moral insanity* ", *is merely another name for the various degrees of inconsistency in action to the disadvantage of one's fellow-beings.* Russian literature bristles with characters displaying behaviour of this sort. Readers of Gorki's *My Fellow Traveller* will find it difficult to see any

[1] H. B. Irving, *A Book of Remarkable Criminals* (1918).

verisimilitude in the character description of Shakro, yet there are no doubt many individuals of a similar type who display what is commonly called " cheek " in an appalling degree.

Consistency Basis of Justice. The *lex talionis* is after all the most logical means of asserting the sovereignty of the consistency principle. A callous nature can be softened only by receiving an equal amount of suffering to that caused. The requirements of our modern criminal system, however, call for other methods of treatment. The preventive view in penology is manifestly based on an expedient rather than an intellectual foundation, considering, as it does, the *lex talionis* a relic of a barbarous age when retribution or revenge pure and simple was the *raison d'être* of punishment. Yet the retaliatory measure dating from pre-Biblical times is still resorted to in premeditated capital offences. We have no uniformity to-day in dealing with the criminal brought to book. There is simply an effort made to protect ourselves against the anti-social marauder, but it cannot be said that the end of justice is served when the perpetrator of a mayhem act, let us say, receives a year's sentence. So long as the man who voluntarily caused the suffering himself suffers less than his victim, justice is out of the question ; and just how confinement for a certain length of time can be compared with the pain and deprivation resulting from the loss of limb is something beyond comprehension. Consistency does not enter here at all.

Philosophers Favour " Lex Talionis." A profound mind like Kant's has not dodged the issue. He definitely clings to the *lex talionis* in his philosophy of law, curiously enough, with a regard for the dignity of the criminal, who would most assuredly forego the privilege. According to that critical philosopher, it would be treating the prisoner as *a means* and not as an end to punish him merely for the purpose of protecting society or deterring would-be criminals. And the criminal like everyone else must be treated as a person ; for the categorical imperative applies to him too. Thus is brought about the paradoxical state of affairs in which the modern reformer who would employ the convict as an instrument is far more welcome to him than the austere Kant who would have the murderer's life taken in order to save his dignity. Kant's penology is, of course, coloured by his supreme ethical maxim ; but at least the conclusion which he arrives at is more in keeping with the dictates of· justice than the prevailing measures of the legal system.

Hegel also discloses a decided leaning toward the consistency principle when he holds the punishment to be a necessary antithesis to the offence. Again, there is the invasion of a strictly practical sphere by philosophical presuppositions. But what should strike us as significant is the fact that thinkers of the highest order, such as Kant and Hegel, were not taken aback at the thought of making the punishment fit the crime.

Let it not be imagined, however, that I am anxious to have the ancient *lex talionis* put into force. There is at least one serious drawback to it. Modern society regards the offender as one of its members, and is therefore eager to protect its left wing as well as its right wing and centre. It does not view with relish the prospect of matching the number of those crippled, maimed and blinded through intentional violence by an equal number of such unfortunates, let alone the colossal complication of establishing the degree of the intent, the nature of the circumstances (provocation, physical or mental state of the miscreant, etc.) as well as the intensity or extent of the suffering.

All these arguments, however, in favour of the prevailing administration of justice should not blind us to the fact that its essence is still the principle of consistency which in its psychological form exists as an urge in man connate with his other tendencies to action and just as universal. If isolated cases of the conspicuous absence of this urge can be pointed to now and then in some criminal, the relative universality of the urge is not on that account to be discredited any more than a case of compléte absence of sexuality would disprove the potency of this instinct in mankind.

NOTE

Elsewhere,[1] the distinction has been made between characters and personalities, in that the former deal with principles, at all times, while the latter are concerned with people and their feelings. The personalities are more impulsive ; the characters are primarily more inhibitive, but their inhibition is only a springboard for action in which their self-interest is subservient to the cause at stake ; hence their instinctive tendencies are for the time being suppressed.

[1] A. A. Roback : *Personality in Theory and Practice*, 1950 (Sci-Art) pp. 288 ff.

CHAPTER XXXIV

CHARACTER AND CONFLICT

Prevalent View. It has been generally held by moralists and psychologists that the man of character is one who has no conflicts, one who has been able to overcome the many struggles of desires for supremacy which mark particularly the *Sturm und Drang* period in life. The settled man is regarded as having won his victory over the besetting temptations cropping up in youth. The older we grow, the less obstructed is supposed to be our contemplated course. In the recent terminology, integration usually implies or presupposes the absence or minimal survival of conflict. Furthermore, it is frequently taken for granted that the man who gives evidence of conflicts in his behaviour cannot be truly said to possess character ; for character is meant to include decisiveness as one of its ingredients.

Outstanding Service of Freud. The concept of conflict, as we shall see presently, is not so new as most popular authors make it out to be. Let us concede, however, that Freud and his disciples have shown the significance of conflicts in our social system, and have directed the attention of teacher, physician, social worker—in short, all those who are concerned with the welfare of the individual to the operation of a mechanism which had been but vaguely understood before their days. Hitherto it was thought that great inner conflicts took place only in the imaginative productions of literary minds. The man in the street was not credited with such mental processes to any appreciable extent ; and the ambitious young man, his mind taken up with arduous endeavours, surely was not suspected of undergoing the anguish of being pulled in two different directions.

It has generally been overlooked by writers that the conflicts do not necessarily have to be between a natural impulse and an imposition of society. There are quandaries of which the average person has no idea. It takes a sensitive soul to understand the sufferings of Novalis or Amiel, and who but the highly cultured can appreciate the qualms of Ernst Renan repeating to himself many times a day the Hebrew phrase " *Naftoulay Elohim Niftalti* " (" I have wrestled the wrestlings of the Lord ") as his faith was being shaken while preparing for the priesthood at the Seminaire St. Sulpice ? [1]

There are conflicts and conflicts. Renan's conflict was of a higher order in the hierarchy than that of most people ; but as psychoanalysis has demonstrated, nearly every one goes through certain crises in which the individual desire contests the authority of the social restraint.

Whether these conflicts are as disastrous as the Freudians claim is another matter which need not be considered here. The question posed is simply this : Has the man of character rid himself of conflicts ? or put in another form : Is the manifestation of conflicts the symptom of characterlessness in proportion to their number and intensity ?

Literary Illustrations of Conflicts. In opposition to the general belief which accepts the affirmative answer to this query, I should wish to point out that just as no military leader can prove, even to his own satisfaction, his prowess unless he takes part in battles, so no man can be accredited with character of a high degree unless his mind is the seat of conflicts, but—and hereto is attached an important rider —he must *recognize the nature of his struggle*, and not be merely in the position of Buridan's ass between the two bundles of hay. Hesitation is not conflict, and the mere lamentation of one's plight is no solution to the problem. Dramatists, in order to draw out all the literary possibilities of their hero's or heroine's predicament, invariably render

[1] E. Renan, *Souvenirs d'enfance et de jeunesse*, chap. v.

their characters sentimental because of the rumination of the same thought in a different phrasing. Particularly is this true of the French tragedians, e.g. Corneille in *Le Cid*. No progress is made in Chimène's conflict between her love for Rodrigue and her abhorrence of marrying her father's slayer, while the audience is being filled with the poetical turns and bouts of the loving pair. It is not the conflict which detracts from the strength of character, and it is not in the speed of the solution that the character is redeemed, but rather in the *method* adopted to solve the conflict ; and it is for this very reason that Hamlet's course in soliloquizing, " To be or not to be " provokes a mild scorn. The resolving of a conflict requires *reasoning not poetizing*, but of course the poet who creates his characters realizes that there is far more beauty and attraction in poetry than in reasoning, hence the somewhat pathological complexion of most dramatic characters.

Types in Whom Conflict is Missing. In actual life conflict is neither pathological nor an indication of lack of character. On the contrary, I should say a person of character, provided he is not devoid of spirit, would find himself passing through many a crisis because of his associations and relationships. *Two types of people avoid inner conflicts*—those who are born to be led, and those whose conscience is so dimmed and their consistency urge so slight that they will allow nothing to stand in the way of attaining their object.

When it is contended that once a man's character is formed his attitude will be fixed for every new occasion, it is forgotten that circumstances may arise which require a different attitude, to which the former fixity does not apply. We are here not dealing with a change in character, for there is no contradiction in reacting differently to an entirely new situation , and still less does the presence of a conflict imply behaviour that is not in keeping with the individual's established principles.

Why Conflict Reduces With Increasing Age. If we go through fewer conflicts as we reach the uncertain age of discretion, it is not because of the growth of character, but rather because usually the man of standing, as he grows older, hedges himself in by assuming responsibilities which make it easier for him to avoid having conflicts. His position is too great a matter to risk losing or his family ties are too sacred to entertain any course of action which would be interpreted as *outré*. The more settled he is, and the more responsibilities he assumes, the less likely is he to be diverted from the conventional routine into which he had naturally slipped, and the result is of undoubted social value. But it would scarcely be right to attribute this absence of conflict to one's self-improvement. Rather does it issue from a certain moral inertia or indolence backed by rationalization and the desire to meet the approval of the collective body of families, viz., society, whose comfort is at stake in the case of individual inner conflicts.

The Safety-valve of the Complacent.—The great formula which conjures away conflicts of all sorts consists of simply the words, " It doesn't pay "—a phrase which at first cômes out articulately but later is supplanted by a toss of the head, a shrug of the shoulders or some other listless attitude carrying the meaning of the original phrase. Of course, the attitude is quite a proper one for many occasions, but there is a real danger of its becoming mechanized so that it crops up no matter what the situation, and thus becomes a ruling motive, banishing from sight every principle worth fighting for. Such a man stands in character below the one who is torn between two opposing impulses, and if psychologists, mental hygienists, social workers, and others do not incline to this view, it is because comfort, success " carry on " has become the watchword and goal of modern civilization. Anything which disturbs the equilibrium of society is frowned upon, even though this social balance is such in appearance only, and in reality sorely needs adjustment. Only in a superficial way is the social end furthered by the lack of individual inner conflict. In a deeper sense, the loss is often greater than the gain, for it engenders a certain moral cowardice and even hypocrisy.

Nor should it be assumed, on the other hand, that I am advocating the cultivation of conflicts in order to have a battlefield for conquest. My chief point is that they should not be studiously and artificially avoided. In due course they are bound to occur, and they must be dealt with on the merit of the opposing sides and not on the strength of a ready-made attitude, the source of which is the protection of one's own interests under the guise of social expediency.

The Use of Conflict.—Not all conflicts are objectionable. Some even may be salutary to the individual in that they tend to preserve the smouldering remains of the poet whom, as Herder said long ago, every man survives. Without conflicts a man might develop reactions with mechanical regularity. Too much has been ascribed to the working of mental struggles. In the hierarchy of possible conflicts, there are normal and abnormal types. A great deal will depend on the content of the clash, on its duration, on the frequency of such occurrences, and, of course, most of all on the consequences. *Conflicts are hurtful to persons with neurotic tendencies,* most assuredly ; but it is not necessary to condemn all conflicts on that account. Even if all mental disorders should have as their immediate cause some inner struggle, it would not follow that all conflicts lead to psycho-neurosis.

The Freudian conception of conflict which makes room for unconscious mental rivalry, totally unknown to the patient except through psychoanalysis, is probably greatly exaggerated. I am unwilling to believe—and not on the strength of any convictions of human dignity—that we are seething with incestuous, homosexual and malevolent desires that are always kept in check by a rigid censor who, however, cannot curb the protean shapes which these repressed desires assume in order to express themselves as best they could. Sex conflicts there are aplenty, but these, with few exceptions, are *conscious* in every sense of the word, and very much so. The unconscious conflicts, the so called Œdipus and Electra complexes as well as the Jungian constructions and interpretations in terms of regression (aspiration to return to mother earth, the womb) are highly speculative and the evidence produced by the psychoanalysts to prove their case does not warrant the conclusion. Dreams, slips, and other manifestations may be interpreted in numerous ways, and can be stretched to meet any theory.

Great Mediaeval on Conflict.—Directing our attention once more to the relation obtaining between character and conflict, we may with profit turn to a passage in the *Eight Chapters* of Maimonides, which shows clearly how some of the problems raised in recent years were taken up in the Middle Ages and disposed of with admirable precision and lucidity. The illustrious son of Maimon evidently recognized that conflicts might arise regarding what we should now call *conventional impositions* as well as in relation to *natural* or perhaps *absolute injunctions*. The individual then is judged according as his conflicts are of the first category or the second. But let us have Maimonides' own words :—

> Philosophers maintain that though the man of self-restraint performs beneficent and worthy deeds, yet he does them while craving and longing all the while for immoral deeds, but, subduing his passions and actively fighting against a longing to do those things to which his energies, propensities, and mental make-up excite him, succeeds, though with constant vexation and a feeling of injury, in acting morally. The saintly man, however, is guided in his actions by that to which his inclination and constitution prompt him, in consequence of which he acts morally from an inner longing and desire. Philosophers

unanimously agree that the latter is worthier and more perfect [1] than the one who has to curb his passions, although they add that it is impossible for such a one to equal the saintly man in many respects. In general, however, he must necessarily be ranked lower (in the scale of virtue) because there lurks within him the desire to do evil and, though he does not do it, yet because his inclinations are all in that direction, it denotes the presence of an immoral trait in the soul. Solomon, also, entertained the same idea when he said, " The soul of the wicked desireth evil " and, in regard to the saintly man's rejoicing in doing good, and the discontent experienced by him, who is not innately righteous, when required to act justly, he says, " It is bliss to the righteous to do justice, but torment to the evil-doer." Thus there is, as would seem, a confirmation in the Scriptures of the teachings of philosophy.

Talmudists on Mental Struggle.—When, however, we consult the Rabbis on this subject we find that they consider him who desires iniquity and craves for it (but does not do it) of greater esteem and perfection than the one who feels no torment at refraining from evil ; and they even go so far as to maintain that the more praiseworthy and perfect a man is, the greater is his desire to transgress, and the more grieved will he feel at having to check it. This they express by saying, " Whosoever is greater than his neighbour has likewise greater evil inclinations." Again, as if this were not sufficient, they even go so far as to say that the reward of him who overcomes his evil inclination is commensurate with the hardship occasioned by his resistance, which thought they express by the words, "According to the labour is the reward." Furthermore, they command that man should

---

[1] The Hebrew word "Shalem" which represents the original term in the Arabic opuscule might easily be rendered as "integrated". In its etymological sense, the word signifies "complete", "whole", "sound".

TT

conquer his desires, but they forbid one to say, " I by my nature, do not desire to commit such and such a transgression, even though the Law does not forbid it." Rabbi Simeon ben Gamaliel summed up this thought in the words, " Man should not say, ' I do not want to eat meat together with milk ; I do not want to wear clothes made of a mixture of wool and linen ; I do not want to enter into an incestuous marriage,' but he should say, ' I do indeed want to, yet I must not, for my Father in heaven has forbidden it.' "

Clearing up a Seeming Contradiction.—At first blush, from a superficial comparison of the two statements [that of the philosophers and that of the Rabbis] one might be inclined to say that they contradict each other. Such, however, is not the case. Both are correct and, moreover, are not in disagreement in the least, as the evils which the philosophers term such—and of which they say that he who has no longing for them is more to be praised than he who desires them but conquers his passion—are things which all people commonly agree are evils, such as the shedding of blood, theft, robbery, fraud, injury to one who has done no harm, ingratitude, contempt for parents, and the like. The prescriptions against these are called *commandments*, about which the Rabbis said, " If they had not already been written in the Law, it would be proper to add them." Some of our later sages, who were infected with the unsound principles of the *Mutakallimun*, called these *rational laws*. There is no doubt that a soul which has the desire for, and lusts after, the above-mentioned misdeeds is defective ; that a noble soul has absolutely no desire for any such crimes, and experiences no struggle in refraining from them. When, however, the Rabbis maintain that he who overcomes his desire has more merit and a greater reward (than he who has no temptation), they say so only with reference to laws that are of a traditional nature. And with reason, since, were it not for the Law, they would not at all be

·considered transgressions. Therefore, the Rabbis say that man should permit his soul to entertain the natural inclination for these things, but that the Law alone should restrain him from them.

And now reflect upon the wisdom of these men, of blessed memory, manifest in the examples they adduce. They do not declare, " Man should not say,, ' I have no desire to kill, to steal, and to lie, but I have a desire for these things, yet what can I do, since my Father in heaven forbids it ! ' " The instances they cite are all from the ceremonial law, such as partaking of meat and milk together, wearing clothes made of wool and linen, and entering into consanguineous marriages. These, and similar enactments, are what God called " statutes ", which, as the Rabbis say are " statutes which I [God] have enacted for thee, which thou hast no right to examine, which the nations of the world attack, and which Satan denounces, as for instance, the statutes concerning the red heifer, the scapegoat, and so forth ". Those transgressions, however, which the later sages called *rational laws* are termed *commandments*, as the Rabbis explained.

It is now evident from all that we have said, what the transgressions are for which, if a man have no desire at all for them, he is on a higher plane than he who has a longing, but controls his passion for them ; and it is also evident what the transgressions are of which the opposite is true. It is an astonishing fact that these two classes of expressions should be shown to be compatible with one another, but their content points to the truth of our explanation. [1]

Thus has Maimonides settled the question.

[1] Maimonides : *Eight chapters* (being an introduction to the tract of Aboth or Ethics of the Fathers), chap. vi.

In the translation of this chapter of Maimonides' psychological essay I have followed both the Hebrew translation of Ibn-Tibbon and the English rendering of J. Gorfinkle, changing a number of terms and phrases in the latter, but adopting it on the whole.

Grappling with the Issue.—What are we to do with the conflicts arising out of the established conventions of society ? " Avoid them " exhort the Puritans. " Sublimate the lower impulses," is the advice of psychoanalysis. The reply to the former is that the broader the personality, the more intellectual the individual, and the deeper his nature, the more difficulty will he have in avoiding the very things which go to make up the warp and woof of his being ; and if he can manage to steer clear of the troubled waters of mental struggles, it is only at the expense of a dull and dreary life which possibly in the long run will prevent him from accomplishing his tasks for the benefit of society. Now, I cannot sufficiently emphasize the need of distinguishing between the *conflict* and its *outcome*. At present I am pleading in defence of the conflict and not on behalf of the pleasurable desire which forms one of the two ingredients of the conflict. Persons with neurotic tendencies, weak-minded people, must of course guard themselves more zealously than others, just as those with digestive difficulties usually avoid rich or heavy food.

The Subterfuge of Sublimation.   As to the injunction of sublimation, of turning our attention to useful ends, thus diverting it from the issue in the conflict, it is not always clear whether the foreign body could be disposed of so easily, especially where the circumstances and the rationalization may help to legitimatize the impulse to be sublimated.   Psychoanalysis has shown that there is much room for improvement in the moral ordering of society, and yet proffers no definite suggestions for its betterment, resignedly implying that the will of the " Leviathan " politic must be done. But as has already been intimated, character does not include the element of obedience. Sometimes it is to be attached to the most dogged resistance ; and, therefore, the psychoanalytic position which is removed from this delicate, but cardinal, point[1]

[1] Flügel's *Psycho-analytic Study of the Family* is the most direct approach to the subject from that angle.

somewhat smacks of hypocrisy ; although apparently for social reasons and since strength of character is comparatively so rare, the Freudian normative or exhortative phase constitutes a wholesome counterpart to its descriptive and explanatory phases. Let us not, however, forget that we are concerned above all with scientific consistency, no matter what the consequences, in which case I cannot help feeling that the device of sublimation, which incidentally has been known and resorted to probably from time immemorial, is not much different from repression. Successful repression *is* sublimation, for surely we do not expect a person after a mental crisis, unless he has actually succumbed to the strain, to keep ruminating about the case. Naturally he seeks to divert his mind with some hobby or work. Conversely no amount of sublimation will succeed in obliterating entirely from the mind an experience over which one has been greatly exercised.

While Flugel, in his 1928 review, attempted to expose my inadequate account of Freudian doctrine when I suggested that psychoanalysis would enjoin sublimation in conflicts between the *amo* and the *veto*, he appears to confirm me in 1945, when he writes ". . . in the doctrine of sublimation it [i.e. psychoanalysis] indicates a satisfactory compromise between the superego and the primitive id impulses may be attained ".[1] Granted that sublimation is an unconscious process, there is no disproof of the possibility that it may be initiated by a suggestion or fiat.

Sublimation is undoubtedly a sound practice, nevertheless character does not hinge on this. The man of the highest type of character and great independence is not one who will consult the majority or all the Mrs. Grundys taken collectively. The light of his reason built on the foundation of consistency will be his only guide ; but he who is not of that mettle will find it a dangerous procedure to adopt any other policy or plan

[1] J. C. Flugel, *Man, Morals, and Society*, 1945 (Internat. Univers. Press), p. 248.

than sublimation. Like many who wish to embark on artistic careers at the risk of losing their all, those who will act as if they were a law unto themselves without having the moral and intellectual wherewithals are sure to come to grief, while yet he who is capable of acting for himself in the face of public censure will be confident of his course, trusting to his own reasoning rather than to the psycho-analytic rule born of expediency.

Freud and Maimonides compared. Freud seems to follow his celebrated predecessor in the Dark Ages, Moses ben Maimon, except that the latter speaks of the law of the Lord, while the former bids us to subject ourselves to the conventions of society. Their counsel is certainly of great advantage, yet strong characters will not always heed it and should not be judged by ordinary conformist standards but in the light of all the circumstances which only posterity can properly evaluate.

This is not to be taken as a brief for libertinism or narrow individualism. *The universal must never be lost sight of whatever the deviation might be from commonly accepted forms.* There is no place here for the gratification of the individual craving, whim, or fancy ; and he who steers his ship on his own responsibility must expect no comfort if through miscalculation he meets with disaster. But then our fearless navigators on the high seas of life should not be censured if they see fit to embark on a new route.

The individual who cherishes a regard for universals in action may not bother much about public opinion, but his conduct need not on that account be subversive of the common good. Even if he does not consult the conventions of society, he still may be a better representative of society than those who blindly follow custom. While *he* helps to shape the course of progress, the latter impede its march by keeping in a rut. The illustrations in the next chapter will elucidate this contrast between consulting the interests of society and merely obeying the behests of convention ; and when the individual and society do not see eye to eye, there is bound to be a conflict, first in the mind, then in the open.

Conditions of Conflict. As was stated earlier in the chapter, two types of people may be said to claim immunity from mental conflicts ; first, the spiritless and phlegmatic, on whose mind the world of sense makes little demand, and, secondly, the unscrupulous and unprincipled in whom the incipient conflict is brought about through fear alone ; and as confidence sets in even this beginning disappears. The *greater the spontaneity, and the richer the experiences the more scope for conflicts.* Intellect is not a negligible factor in inducing the inner conflict. Both intellect and affectivity on the subjective side and the potency and variety of the circumstances on the objective side are responsible for the extent of the inner struggle. It is significant that in the Great War the conscientious objectors, who certainly must have had their mental conflicts before ultimately deciding on the final step, were as a group far more intelligent than any army group, not excepting the officers, as shown by the test scores.

To be sure, sex conflicts do not belong to the same category, nevertheless the formula holds here too. Given a person with an independent spirit, high affectivity and favourable circumstances, and the conflicts will not be wanting.

When are Conflicts Unconscious ? I am not disposed to dogmatize about conflicts being invariably conscious. In juveniles it would seem from Healy's *Mental Conflict and Delinquency*, Jung's *Über Konflikte der kindlichen Seele*, and van Waters' *Youth in Conflict*, that there are numerous cases of unconscious mental conflicts ; and probably many neurotics are to be classed in that category, lacking insight into their own affairs. Those with the child's disposition are particularly to be noted as possibly coming under that head. But how far would this concession go to prove that the operation of conflicts is a factor in character ? The evidence in the first place would point in the direction that the more character, the less likely are the conflicts to be of an unconscious kind, so that in all probability the question of unconscious conflicts would not enter into the evaluation of character, our assumption being that one of the by-products of a fully fashioned character is the insight into one's own conflicts. And in order to avoid misunderstanding, it may be stated that mental conflict is not to be identified with desire or with sentiment, or with complex. As that psychological writer Anatole France bears witness in his thinly disguised autobiographical sketch *Le Livre de Mon Ami*, " not a few are filled with a longing for a something which seems always at hand yet . . . to be found nowhere." The dawn of that vague desire in adolescence needs no further documentation. A mental conflict, however, as an opposition between two elements cannot be placed on the same level as a simple desire or longing. Complexes [1] may also be and most frequently are of an unconscious nature until analysis is begun, but again these are not to be confused with conflicts, even if they play a part as accessories either before or after the fact.

Finally, supposing we grant that unconscious mental conflicts are plentiful even with those who otherwise give evidence of a high degree of character, one fails to see how anything of which a person is unconscious can justly be held to his disadvantage, an argument which Hadfield seems to hint at but does not fully develop. Surely one cannot suffer in esteem for an unknown process any more than for an incipient pathological condition, unless the inference to be drawn is that every person must at regular intervals consult a psychoanalyst in

---

[1] Some writers would appear to draw a distinction between sentiment and complex on the basis that the former is something conscious and the latter unconscious. The distinction is surely there but not on this ground, for both may or may not be in consciousness. We should rather note that the *difference* lies in the fact that a sentiment is of a social origin and contains an intellectual ingredient, while a complex is an individual and purely affective factor.

order to have the hidden complexes brought out to the surface—or perhaps to have non-existent complexes planted in the individual by means of suggestion.

The Upshot.—In this chapter it was brought out then that the widespread view [2] that conflict and character vary inversely is not justified, that conflicts arise in men and women of the highest character, and that the richer the experiences, the wider in scope are the conflicts. As to unconscious conflicts, even if such should occur in the normal adult, their relation to character may subserve a diagnostic but not an evaluative purpose. In other words while we should probably be able to establish after a correlational study the fact that those whose mind is the seat of unconscious conflicts are not such as would possess character in any distinctive sense, we are in no way entitled to the conclusion that because of such unconscious conflicts, an individual's character is to be called into question.

[2] This doctrine, which seems to be a corollary of the Freudian system, has been made the fundamental thesis of Holt's conception of ethics as outlined in his *Freudian Wish*, and not only forms the gist of Givler's *The Ethics of Hercules*, but is implied in the diametrically opposed school, represented chiefly by McDougall (cf. his *Social Psychology*, pp. 261–263, sixteenth edition).

CHAPTER XXXV

CHARACTER AND ADJUSTMENT

I

No Adjustment Without a Standard. So great is the force of inertia and so negligible the desire for critical analysis that after a generation of sharp opposition, the term adjustment is still in vogue and employed as a sesame to the solution of all problems between the individual and society. Little boots it that the word adjustment is devoid of significance apart from a *standard*, still less does it seem to matter that the environment, milieu, society, and other standards, to which the adjustment is customarily held to be made, is something elusory in definition, the panacea has such a firm hold on the enlighteners of the public that it scarcely can be abandoned.

Objections to Environmentalism. Spencer it was who cast a spell over the naturalistically inclined ; and since his day the concept of adjustment in conjunction with the doctrine of evolution has served to set at ease many an optimistic mind. His critics were not behindhand in detecting the circularity of his procedure, but so far as I am aware, he did not take them seriously.

It has been pointed out, for instance, that an amoeba is just as well adjusted to its environment as man is to his, that adjustment as such can but have reference to a shifting standard, that furthermore an environment is one thing to one person and quite a different thing to another. The followers of a pure naturalism were obdurate in their representations, and their descendants to-day have even grown so bold as to ascribe nearly all the makings of personality, especially character, to environmental influences. When it is brought to their attention that in a family where the children are reared in the same way and attend the same school, they may yet manifest different groups of tendencies, these advocates of an environmental outlook or bias deny that the environment is the same under the conditions outlined, contending that the children still have lived in their own individual environments. Discounting the negligible number of important variations due to sheer accident, we should have to accept the conclusion then that it is the child *who picks his environment*, and even in these fortuitous happenings which may have affected him so as to give a different twist to his future, we can in no way be positive as to whether, had the same event or events occurred to his brother or sister, it would have affected them in the same way. We have more reason to suppose that the reaction would be different, just as the environments, though the same, are held to be different, and for the same reason, viz., that each individual has his own personal idiom.

The Social Bias in Adjustment. So much for the background of this chapter. It is now possible to deal with the relation between adjustment and character as discussed by various groups of social workers in the broad sense of the word, men and women who are concerned with the welfare of the individual, and whose criterion of character is derived from the average person as the main constituent of society. Character becomes for such writers and teachers a pragmatic function which renders possible social organization. Everyone whose behaviour allows of the smooth working of this organization is regarded as possessing character. The anti-social individual, the recidivist is lacking in this essential. One who can adjust himself to the demands of society can acquire character; one who does not, or cannot, so adapt himself is necessarily defective. He will be experiencing difficulties in the form of conflicts either with those he comes in contact with or will be enduring mental struggles within himself; and these difficulties largely are regarded by the adjustment schools as symptomatic of a weak character. Thus, mental health, success and efficiency enter in, even if only as negative criteria of character.

Evolution of Society Result of Maladjustment. No doubt there is a certain value in this point of view, but I feel that the great events in history do not justify it as scientific, as representing the truth. The trouble is that in everyday life we do not meet the negative instances which are crucial to the question at issue, whereas the cases which help to form the adjustment criterion are practically all of a kind to confirm the notion that he who finds it difficult to adjust himself possesses less character than the typical sales manager, Rotarian, Elk, Lion, Christian Scientist, etc., who always appear so satisfied with the world and with themselves. On the other hand, the chronic grouch, nag, who is always disgruntled, does seem to be in the wrong, especially as his problems come up for discussion at institutional staff meetings. Let us not forget, however, that *society has evolved to a great extent through the efforts of those who were unwilling to conform to the society of their day*, and in this very dissenting have they revealed their high character for which their memories are universally honoured.

Bearing of History on Problem. A long list of reformers may be drawn up who in no way could be said to have adjusted themselves to the conventions of their day and who, because of their non-conformity, paved the way for greater freedom and more reasonable institutions. When Luther nailed his ninety-five theses to the door of his chapel, when Pinel unfettered the miserable lunatics kept in dungeons, when Wilberforce plunged into the struggle for the abolition of slavery, there could hardly be a question about their adjusting themselves to society. Their characters shine forth through the pages of history in undiminishing splendour not in spite of their conflicts but rather because of them. Had it been an easy matter to defy the Roman Catholic Church or to secure humane treatment for the insane, our estimate of the work of Luther and Pinel would not be nearly so high.

It is not my intention to prove that dissatisfaction with one's environment or maladjustment is indispensable to, or concomitant with, strength of character, but rather to indicate by means of well-known instances that adjustment is not an essential in the ingredients of character and should not enter in as a factor for its evaluation. We are not concerned with the problem of moral exhortation but with a question of scientific analysis ; and we have not yet forgotten the words " And the truth shall make you free ".

Begging the Question. The policy of adjustment—for after all it is rather a policy than an ideal—at bottom hinges upon this consideration. If we adjust ourselves to the conditions of, let us say, society, assuming that this has a definite meaning, progress would be less impeded than if we were unadjusted, and clamoured for personal rights and privileges. Such is, of course, undeniable, but the crux of the question lies in the *mental facts requiring adjusting* ; and the governing feature of the outcome, whether desirable or not, attaches to the *character* of the adjustor. The lowest denominator is not adjustment but something such as *reasonable inhibition, where the personal or individual end is subordinated to a universal principle.* It is true that in the common run of men the temptation is strong not to adjust themselves in this fashion, but what if they do not inhibit their instinctive urges, do they not adjust themselves, nevertheless, when choosing the less desirable course of action ? Is the callous family deserter who, in order to carry on a romance with an inamorata, free from all responsibilities, makes his escape to a distant country where he is beyond the reach of the law—is such a one any less adjusted than the person who through inner conflicts decides to bear his cross with equanimity ?

Attempt to Split the Difference. But perhaps finally a distinction will be drawn between a *psychological* adjustment and a *social* or an *ethical* adjustment, in which case the significance of the term adjustment for our purpose dwindles to nothingness, and we are once more on a platform of values unaffected by mere biological trimmings, serviceable to be sure in their own sphere, but of little consequence in the question at issue.

Were we even to grant the validity of the distinction, instances may be cited which derive their approbation not from a social adjustment but rather from an inhibition in order to satisfy a principle.   Let us take the following anecdote from the life of Sir William Napier, as related by his son and cited by Smiles in his famous essays on *Character* :—

" He was one day taking a long country walk near Fresh-ford when he met a little girl, about five years old, sobbing over a broken bowl ; she had dropped and broken it in bringing it back from the field to which she had taken her father's dinner in it, and she said she would be beaten, on her return home, for having broken it ; when, with a sudden gleam of hope, she innocently looked up into his face, and said : ' But yee can mend it, can't ee ? '

" My father explained that he could not mend the bowl, but the trouble he could avert by the gift of sixpence to buy another.   However, on opening his purse it was empty of silver, and he had to make amends by promising to meet his little friend in the same spot at the same hour next day and to bring the sixpence with him, bidding her, meanwhile, tell her mother she had seen a gentleman who would bring her the money for the bowl next day. The child, entirely trusting him, went on her way comforted. On his return home he found an invitation awaiting him to dine in Bath the following evening, to meet some one whom he specially wished to see. He hesitated for some little time, trying to calculate the possibility of giving the meeting to his little friend of the broken bowl and of still being in time for the dinner-party in Bath ; but finding this could not be, he wrote to decline accepting the invitation on the plea of ' a pre-engagement,' saying to us, ' I cannot disappoint her, she trusted me so implicitly.' "

Now an advocate of the adjustment school would scarcely be able to approve of such a fuss over a promise given to a little girl. In this case the adjustment called for would be to banish the incident from the mind and attend to the more important thing, viz., the dinner party. Certainly it would be easy to find a way out of the obligation. (1) It was not Sir William's fault if the little girl dropped the bowl. (2) Probably his promise would not have been taken seriously by the parents. (3) Her parents could not reasonably punish her for an accident. (4) If that is the treatment she expected at their hands, she must have been inured to it by this time. These and other excuses might be conjured up in addition to the peremptoriness of the call. Yet the promise to the child counterbalanced all the bids of the adjustment attitude ; and it is the winning out of the principle which calls forth our admiration. Such is the stuff character is made of.

One more illustration from the same book ; this time in connection with the generous spirit of the great Laplace. The young mathematician Biot had read an important paper before the French Academy on a certain type of equations :—

" The assembled savants at its close felicitated the reader of the paper on his originality. Monge was delighted at his success. Laplace also praised him for the clearness of his demonstrations, and invited Biot to accompany him home. Arrived there, Laplace took from a closet in his study a paper yellow with age, and handed it to the young philosopher. To Biot's surprise he found that it contained the solutions, all worked out, for which he had just gained so much applause. With rare magnanimity Laplace withheld all knowledge of the circumstance from Biot until the latter had initiated his reputation before the Academy ; moreover, he enjoined him to silence ; and the incident would have remained a secret had not Biot himself published it, some fifty years afterwards.''

II

Relation to Normality. The adjustment criterion of character is valid for application only in that sphere which is bounded by average behaviour, by mediocrity. Adjustment spells normality and normality, of course, forms the great bulwark of society. The abnormal and the poorly adjusted disturb its equilibrium, and usually belong to the anti-social class. Naturally then the social conception of character would require proper adjustment as a *sine qua non* of this prized complex of qualities.

Abnormal Determiners of Normality. On the other hand, however, there is such an event as exceeding the bounds of normality, thus falling, in a sense, into the category of abnormality and yet enjoying the possession of character. Such malcontents and maladjusted souls cannot be seen except through their own light *for they determine the normality of future generations.* Hence it would be little short of absurd to appraise them unfavourably for deliberately raising the standard of appraisal through their actions. Surely they cannot be expected to point the way to a new road and at the same time rest on the old and beaten path.

Concept of Normality. The question as to what is the normal has now for many years been a perplexing one. William James strikes directly at it in his *Varieties of Religious Experience,*[1] and Kronfeld in a recent book points out three more or less unsatisfactory uses of the word,[2] (a) deviation from the average, (b) ethically ideal or socially adaptive, (c) conformable to law.

It occurs to me that the stumbling-block consists in the extension of a term valid enough in the biological sphere to

[1] W. James, *Varieties of Religious Experience,* p. 15.
[2] A. Kronfeld, *Das Wesen der psychiatrischen Erkenntnis,* pp. 425–426.

a realm in which it must be governed by different criteria in order to enjoy its significance. A pathological condition is abnormal even if it strictly conforms to natural law, because it is plainly to the detriment of the individual. The same pathological condition in the individual may not be abnormal at all when viewed in the light of the vistas which this illness has led to. For the individual, Luther's experience of illumination was symptomatic of a morbid state ; for mankind, inasmuch as it led to greater individual freedom in thinking, it was wholesome, and nothing wholesome can be thought of as abnormal.[1] Viewed from the standpoint of the organization of the Roman Catholic Church, his open heresy was certainly an abnormal feature of his behaviour, and on more than one occasion was he charged with being the victim of the devil. But who to-day would be so abnormal as to entertain such an opinion of Luther's conduct and state of mind ?

It is usually taken for granted that society knows what is beneficial for it, what would lead to the progress of mankind, but that is just the point yet to be proven.

Different Spheres of Normality. As I view the situation, *normality in the accepted sense* as adjustment or adaptation is a quality which is applicable in *restricted spheres where values are not involved.* We are within our rights to consider a bodily temperature of 105 abnormal, because such a condition has always been known to go with illness, and while conformable to natural law, it is in effect the cause of discomfort, pain, and eventually death, and therefore abnormal, inasmuch as it is deleterious to the organism. The indications are clear both subjectively (introspectively) and objectively. If, however, an organ should function differently in a certain individual than in all others, without showing any ill effects, the only sense in which the word abnormal could be applied

---

[1] Cf. also James's significant utterance " For aught we know to the contrary, 103° or 104° Fahrenheit might be a much more favourable temperature for truths to germinate and sprout in, than the more ordinary blood-heat of 97 or 98 degrees ".

uu

here would be in that of being different from the average-
really the schoolboy view of normality.

Now it matters little whether an individual's act will be
designated as normal or not in this sense. In fact, if anything,
this type of abnormal behaviour might be matter for elation
and emulation. But can we really, in any significant sense,
hold a person to be abnormal for not thinking as the majority
does and acting consistently on his belief ? The answer would
certainly depend on whether the conduct in question harms
anyone directly or not. It is decidedly abnormal to entertain
murderous views, but is it abnormal to reject the sanctity of
certain political or religious dogmas or to dispute the
desirability of certain institutions or customs ? It might have
indeed been abnormal to show evidence of rank dissension,
were one opinion held by all intelligent people throughout the
ages on such matters, just as in respect of theft, lying, robbery,
hypocrisy, cruelty, etc., but the *counting of the heads in a
given age or society cannot determine the absolute normality
of a certain type of behaviour*, and for that reason no one should
be condemned as *lacking in character if unable to adjust
himself to his environment*.

Explanation of " Absolute " Normality. I am aware of the
novelty of this phrase. I mean by *" absolute normality "* a
*quality attaching to behaviour which, in the course of ages, will
be adjudged as reasonable*. Vision is the great determinant of
absolute normality. With the man of vision, the present is
extended into the future and circumstances are transcended
by the towering rock of ages—Reason. No one, of course,
except a prophet can foresee what might be thought right a
thousand years hence, but the man of vision will be able to
sense the direction which reason is bound to follow ; for its
course is *orthogenic*, and what relapses it does suffer are all
confined to definite localities, periods, and the masses, but
do not apply to that *great commonwealth of thought which
knows neither time nor place*—the commonwealth constituted

by the great minds in philosophy who seem to be united at least by the uncommon bond of tolerance, no matter how divergent their views may be in metaphysics, religion, or other spheres of human endeavour. *If counting the heads is a valid method of evaluation, then the heads should be those of the intellectual leaders* and not of the general run of humanity at a given age, the rank and file of society.

Is Suicide Normal? The ridiculous attitude toward suicide is one of the illustrations that may be cited here. It is true that society ought to protect a foolish individual even against his own folly ; and many suicides take their lives only in a moment of despondency, but to punish a person for adjusting himself to the world by renouncing it after due deliberation is a preposterous measure in spite of the fact that it is still in force. Sooner or later, however, the world, that is to say, the intellectual middlemen who derive their ideas from men of genius and dispense them to the masses by way of the press, the popular book, the pulpit, and the lecture platform, until legislators see fit to act on the information, will become impressed with the inescapable logic of Hume's and Schopenhauer's argument [1] to the effect that while suicide may be a mistake it is far from being a crime.

Taking one's own life, then, is a *relatively* abnormal act, but it is not such absolutely ; for no amount of quibbling can confute the rational position that it is reasonable for an individual who is, let us say, suffering from an excruciatingly painful and incurable disease to liberate himself from his tortures by dying at his own hand. Nor will suicide become more normal, if its rate, which is steadily growing in our

---

[1] " It is a great disgrace to the English nation," observes Schopenhauer, with reference to Hume and his famous essay *On Suicide*, " that a purely philosophical treatise, which proceeding from one of the first thinkers and writers in England, aimed at refuting the current arguments against suicide by the light of cold reason should be forced to sneak about in that country as though it were some rascally production until at last it found refuge on the continent."

over-civilized world, increases tenfold.   Its rationality co-
efficient will not have changed one whit.

War Decidedly Abnormal.   War, on the other hand, which
has been a normal phenomenon from time immemorial,
is on the principle set forth in this essay *abnormal* ; and were
the masses more intelligent and the rulers (both nominal
and factual) less selfish and impulsive, the nefarious practice
of annihilating in the most brutal manner innocent people,
simply because their immune and invulnerable rulers were
aggressive, would actually be accepted as decidedly abnormal,
especially after thousands of years of harrowing experience.[1]
Here is a case where the raving prophets of Israel were endowed
with a power of vision which was denied to Plato and Aristotle
who thought the highest type of courage was that shown by
a soldier on the battlefield, and a military death the most
beautiful sacrifice.   It is no reflection on these two *colossi*
of antiquity that they were permeated with the spirit of their
time and their people, just as their views on slavery, while
betraying a lack of vision in this respect, do not detract
from their unsurpassed greatness as teachers of mankind.

Supremacy of Reason.   The sovereignty of reason which
*consists of the accumulated approval of the majority of thinkers
throughout the ages* is not in danger of being impugned because
of occasional dissension among its aristocracy.   Liberty of
thought and freedom of action without prejudice to others
are what all great intellects have striven for, even when they,
as in the case of Hobbes, contradicted themselves by
championing the cause of political autocracy.

Again, let me point out that my meaning is not that reason

---

[1] Another illustration :   the burning of heretics in the fifteenth
century in Spain and two centuries later the hanging of " witches "
in Salem was evidently considered normal by the people of the time
or else they would have risen against such horrors, but how revoltingly
abnormal the *auto da fè* must appear in the perspective of rational
thought.   Many such other relatively normal acts, statutes, edicts,
practices, etc., might be cited which must be appalling to contemplate.

derives its supremacy and measure of finality from the approval of great minds, but rather that its own inherent force invests it with universal validity and objectivity ; and therein is grounded the concept of absolute normality.

Distinction Between Ideal and Absolute Normality. At this stage some readers will exclaim : " But why not state that the normal is the ideal and save words ? " My answer is that I do not identify the two. An ideal is *ex vi termini* a pious wish, never realized ; and, besides, we never can see so far ahead as to be able to tell with certainty that the blue bird will after all not turn out to be black. Furthermore the ideal implies an *object or situation remote in thought : the normal is merely an attribute or adjunct to be attached to that which is already before us.* To be sure, the absolutely normal moves in the direction of the ideal, so far as we can foresee it, but it essentially deals with the practical present. We can ask significantly of any act or event whether it is normal in the *sense of conforming to reason*, but it is only of theoretical importance to ask about a situation whether it is ideal.

After this somewhat digressive exposition of " absolute normality ", it is scarcely necessary to add that the normality which is usually referred to in speaking of conduct and character traits is of the *relative* kind which is dependent on the time and place of the judge and the person judged. It is this narrower criterion of normality, which unfortunately is generally accepted, that has been a thorn in the flesh of so many noble minds to this very day.

Man of Vision Sneered At. No Socrates is put to death nowadays for enlightening the youth. No Timothy is banished from the state any longer for adding new strings to the lyre or for introducing new musical forms as that ancient rhapsodist of Miletus was said to have suffered at the hands of the Lacedaemonians, but still the spirit of intolerance hounds the reason-inspired individual who refuses to be swayed by the idols of the market place and the dogma of the crowd. If such an individual is not crucified, burnt at the stake, stoned, imprisoned, or banished, he at least must endure the opprobrium and sneers of the common people because they cannot soar to his heights ; and he is convicted not only of maladjustment but of characterlessness.

Eccentricity *per se* **Undesirable.** Perhaps we need not go so far as the great apostle of personal liberty, J. S. Mill, who would make a virtue of non-conformity and eccentricity, saying, " Precisely because the tyranny of opinion is such as to make eccentricity a reproach, it is desirable, in order to break through that tyranny, that people should be eccentric. Eccentricity has always abounded when and where strength of character has abounded ; and the amount of eccentricity in a society has generally been proportional to the amount of genius, mental vigour, and moral courage it contained. That so few now dare to be eccentric marks the chief danger of the time." Yet even if we should hold that eccentricity is not to be flaunted simply for the sake of stirring up the stagnant pool of custom but should rather be made manifest only when a principle is involved, Mill's vigorous deprecation of the philistine attitude which, alas, has invaded our social sciences, both theoretical and applied, has much to be said in its favour ; and it is even truer to-day than it was in Mill's generation that " the man, and still more the woman, who can be accused either of doing ' what nobody does ' or of not doing ' what everybody does ', is the subject of as much deprecatory remarks· as if he or she had committed some grave moral delinquency ".[1]

Not a Matter of Proportion. What if there is one fine character to one hundred characterless people among those who cannot easily adjust themselves to conditions ; the exception is a crucial one in view of the circumstances and consequences to progress. We are dealing here not solely with quantity but with quality as well, and one Socrates,

[1] J. S. Mill, *On Liberty*, chap: iii.

one Savonarola, one Giordano Bruno, one Thomas More is sufficient to controvert the whole philosophy of the adjustment school of character, gathering its support mainly from the fact that maladjustment in the form of illicit desires, jealousy, revengefulness, contentiousness, and other such undesirable states, leads to anti-social behaviour. Maladjustment is not enough to warrant condemnation. It depends on the nature of the difficulty, and each case is to be judged separately.

This prepares us for the question which might naturally be asked at this point, viz., How is one to know whether the reaction arising out of a defective adjustment is a symptom of character or of characterlessness ? And furthermore will not every malcontent who deviates from the conventions of society be entitled to the consideration that some day, with changing forms and conditions, he or she may still be highly esteemed for actions which, because of a narrow point of view, are now regarded as reprehensible ?

Purpose and Circumstances to Settle Issue. The answer to this di-phasic question is simply this : we endeavour to get at the purpose of the person we are judging, and in order to accomplish this end we must bear in mind all the circumstances. George Sand and George Eliot were contemporaries who bore striking resemblances to each other. Not only did they both write fiction, not only did they choose to be known by a masculine *nom de plume*, but they have been in addition strictured for a similar weakness, viz., lack of chastity. Nevertheless there was a world between them ; and George Sand's reputation will remain coincident with her character in this respect, while George Eliot will be looked upon as a pioneer whose course counted considerably in removing the unjust restrictions against persons who sought to be absolved from intolerable marital ties. Taking the law into her own hands, she, by virtue of her influence as a famous writer, was partly instrumental in bringing about a change in a judicial system which had been granting special dispensations to the rich as against the poor and to men as against women. The promiscuity of George Sand achieved nothing except the gratification of her own desires. The liaison of George Eliot served as a powerful argument against a narrow-mindedness which well-nigh bordered on hypocrisy.

Danger Element Subordinated to Truth. We need fear little that such an opinion might lead to rash deeds on the part of the youth, on the ground that each one could look upon his questionable act as that of a reformer who would open the eyes of the world.   Science is no guardian over fools. Just as each experimenter with TNT, just as each aviator must assume full responsibility for his endeavours, so every person who steps beyond the chalk-mark of social convention is doing so at his or her own risk.   One might as well be asked to exaggerate the dangers of aviation as to place the taboo on discussions regarding the moral legitimacy of disagreeing with established custom.

III

A Serious Delusion. It is not difficult to account for the popularity of the adjustment theory especially at this time with the increase of institutions for the improvement and care of the individual.   Spencer's phrases " Social Statics " and " Social Dynamics " tell the whole story.   There is a caressing thought in certain quarters that man can be governed and repaired when not functioning in the normal way just as if he were a bit of machinery.   Our juvenile institutions, family welfare bureaus, psychopathic hospitals, mental hygiene stations, etc., are partly committed to this notion.   Here a crank is turned, there a screw tightened, a gear adjusted at another place, and the mechanism can again take care of itself; and if adjustment is the fundamental of character, then might one assume that a person of a sub-normal character can after a certain period of institutional care develop into a fine type of character.   An adjustment of some kind surely does take place ; to deny therefore the efficacy of our above-mentioned institutions would be gratuitous and in bad grace, but the cases of relapse and second and third commitments are too numerous for us to shut our eyes to the gravity of the problem, a problem which affects not only those primarily afflicted with the deficiency but their victims in marriage, or even acquaintances and strangers. After the delinquent is put on probation and pronounced reformed, or the psychopathic patient is discharged as cured, the happiness of at least one other person is jeopardized, and the commercial phrase, sanctioned by lawyers, *Caveat emptor* is no consolation for those who have been duped or attacked.

Perils of Artificial Adjustment. The personal attitude adopted by our social machinery is, of course, not to be deplored, and adjustment no doubt has its rightful place in the therapeutic and the penal order ; but sometimes it seems as if we were adjusting society to the individual and not *vice versa*. We take a personal, one might almost say a paternal, interest in the defective, deranged and delinquent, forgetting that we have obligations also to those who have suffered or will inevitably suffer as a result of the protection society is giving to the characterless. Absent though these past and potential victims are, they are yet real, worthy of our consideration at least in a measure equal to that accorded to the unfortunates taken under the wing of modern reform tendencies.

We can well understand that the business of the hospital staff is to cure, that of the probation officer to plead for certain prisoners, and perhaps it would not constitute contempt to add that it has become more and more the practice of juries, and especially judges, to be lenient with criminals (though often unduly severe with those guilty of a political offence or violation of one of the statutes). There is nothing blame-worthy about a man who always thinks of his charge first without taking the trouble to look at the obverse of the medal.

But the adjustment is made on behalf of one individual at the expense of those whose self-adjustment has cost them a long and painful effort. The policy of adjustment which has undeniably been growing in recent years has brought about an unjust levelling result with the democratic principle carried into the depths of institutional life. It is true that society is constantly adjusting itself to the conceptions of superior individuals, but the tendency, as the great masses usurp more and more power unto themselves, is to adjust society to the needs of the inferior, so that an *idiot savant*, because of his skill or opportunities in some one line of entertainment, no matter how brutal or vulgar, is often looked upon as a hero and is literally worshipped by millions of both chronological and mental juveniles.

Conclusion.   To revert to the main issue between adjustment and character, we may summarize the gist of the chapter by saying that the relationship is if anything inverse, i.e., if we so much as grant that adjustment can be a criterion at all in view of the loose moorings. Adjustment may be said to be indicative of prudence ; it may certainly lead to success, but it does not reveal the earmarks of character. What person does not know that just by so small an adjustment as scattering compliments, one may derive a great deal of material benefit ?   And furthermore, cajolery is by no means frowned upon as a practice.   Indeed, society rather looks at it with approbation, yet he who has intentionally thus adjusted himself, no longer can claim to possess character. In a word : far from character depending on adjustment, the adjustment is a function of one's character.

CHAPTER XXXVI

Components of Environment. The perennial question whether heredity is a more potent factor in the make-up of an individual than his environment is one which would naturally be asked with reference to character. But first of all, let us determine what elements enter into the so-called environment which might exercise its influence in modifying one's character. It would scarcely be necessary to present a full list of these possible factors. Only several of the most important will be dwelt on here.

Bacon, as we have seen in Chapter VIII, was of the opinion that many circumstances conspire to alter the original constitution of man. Without taking the trouble to substantiate his statement, he mentions such factors as prosperity and want, climate, condition of health, social status, honours conferred, and several others. It is curious that he did not think of the effect of food on character, and also that he only implied the incidence of occupation. A number of these conditions and qualities which Bacon enumerates are not within our scope, for they are coeval with character and can therefore not determine any change, or rather they cannot be regarded as environmental. Among these are noble or humble birth, sex and appearance.

Two General Positions. There have always existed two different points of view with regard to the modification of character. One may point to the transcendentalists, in the wide sense of the term, who, like Emerson and many others both before and after him, believed that the very essence of character consisted in remaining unshaken in face of

circumstances.   On the other hand, there were the environmentalists even in the days of antiquity who would make
the vicissitudes of life the barometer of character.   In recent
German books a compromise is struck by referring to both
endogene Charaktere and *Schicksalcharaktere*.   The latter are
governed by circumstances and exhibit a different set of
reactions than do the endogenous characters.   It is possible
also to base this division on the assumption that there are
in each one of us both unmodifiable and modifiable constituents
combined in different proportions.

Health.   What, then, are the turns of circumstance which
would be most apt to affect our character ?   Disease seems
to be the one most frequently referred to in the literature.
Thus Azam, as we have seen in Chapter XII, cites cases
purporting to prove that a cheerful and agreeable person
may turn into a morose grumbler or whiner.   Janet, too,
speaks of the modifications of character in hysterical patients,
but from the examples adduced, it becomes apparent that in
common with other French writers, he understands the term
character to embrace all the elements of personality, including
intelligence and conduct in the widest sense.   " The character,"
he says, " depends mainly on the primitive intelligence
of the patients, on the surroundings in which they have lived,
and on their education . . .   We should not attribute to
any malady traits of character which would have been exactly
the same independently of the malady.   We must, therefore,
describe only the modifications of character ;   the transformations which the malady has evidently brought with it
in the conduct of patients." [1]   And what modifications does
he finally produce ?   Modifications of intelligence and of
acting, as well as of the emotions.   " Hystericals, above all,
lose quickly social sentiments, altruistic emotions, perhaps
because they are the most complex of all." [2]

[1] Pierre Janet, *The Mental State of Hystericals* (1892), Eng. Trans.
(1902), p. 198.   [2] *Loc. cit.*, p. 208.

Neurosis and Character. It has already been remarked that there is no advantage gained in the indiscriminate use of the word character so as to encompass all possible qualities other than the physical. What takes place in the hysteric or neurotic is probably a *progressive degeneration of character* as a result of three-fold disturbances: (*a*) irregularity of instinctive function, (*b*) defect in the inhibitory system, and (*c*) the inapplicability of regulative principles. Instead of a degeneration, a temporary or intermittent paralysis of the various character functions may give rise to the puzzling behaviour of the patient ; but it is quite in order to ask whether a person displaying such marks was ever the possessor of a well-knit character, to begin with. If character is that human trait-complex which resists the onslaughts of circumstance, can we credit the individual who has undergone a change in character with that degree of integration which it is customary to attribute only to those who have not allowed themselves to be overturned in the struggle against destiny ? Must we not be led to the conclusion that the very tendency toward hysteria, or indeed any nervous trouble, is in itself a symptom of a comparatively low order of character ? Whatever eccentricities might be discovered in some of the great figures of philosophy, would it be easy to picture Socrates, Plato, Aristotle, Spinoza, Hume, Kant or Fichte as hysterical ? May we not therefore express the suspicion that with highly neurotic individuals it is not so much a matter of their character having undergone a change as of their *collapse* at the first serious onset in consequence of their defective constitution which lacked, in the first place, adequate organization material for unifying the various character elements ? Our earlier conclusion, " *There is no character to the insane,*" may be amplified to leave room for the codicil ˙ and very little to the typical neurotic ". One is reminded here of the important finding by Mott and others to the effect that war neuroses were almost confined to those who were on the lower intellectual and moral levels.

The Ductless Glands. Some remarkable accounts of personality changes, in a few instances due presumably to endocrine alterations and, in others, to a serious shock, are related by Berman in a recent book where he puts forth the claims of endocrinology less blatantly than in his previous work. " A change in the glands of internal secretion, an injury of certain portions of the nervous system or a specific experience or experiences are what we find, as a matter of fact, without prior theoretical considerations, in studying instances of personality transformation. It is upon glands, nerves, and experiences that we can put our finger in particular cases as the causes of such mutations." [1]

But even assuming that Berman is justified in his conviction that the three factors mentioned are responsible for the modifications in personality he described, we cannot be quite certain that the endocrine functions are the *immediate* causes of the changes. Berman himself senses the difficulty when he admits " that it is sometimes extremely difficult to trace the chain of sequences and to say which come first, an alteration in the endocrine glands, a deeply undermining modification in important mechanisms of the nervous system, or a shifting and shaking of the foundations of experience ". He recommends applying " various criteria and tests " to determine the distinctions, but as he has not specified them, the query still holds.

Aside from this, however, we must again recall the fact that personality is not to be identified with character and that even a change of personality does not necessarily involve a modification of character as we understand it here.[2]

Food. It may seem needless to undertake proving that the kind of food one assimilates has no bearing on the develop-

---

[1] L. Berman, *The Personal Equation* (1925), p. 102.
[2] *Vide supra*, chap. ix.

ment of character, yet some belief or other in such a connection has existed at all times. Environmentalists, not merely of the materialistic type, have often been heard to contend " Tell me what you eat and I shall tell you what you are ". This view has taken on its crystallized form in the convenient pun, *Der Mensch ist was er isst* (" A man is what he eats "). It has been thought that coarse foods tend to develop a coarse personality, and that the daintier dishes contrariwise would refine the person who partook of them. How often have the Hindus been pointed out for confirmation of this rule, which was to be further reinforced by the citation of the eating practices of the Esquimos ? Among the many American quackeries may be found a special brand devoted to food fads. One of these modern superstitions preaches that " eaters of lamb meat are of gentler dispositions " (than eaters of beef or pork, I suppose). Recently this claim on the part of food-centered theorists has, in a modified form of course, received some support in endocrinological circles. To quote Berman again " Researches of chemists extending over the last hundred years or so have demonstrated two very important facts : first, that all living things have practically the same chemical composition ; and second that the composition of animals, including human beings, is essentially that of the food they eat ",[1] and in another paragraph, " We are such things as our foods are made of ".

Moral of the Human Ass. That prince of satirists, Lucian, little dreamt when writing his story of the ass [2] who, after regularly helping himself to the epicurean menu of a chef in the employ of a wealthy Greek, began to perform actually human stunts—that nearly eighteen centuries later scientists would discover a grain of truth in his farcical fable. There is one important feature, however, which we must not forget

[1] *Loc. cit.*, p. 144.

[2] This story, *Lucius or The Ass*, which may be spurious, is reminiscent of a similar tale, " The Golden Ass," by Apuleius.

as applying seriously to the issue on hand. That ass of Lucian, originally Lucius, must have had a non-asinine character to begin with if he preferred human food to that commonly acceptable to asses, and particularly since he was able to hoodwink his master and gorge himself with stews and sauces and wines without being discovered.

Character-Type and Choice of Food. It is really this circumstance which possibly provides the key to the whole situation. Each person chooses the food conformable with his constitution ; and if there is a degree of correspondence between character and food, the reason probably lies in the fact that there is a *tertium quid comparationis*, which mediates between the two distinctly-related entities. My observations may be altogether too meagre to base any judgment thereon, but scant as they are, they lead me to think that the sugar-loving and candy-eating people are mostly those who come under the " primary functioning " category (Chapter XIV) and that the more persistent, less fickle, more reliable individual, while not shunning sweets, does not indulge in them as a food. One might have argued then from this correlation that the ingestion of sugar is apt to develop such a character, while what seems more plausible in the event of a decided concomitance is that a person with such and such traits would have certain food predilections. To be sure, when a starveling becomes a sybarite, the change will not be without its effects on the individual's character, but if we stop to reflect on this case, we should at once realize that the changed condition has no more than released the original nature of that individual, or else the changed habits had come about *pari passu* with a transformed point of view, in which event the change is primarily not one of character but of intelligence or belief. Sudden affluence will never effect such a metamorphosis in the character of a man of worth as to cause him to cast all principles to the wind or to join that half which " doesn't know how the other half lives ".

In sum, there is no evidence to indicate that food is an appreciable factor in the shaping of character or its modification.

OCCUPATION AND CHARACTER

What Determines our Calling ? The vocational influence on character did not loom up as a problem in characterology until recently. Baumgarten approaches this subject thoughtfully in a brief paper [1] where she points out that the matter of determining the relation between character and occupation is beset with obstacles. On the occupational side we lack a serviceable classification, while on the other side we disagree as to the concept of character. It is her belief that the inclination toward a certain activity as expressive of one's personality is a much underrated factor. To rely on the testimony of the individual in question would not be scientific, because often the motive is unbeknown to the person. Furthermore in every profession or vocation there is scope for a division of labour or functionalization in accordance with the urge of the individual. In medicine, one may be a surgeon if sadistically inclined, or engage in research work if of the peace-loving disposition, or again, if of the active sort, the yearning for administrative or executive duties may be gratified. The division between active and passive characters and between sociable and unsociable natures is made in the interest of a classification of occupations on the basis of inner urges. Sympathy and love of mankind are the mainsprings of many occupations. The physician, the nurse, the teacher, especially of defectives, the missionary and the politician who represents radical views, for which he is likely to be persecuted, come under that head, according to Baumgarten.

On the other hand she sees in the usurer, the police inspector, the detective, the prosecutor, the judge, the

[1] F. Baumgarten, " Charakter und Beruf " : *Jahrbuch der Charakterologie*, 1926, vols. ii–iii.

warden or governor of a jail, the vivisector in science, the caricaturist, the surgeon, the trapper, the butcher and many others whose duty or *métier* is to cause pain or execute restrictions—a sadistic element, a quality of malevolence. Even masons and woodchoppers are regarded as taking pleasure in their work of hammering or cutting down.

A Disputable Point. There is an element of truth in Baumgarten's observations, yet it is not at all safe to say that the two divisions are fundamental. Even an inquisitor, as Victor Hugo has so persuasively, though not convincingly, drawn him in his *Torquemada*, may be a benevolent creature in many respects ; and the attitude which the sheriff or the hangman takes towards a convicted prisoner does not emanate from a tendency to gratify their malevolent propensities but rather from the feeling that they are dealing with an enemy of mankind who must suffer for the pain which he has inflicted on others.

Job merely Helps to Reveal Traits. The converse question as to how far character is affected by vocation is one which offers an even better opportunity for fallacious reasoning. Baumgarten quotes Aschaffenburg's obvious conclusion that various species of crime are dependent on the type of occupation. It is certainly well known that cashiers in banks are more susceptible to defalcations than others, that lawyers are often guilty of embezzlement, that government officials will not always withstand the temptation of receiving bribes. Do these facts prove that character is debased because of such occupations, or on the other hand, as Baumgarten implies, that some vocations are apt to ennoble the character of those who have adopted them ? We should grant that when a characterless person falls into an occupation which taxes his inhibitive tendency, his sordidness will be increased. A man of integrity, however, will only give a more pronounced form to his character when placed in difficult positions.

The upshot of the article, viz., that character is a greater influence on vocation than vocation is on character not only seems acceptable but might be amplified by the statement that there is an inverse ratio between the two factors, so that the more highly integrated the character, the less will it be affected by the occupation, and *vice versa.*

HOME AND SOCIAL INFLUENCE

The power of social agencies for building character has been stressed by educators, reformers, clergymen and writers of various schools of thought. While this influence cannot be denied, it is probable that the environmental bias in educational circles has resulted in overestimating the effect of non-hereditary factors. If education and discipline were of no consequence in training individuals to give preference to certain tendencies and not to others, there would be no point in correcting children. We should then leave them to their original natures and people the world with a race of savages. On the other hand, it is well known that the most rigid supervision will not prevent some youths from engaging in culpable pursuits.

Part Played by the Mother. One of the agencies singled out for special distinction in developing character is undoubtedly that of example. Smiles, in his famous book on Character, has devoted a whole chapter to show that many great men were inspired to live a noble life by the example and the exhortation of their mother, while Byron's weaknesses of character were in large part due to the attitude his mother had taken toward him and her display of temper. Smiles infers that the home influence must have played a very large part in shaping the character of these men, for in some of the cases he cited, the father was a worthless man ; hence the moral maturation of the son must have taken place thanks to the constant care of the mother. It did not occur to the good Smiles that the famous men he mentioned may have *inherited* their good qualities from the mother,[1] so that while the home influence is to be taken into consideration, it by no means furnishes the key to the situation.

Companionship. We hear so much about the influence of immoral associates and the fact that the road to the gallows or the electric chair leads off from the nest of evil companionship : but what famous man, reared in the slums, has not had embryo thieves and robbers, if not murderers, for his chums ? Naturally as he grew older he would part company with them ; and the reason why the profligate who pleads that his life has been ruined by anti-social comrades did not sever connections with them is simply that "birds of a feather flock together". Nor do we have to go far to seek the reprobate who was surrounded with all sorts of good influences in his childhood and youth, and yet found his way to the scum of the earth.

Few people in a civilized community have had more evil agencies than good influences bidding for their attention. To say that they are weak characters because they did not follow the latter rather than the former is only another way of stating that they are characterless.

Circumstances Count only with Average Person. To conclude, then, we may glean from the foregoing that while environmental influences must be reckoned with as factors of character, their effect is not marked at the extremes, i.e., where an individual is either anti-socially predisposed or, contrariwise, possesses the makings of character, with a strong consistency urge dominating the elements. The average person is more susceptible to the play of circumstances, but even with the man in the street, heredity or innate qualities (inhibitability) are of greater weight than mere environment.

[1] This comparatively simple problem is still in the speculative stage, and yet its solution, which I hope to undertake in the near future, is bound to shed much light on a variety of social phenomena and is apt even to serve as a guiding post in the settling of delicate questions which come up in everyday life.

CHAPTER XXXVII

THE SEAT OF CHARACTER

With the rise of physiological psychology it has become customary to look for the location of every mental process which merely suggests the possibility of localization. Descartes' futile search for the seat of the soul has not served to discourage the efforts of psychologists and physiologists to connect the mental phenomenon and the physiological process in a definite place in the nervous system.

The influence of phrenology had made itself felt prior to this co-operation between physiology and psychology. Traits were localized as readily as organic functions, and the whole cerebrum became the abode of character cut up into bits and pigeon-holed into tiny compartments.

Cerebellum Hypothesis of Luys. The phrenologists, however, were not dealing with character as such, and if asked to name the seat of character they would probably simply point to the head. Azam in this respect was more ambitious. Following Luys, from whom he quotes several passages, he seems to favour the hypothesis that character resides at the base of the brain and in the parts which receive the irradiations from the cerebellum. Luys had written that it " is the cerebellar innervation which gives our movements continuity and energy ". Seeing that patients whose cerebellar region is impaired are subject to a motor disorder, for instance not being able to shake hands, he concluded that " there is therefore a lively active and unconscious force irradiated from the cerebellum which gives our physical operations the slowness or energy with which they are endowed ".

Several cases, cited by the same physician, who is further quoted by Azam, would indicate that a compression of the corpus striatum might lead to depression, while the atrophy of this organ begins to manifest itself through the embittered and violent temper which a patient would develop in spite of his former gentleness and amiability.[1] Again we note that the term character is used here in a miscellaneous sense, and the observations of Luys do not prove anything. One might expect that a suffering person would after a long period of affliction grow to be depressed, grouchy or irritable, without attributing this change in attitude to the condition of the cerebellum.

Can a Complex Function be Localized ? It appears that the French physicians who wrote on this subject were not particularly anxious to analyze their task. The question whether such a complex function as character can be localized altogether deserves priority over the problem of its location. Without the nervous system, naturally no character ; without the brain, no character. We may go further and point out that since character involves knowledge, then we could have no character were it not for the cortex, but does this mean that the cortex is the seat of character ?

Confusion of Issues. The question as to the abode of character is not unequivocal as it is generally discussed. In the first place, it may be understood in the sense that without that particular organ in which character is supposed to reside, there would be no such thing as character. The seat in this case really connotes the *physiological ground* or *substrate* of character. As compared with this phase of the question, the query as to the *location* of character has little significance, although it may appeal to our curiosity. These two different senses again are to be distinguished from another which asks after the *correlate* of character in external organs and behaviour, and thus assumes the symbol to be

[1] E. Azam, *Le caractère dans la santé et dans la maladie* (1887), p. 212.

the ground. Popular character analysis has much to answer for in propagating this view. It is supposed, for example, that one with a peculiarly shaped ear or an ill-formed mouth is the bearer of a certain character because of these irregularly formed organs.

If we knew more about mental and physical correlations, we should discover probably correspondences in the most minute parts of the organism. We might expect such correspondence on the principle of the uniformity of nature ; but should we then be justified in holding that the seat of character is in the toe-nails or the lines of the palm ?

" Chemique " as Basis of Character. The modern votaries of endocrinology seek the location of character in 'the ductless glands and incline to view the chemical constitution of the organism as the ground of character. Anyone who is committed to a strict psychophysical parallelism will most probably accept this conclusion, which must be rather obvious but not very enlightening. Intelligence too is grounded in the chemical constitution of the nervous system ; for in the last analysis differences in the quality of nerve substance are differences in the physico-chemical make-up of the nerve fibres and their connections. The seat of character would be the body as a whole, but evidently this diffuse allusion cannot satisfy us.

The popular linking of character with the spine, as evidenced in the phrase " to have no backbone " is interesting but need not divert us from the track. The " backbone " in this connection is only a symbol of firmness, the physical quality suggesting the mental. The jelly-fish, for this reason, is singled out as the organism with the least claim to possessing character.

The French physician who thought that the cerebellum was the seat of character must have narrowed down the concept to some composite of energy and motor ability. The function of the cerebellum was long supposed to have been that of motor co-ordination, but what has this to do with character as the people have understood this word for ages ? And in what way can an autopsy on a patient reveal the inherent connection between character and the operations or the condition of the cerebellum ?

Optic Thalamus as Personality Centre.—Walter [1] is inclined to link the optic thalamus and the brain stem with the more distinct function of personality, but it is difficult to see any supporting evidence for this conclusion except that Head has regarded the thalamus as the elaborative centre of affective qualities, while Kleist has emphasized the rôle of motor expression in the realization of psychic functions, and the brain stem is supposed to be the centre of the motor system. Obviously all this has little to do with character, although the question posed toward the end of the article (which is practically devoted to the discussion of brain localization) reads : " Can we now at least in this sense speak also of a localization of other phases of the personality, which fall in the sphere of the emotional, that is to say, the feelings and the will ?"

ANALYSIS OF CONCEPT PRECEDES QUESTION OF LOCALIZATION

It seems to me that before the question of the localization of character can be legitimately put, it is necessary to examine just what is involved in the concept. To be sure, intelligence has its place there ; for at least the knowledge of right and wrong is a *sine qua non* of all conduct which allows of appraisal. Certainly an imbecile cannot be said to exhibit character in a well-defined form, even if his obedience, kindness and perseverance are manifest. The mechanical nature of his behaviour causes us to call in question the application of the term " character " to his traits. Intelligence then is one of the essentials to be presupposed.

[1] F. K. Walter, " Die materiellen Grundlagen der geistigen Persön-lichkeit " : *Jahrbuch der Charakterologie*, 1924, vol. i.

Location of Inhibitory Mechanism. Inhibition, we shall remember, was set down as the core of character. Now the inhibition is of instinctive tendencies, but it is not at all clear that the inhibitory mechanism resides in those parts of the brain which preside over the instinctive tendencies, even if we should be certain about the habitat of the latter. The ground of character is to be sought in the *nervous organization which governs the inhibitions,* and partly also in the strength and weakness of the various connate urges. Thus, a person with a strong materially acquisitive instinct will be apt to suffer more breaks in the inhibitory mechanism when the reaction is to money matters. The individual with an oversexed constitution is apt to succumb easily in matters which affect this weakness.

The location of our instinctive mechanisms is still a mooted point. The sex instinct is, of course, linked up with a definite organic apparatus, but is the acquisitive instinct in any way connected with the hunger impulse ? At any rate, the question of the seat of our instincts is subsidiary to our present problem; for the *essence of character is the inhibition of the instincts,* and unless we assume that the instinctive urges are checked largely because of their low intensity, and similarly are difficult to inhibit because of their relative strength, we should still be on our search for the physical basis and location of the inhibition.

Motive Force of Inhibition. Furthermore, it must be understood that inhibition is but an abstract principle. The inhibition of the extensor or flexor muscles is something entirely different from the inhibition of an instinctive urge. The object of the inhibition is of paramount importance. But even of greater significance is the motive force of the inhibition, i.e. whether it is a mere automatic affair or a desire or an idea or a principle.

Our problem thus becomes so complicated that one might ask whether it is of value so much as to consider it. Its value,

I believe, lies in breaking up the ground, in aiding us to
re-connect parts which had been wrongly joined together
in the popular mind, and thus to reconstruct the common
notions of character. We should moreover not lose sight of
the fact that our own results might be checked up by noting
the possibilities of a complex problem. To take an instance :
if we should be disposed to regard a person's general
inhibitability as a mark of character, and in turn a function
of the speed of nerve processes, or of the arresting force of
the synapses, then the dynamic person, whose movements
are explosive, can scarcely compare in character co-efficient
with the person whose inertia leads him to stop and ponder
at every move. Or, might we resort to the alternative
interpretation that a dynamic genius like Luther was moved
to inhibit his instinct of self-preservation by an *idée fixe* ;
that, in other words, the strength of his belief in his mission
was sufficient to counterbalance all fears which he might have
harboured for his life and safety ?

The Dilemma. In this event, either we should be compelled
to attribute character to every individual obsessed by an idea
the pursuit of which is carried to an unusual extent, even if
not to realization, or else we should not be ready to endow the
great German reformer with a high order of character.

Safety Devices for Avoiding the Dilemma. There are,
however, *two criteria* which may serve as guides. In the
first place, the *inhibition typifying character is of a distributive
kind, affecting all instincts in greater or less degree.* The person
with an obsession which leads him to make many sacrifices
will easily be recognized as such. The connection between
his behaviour and the autistic ruling idea will be obvious
at every step. Secondly, *the idea or principle underlying a
man's rigid inhibition must,* according to our whole doctrine,
as will be remembered, *prove eminently rational, one which
aligns itself with the progress of humanity.* To such an extent,
at least, must we count ourselves absolutists as to discriminate

between the rational and the irrational, between a social value and an individual ambition ; and on this basis, can we decide between Napoleon's ruling passion and Luther's striving for reformation. The warrior who is battling for an illusory cause may *think* he has right on his side, but he who is in the vanguard of progress *knows* that his cause is just. His character is calibrated through the instrument of insight, which sets him off from other energetic men who, even if they built more wisely than they knew, may still have lacked vision as regards their special endeavour.

We thus come back to the previous thesis, which is this : that if the question of the seat of character is asked, we must look for the answer in the *direction of the physiological condition of general inhibition and in specific phases of intelligence, for instance insight,* especially as to the relation of the ego to others ; for without this quality no consistency principle in action is possible, although the psychophysical ground of this action consistency is by no means clear even in the presence of this quality.

Piéron tends to make short shrift of the attempt to localize personality when he writes :

It is certainly absurd to look for a cerebral seat of personality, which objectively is an expression of the law of the unity of nervous functioning, and subjectively appears as a complex feeling, the result of a certain mode of mental functioning and formed under the influence of social education.[1]

Yet a few pages farther, he concedes that various writers are in close agreement in recording that disorders of character predominate in the frontal region ; from which stem abulia and apathy, but also impulsiveness and irritability, the power of inhibition being diminished.

[1] H. Piéron : *Thought and the Brain*, 1927 (trans. by C. K. Ogden), p. 44 (Kegan Paul).

To seek to deposit character in the cerebellum as Luys and Azam were doing, or with some of the more enthusiastic exponents of endocrinology, to make character depend on intra-visceral pressure,[1] or to claim the autonomic nervous system for its abode, as implied by Kempf [2] not only over-simplifies the issue but marks a futile attempt to localize something which, because of the complexity of the case, does not permit of definite localization. What we must ask for is not the seat of character but its physiological conditions.

[1] L. Berman, *The Glands Regulating the Personality.*

[2] E. J. Kempf, " The Autonomic Functions and the Personality " in *Nervous and Mental Disease Monographs*, No. 28.

CHAPTER XXXVIII

After treating character and temperament separately, except when it was necessary to expound the doctrines of writers who used the terms interchangeably, we may be expected to show the relationship, if any, between the two, on the view that character is the inhibition of instinctive tendencies in accordance with regulative principles. The question then is : how does temperament affect character ? In other words, is the sanguine individual likely to possess greater character than the phlegmatic or the choleric individual ?

Temperamental Assets and Liabilities. From the angle of the man in the street who judges character by conduct according as it falls in with his own desires or not, the sanguine person, because generally the most amiable of the quartet, would be best appreciated, at least until a serious breach had been committed. The choleric individual is usually disliked because of an irascible disposition which is apt to make underlings, especially, uncomfortable. The phlegmatic temperament is often regarded as colourless and therefore without character. Finally, melancholic people are thought to be too ineffectual and too deeply absorbed in themselves to possess character in any pronounced degree.

As a matter of fact, however, each of the four temperament-types has both its advantages and disadvantages. Even the choleric frequently manage to surround themselves with loyal friends. This fact is somewhat puzzling and in the light of modern theories, particularly that of psychoanalysis (father complex, as in Freud's *Group Psychology and Analysis of the Ego*), it would not be difficult to offer ingenious explanations. The simplest one which occurs to me is that a choleric man is not infrequently one who will protect a friend and fight for him tooth and nail. Of course the masochistic interpretation of the master-slave relationship is not excluded. But before we betake ourselves to the obscure regions of the unconscious, I think it is a sound methodological principle to exhaust all the simpler and more tangible explanations.

 The sanguine can accomplish more than, let us say, the melancholic who are, with few exceptions, inhibited from action, but at the same time they are more susceptible of undoing the good they have brought about, by their lack of persistence. The character of the phlegmatic is supposed never to acquire sufficient strength to manifest itself in decisive matters; and the melancholic person is surely lost in trains of thought and depths of feeling, so that action is out of the question.

Applying the Rule. To the lay mind, character is typified solely through action. Portentous deeds become for the average educated man and woman the touchstone of character. From the standpoint presented in this book, those possessed of the more inhibitive temperaments, i.e. the phlegmatic and the melancholic, are more apt to have the makings of character in them than the sanguine and the choleric, inasmuch as they would find it more compatible with their temperamental constitution to inhibit their instinctive tendencies; but on our own premise, if the choleric individual conquers his irascible impulse and the sanguine person curbs the constant craving for change, which I should regard as an instinctive urge, they have attained a higher level of character, at least with regard to these traits and the behaviour which the traits govern, than have the other two temperamental types.

We must Start on Neutral Ground. Because of the compensations among the temperaments, it would be best to treat each of the traditional types as equidistant from the centre of character. What the phlegmatic lack on the positive side, they make up on the negative side, and similarly if the choleric man experiences greater difficulty in checking his anger than does his phlegmatic friend, he may find it a good deal easier to advance in the face of danger, thus inhibiting his instinct of escape (self-preservation).

Achievement No Criterion of Character. We cannot countenance the popular belief that actual achievement in history is the only genuine index of character. No better illustration will serve our purpose in pointing out the fallacy of such a notion than the characterial comparison of the four great pillars of the Reformation, Reuchlin, Erasmus, Luther and Melanchthon. Of this glorious quartet, Luther will almost invariably be singled out as the greatest. Perhaps as a genius who combined the necessary qualities for the realization of an epoch-making event, he stands out head and shoulders above the rest, but I, for one, should not be willing to admit that his character transcends those of his associates, without whose indispensable aid he could, with all his dynamic qualities, his indomitable zeal and dauntlessness, scarcely have attained his end. Luther's positive characteristics overawe us, but we must not forget to take many circumstances into account, not the least being his powerful bodily frame, his almost fanatical conviction, and of course the protection of the Elector and the political situation of the day.

Luther Matched by Bruno. Another monk took a stand against the teachings of the Dominicans—the frail and unprotected Giordano Bruno—and effected no revolution in the domain of religion. He was burnt at the stake in the prime of life. Bruno by his very melancholic temperament was precluded from achieving greatness in the arena of action, but he attained the highest degree of character by dint of his inhibitions (he deliberately did not heed the warnings of the Church dignitaries who ordered him to retract his philosophical views and forbade him to set forth his heresies, as his teachings were then regarded).

To return, however, to the three great humanists mentioned together with Luther : Erasmus most probably would be criticized as an undecided man, one with changeable ideas, perhaps due to a sanguine temperament, but more likely to the natural dislike of precipitate action, especially where new aspects keep constantly appearing and successively reinforcing each of the two sides of the controversy. The strength of Erasmus's character lay then in his remaining true to his own convictions in spite of the pressure brought to bear on him by Luther and the Reformers on the one hand and the Catholic magistrates on the other.

Character of Erasmus. No better description of the conflict the famous scholar was compelled to undergo and his steadfast adherence to the regulative principle of truth can be obtained than in Erasmus's own account which follows :

Hercules could not fight two monsters at once ; while I, poor wretch, have lions, cerberuses, cancers, scorpions, every day at my sword's point ; not to mention smaller vermin—rats, mosquitoes, bugs, and flies. My troops of friends are turned to enemies. At dinner-table or social gatherings, in churches and kings' courts, in public carriage or public flyboat, scandal pursues me, and calumny defiles my name. Every goose now hisses at Erasmus ; and it is worse than being stoned, once for all, like Stephen, or shot with arrows like Sebastian. They attack me even now for my Latin style, and spatter me with epigrams. Fame I would have parted with ; but to be the sport of blackguards—to be pelted with potsherds and dirt and ordure—is not this worse than death ? There is no rest for me in my age, unless I join Luther ; and I cannot accept his doctrines. Sometimes I am stung with a desire to avenge my wrongs ; but I say to myself : " Will you, to gratify your spleen, raise your hand against your mother, the Church, who begot you at the font and fed you with the word of God ? " I cannot do it. Yet I understand now how Arius and Tertullian and Wickliff were driven to schism. The theologians say I am their enemy. Why ? Because I bade monks remember their vows ; because I told parsons to leave their wranglings and read the Bible ; because I told Popes and Cardinals to look at the Apostles, and make themselves more like to them. If this is to be their enemy, then indeed I have injured them.

The Prowess of Reuchlin. Reuchlin, the father of Humanism, has still less to recommend him—from the popular angle— as a rival to Luther in matters of character. He might have been regarded as a pure scholar who in a phlegmatic vein was content to bring out manuals, grammars and lexicons, unmindful of the great issues about to be fought out in the next generation. But the opportunity came for this seemingly phlegmatic man to disclose his grandeur when he was approached by the despicable Pfefferkorn with a royal mandate to have the Talmud and other sacred books of the Jews burnt. Reuchlin was not philo-Semitic in his sentiments, nevertheless he could not allow such a monstrosity without bringing to bear all his weight on the opposing side. The danger of such opposition can scarcely be realized nowadays; yet when Reuchlin, in company with other authorities, was asked to present his expert opinion as to the desirability or obnoxiousness of these books, he dared to pronounce himself in disfavour of the Dominican project, only to be ruthlessly attacked, summoned for trial and persecuted in various ways because the nefarious scheme of the obscurantists was defeated through his sense of justice and adherence to principle. While it is true that Reuchlin was hardly in jeopardy of losing his life or freedom, his perturbed days as a result of repeated trials, constant defences, both before the tribunal and in writing, and the forced travelling drained his energy and saddened the last years of his fruitful life.

YY

A Great Melancholic. Philip Melanchthon, otherwise known as the Praeceptor of the Reformation, is another instructive example for our purpose. One glance at his portrait executed by Dürer is enough to convince the judge of human nature that he has before him a melancholic type. In Sigaud's classification, Melanchthon would doubtless fit in under the " cerebral " rubric. His character has often been extolled to the point of saintliness. He was said to have been the personification of meekness, of affability, and of justice. But a biographer like Ellinger is not eager to idealize his subject. In this German writer's bulky life of the celebrated reformer, our attention is called to several weak traits which Ellinger endeavours to minimize on the ground that Melanchthon was a *Gelehrtenatur*.[1] Certainly we can appreciate the fact that the scholar will not spontaneously engage in a prolonged warfare with the mighty. A person with such a bent is inclined to make room for compromises, not only because he is usually deficient in the physical energy necessary for protracted combats, but because the drive for knowledge and recognition through intellectual achievement is greater than that for power acquired through force, and also because the theoretical man sees enough of both sides of the issue and is influenced far more by the *status quo*, in his practical measures, than the man of action, whose opinions and conclusions on public matters are bound to seek an immediate outlet in execution.

The case of Melanchthon is more striking. In his youth and early manhood he appears to have manifested a choleric temperament, and his irritability and sensitivity are noticeable in the features and expression of an earlier portrait. The irascible scholar had undergone a rigid self-discipline in order to keep his temper in check, and to take a sweeter view of life than was his wont—a moral exercise which prepared him afterwards for his mission as a mediator or, perhaps better, an intermediary.

[1] G. Ellinger, *Philipp Melanchthon* (1902), p. 593 ff.

Character Estimate of Luther. If Luther stands out as a tower of strength and courage, as an uncompromising champion of what he considered to be a just cause, he falls below Melanchthon in tolerance, in considerateness of other people's feelings ; and if the latter is not on a par with his more glorious grand uncle in respect of force of will, determination, and the dynamic qualities of character, which usually depend on a vigorous and robust constitution, let us remember on the other hand that Luther's acerbity, his dogmatism, high-handedness and relentlessness somewhat detract from his heroic halo. Had Luther not been successful in resisting the Papacy, most likely his personality, and with it, naturally, his character, would not have loomed so large in the annals of history, while Erasmus's sterling traits would have shone with undiminished splendour throughout the ages, as would Reuchlin's and Melanchthon's characters.

An attitude like Melanchthon's, who, when besought by his aged mother, in the heat of the religious controversy which was then raging, to tell her whether she ought to change her form of worship, encouraged her to go on believing and worshipping in her usual manner—an attitude like this was quite foreign to the temper of Luther and bespoke a form of high-mindedness rare even in our own day.

It is not my purpose, however, to compare Luther with his associates. Each of the pillars of the Reformation, in spite of temperamental differences, exemplified a high degree of character in the sense of inhibiting instinctive tendencies. Luther, by taking the initiative in his defection from established forms, inhibited of course the most powerful set of instincts, but the other three showed their stamina on more than one occasion, when the offensive was taken against them. Besides, Melanchthon is known to have curbed his instinct of pugnacity to the extent of appearing gentle in his demeanour. Possibly in the process of overcoming his quick temper he was drawn into a state of melancholy by way of compensation, yet this depression, from which he was beginning to suffer in middle life, cannot be held against him.

As Regards Character—All Temperaments on an Equal Footing. Our conclusion must be as follows then : while there is in all probability a relationship between character and temperament, there is no ground for supposing that any single one temperament is apt to favour a high or a low character. In evaluating character, we are ordinarily disposed to place most weight on action, but the justification of this tradition rests on the fact that character can be judged only through overt acts—only then is it put to the touchstone. The popular notion seems to link character with success, efficacy, execution of a difficult task, which I conceive to be merely incidentals so far as the central issue is concerned, although the consequences for the world may be of untold importance. Achievement through character and character itself are two different things. Undoubtedly a great effect adds to the aura of character, embellishes it, but, if we are to keep our quest clearly in mind, it is necessary to perceive that it does not add to the *value of the character as such*. Character is to be judged on its own merit, and not by some external criterion such as benefiting humanity, a criterion which would bring us perilously near a utilitarian conception of character. That a great character will benefit humanity is a corollary which emanates from the nature of the case (fine insight or vision, inhibition in conformity with regulative principles), but we are by no means warranted in concluding that character derives its value because of the benefits that accrue to mankind as a result of it. The legendary geese that saved Rome from a catastrophe some two thousand years ago, have unquestionably benefited not only the metropolis of the world at the time but presumably mankind, but we cannot bring ourselves to ascribe character to these alert and faithful geese.

CHAPTER XXXIX

CHARACTER AND THE VALUES

Shutting our Eyes to the Values would be Ostrich-like. It was a difficult task to steer clear of ethical discussion in a subject which has always been inseparably bound up with morality, serving, in fact, as its coping stone. Character was conceived of as the fountain out of which emanated moral acts, and conversely, an unbroken succession of moral acts was regarded as the outward expression of character. In our presentation, little attention was given to the moral phase of character. We were not concerned with the problem of character-education, with exhortations or maxims. Only the psychology of character was covered in this essay; and in order to keep the issues clear before us it was necessary to avoid complicating the material with questions from other disciplines. Religion, free-will, the good, the true and the beautiful had all to remain in the background. We cannot afford, however, to ignore in our discussion the subject of value altogether. To speak about absolute principles regulating our inhibitions is already to commit oneself on this question; and yet this absoluteness must be insisted on.

Absolute Principles Presupposed. So soon as we begin to make concessions on this point, we lose our standards and consequently our regulators. Our inhibitions then become devoid of meaning with the result that character is no longer amenable to measurement or estimation, no matter how rough the criterion. By absoluteness, on the other hand, is not meant that the principles are of cosmic proportions, that, in other words, there is justice in the world with or without humanity or that truth is a function of the universe. It is sufficient to modestly make this absoluteness coeval and coextensive with humanity. Whether these principles have originated with man or with a Deity, they are binding ; for our whole cultural structure presupposes them. Not only morality, but all science and art would be in the most precarious condition, destitute of a *raison d'être*, unless the sovereignty of the values were taken for granted. If ideals were mere illusions, and fairness or rightness had no superiority over unfairness or wrongness, then should we be compelled to exclaim with Ecclesiastes " Vanity of vanities ; all is vanity ! What profit hath a man of all his labour which he taketh under the sun ? One generation passeth away, and another generation cometh, but the earth abideth for ever." Forced to this conclusion we might as well give up doing anything which is not for our immediate pleasure. No scientific labours for the benefit of posterity would be undertaken unless the scientists had faith in progress ; and progress *ex vi termini* implies a standard, if not an ideal ; else we should never be certain that our movements and reforms are unlike those of the rotations of a rat in a rotating cage.

Principles Ultimate in Spite of Abuse. We need not go so far as to wonder about the duration of the race and therefore of the values which obtain in the sphere of mankind. Absoluteness does not necessarily mean eternity. Nor are we to suppose that all human beings must be imbued with the grandeur of the regulating principles for the latter to possess the mark of absoluteness. Quite the contrary : truth and justice go a-begging. They are recognized well enough but are not accorded the treatment they deserve. Did not the greatest observer of human nature perhaps of all times bitterly lament " the world's way " which causes

Needy nothing to be trimmed in jollity
And purest faith unhappily forsworn
And gilded honour shamefully misplaced,

And maiden virtue rudely strumpeted,
And right perfection wrongfully disgraced
And strength by limping sway disabled,
And art made tongue-tied by authority,
And folly, doctor-like, controlling skill,
And captive Good attending captain Ill ?

Rare indeed is this article we call justice. Just as often as not is the truth in worldly affairs conspicuous by its absence. But does this rareness make it any the less valuable ? If anything, one should opine that its value is thereby rather enhanced. What if not a single person could be found to have faultlessly inhibited all his instinctive tendencies at the behest of the ethico-logical principles, we must remember with Ben Jonson that

In small proportions we just beauties see ;
And in short measures life may perfect be.

Pernicious Influences of To-day. We must be ready to admit that our regulative principles are only relatively absolute. What do human values amount to in eons of time ? But there is a world of difference between relative absoluteness and absolute relativity. Unfortunately the intellectuals of to-day are too prone to accept as their standard a point of view which from its very nature is *ab initio* without a foundation, and is therefore no standard at all. Psychological textbooks teem with nihilistic theories and analogies. The wheat and the chaff are all treated alike in cynical fashion. Complexes and rationalizations are to explain the most admirable achievements ; and the genius and the prize fighter are accorded the same place in the social order. How many times do we hear it said in mechanistic circles that this or that man of eminence has mounted to the pinnacle of fame because of some physical disability which kept him from indulging in social activities ! We may some day expect to find Kant belittled on the ground that had he not been narrow-chested, he might not have engaged in philosophical pursuits and thus not have written his great *Critique*.

An Excuse for the Incapable. This whole trend of thought seems to be a defence reaction on the part of mediocre people who wish to imply that not natural endowment and an inner impulse to seek truth are responsible for cultural productivity of a high order, but a deficiency in a certain direction which they cannot be charged with. Their normality then is to be taken as the excuse of their lack of achievement. Had they been able to isolate themselves from the rest of the world— we are to understand—were they so asthenic as to be kept from participating in various sports and games, they too would have cultivated their minds to the utmost and might have fared equally well in their endeavours.

Application of Democracy in Sphere of Values Questioned. The spirit of democracy, legitimate in the sphere of politics, has now permeated the interpretative world in such a way that one person or trait is set off against another, as if it were the number and not the quality which counted. A facile writer will reduce the spineless resignation of a mollycoddle and the deliberate withdrawal of a man of character from a certain activity for the purpose of espousing a worthier cause—to the same denominator. "The sour grapes complex" is the glib explanation offered in both these totally disparate cases.

Superficially the reaction is the same. In content there is a wide divergence. If we keep on whittling away mephisto-phelically our principles, standards and values, we run the risk of destroying the significance of the very statements used in this belittling process. In fact these levellers of values never permit themselves to be thoroughgoing in their sweeping reduction. Somehow they find a loophole open to introduce a standard of their own in a different garb, whether this be society, sublimation, integration, adjustment, etc.

Their attitude is redolent of the Greek epigram by an Etonian friend of the celebrated Porson, who Englished it as follows :

> *The Germans in Greek*
> *Are sadly to seek ;*
> *Not five in fivescore,*
> *But ninety-five more,*
> *All save only Herman[n],*
> *And Herman[n]'s a German.*

Rationale of Sublimation. To illustrate : a colleague who frowned at the seemingly reactionary emphasis laid on absolute principles in the essay [1] which forms the basis of this book, nevertheless to my surprise, subscribed to the general thesis of inhibition as the chief factor in character. " But," said he, " instead of inhibition, let us talk of sublimation in the Freudian sense." Now sublimation, as Jones defines it, is " the deflection of the energy of a sexual impulse to a non-sexual and socially useful goal ".[2] Since the sexual impulse is the manifestation of one instinctive mechanism only, it becomes clear that sublimation cannot satisfy our view which demands the distributive inhibition of all instincts in accordance with a regulative principle. If sublimation applied to all instinctive dispositions, as some non-Freudian writers have suggested, there would appear some ground for disregarding the difference in terminology and resorting to the psychoanalytic position. One fails to see, however, why sex energy as such should be deflected, when it does not interfere with the fundamental principles.

Social Utility as Court of Appeal. So much for the major line of attack. There is, however, another issue involved here which is more pertinent to the relation between character and value. Those who dispense with ideals and ultimate or

---

[1] A. A. Roback, " Character and Inhibition " in *Problems of Personality.*

[2] E. Jones, *Papers on Psycho-Analysis* (revised ed.), p. 692.

absolute principles imagine that they elude the problem altogether by studiously avoiding the use of such words as "higher"
and " lower ", or even " desirable ". Sooner or later they
realize that in summing up the situation and setting down
practical conclusions in their capacity as teachers or mentors,
they cannot employ in their injunctions a verb alone. The
verb must be qualified so as to imply a standard. Sublimating
implies such a standard, viz., social utility, but the defect
of this standard is first, that it cannot be applied objectively ;
that is to say, one may discover uses where there are none,
and conversely, one may fail to find uses where such are in
evidence to others ; secondly, there is no reason why social
utility should be erected into a fundamental principle any
more than justice or truthfulness.

There is no logic except that of the acceptance of fundamental principles which would compel a man to adopt the
standard of social utility. If he did not believe that he ought
to help further human progress, the philosophy of psychoanalysis would be of no avail to impose upon him the
deprivation entailed by sublimation, whatever the compensations might be.   It may, of course, be contended that only
through sublimation can mental conflict be reduced to a
minimum, that only through prudence is the average man
enabled to keep out of the clutches of the law. But this does
not always hold, and even if it did, the standard would not be
social utility, but individual welfare.

Evidence on Sublimation Flimsy. Furthermore, the position
that there is a positive relation between sublimation
and social achievement may be challenged on empirical
grounds. It is not likely that Benjamin Franklin would have
accomplished much more if he had sublimated his sex
impulses. And we cannot be certain that Shakespeare,
Goethe or Wagner would have been greater geniuses if they
had remained celibates. If Flaubert and George Sand had
changed rôles with regard to sublimation, perhaps the author

of *Madame Bovary* would have written more and his literary counterpart might have been more restricted in her productivity.

Integration—the New Watchword. Considered from all angles, then, sublimation cannot be held to be a condition of character, nor does it provide us with a practicable standard for judging character. Similarly all other relativistic standards like social adjustment or integration cannot serve the purpose. Integration at best may be a result ; it is neither a condition nor an aim. Why the more integrated man possesses a better character than the less integrated individual can be understood only in terms of fundamental principles, realizations, ideals, strivings, purposes.

Integration in itself is a relative term. Suppose we speak of a machine as perfectly integrated when its parts are so assembled as to be useful in turning out a certain product. Yet the machine becomes more interesting, invested with greater character, figuratively speaking, if it can be put to more uses than one, let us say by a collapsing device. To be sure, it is possible to regard such a machine as a more highly integrated piece of apparatus, so that we might have a hierarchy of integration. But on the other hand it is possible to hold that such devices render the machine subject to interference among the parts and therefore make it less integrated. In other words, from the point of view of integration, the simpler it is, the more typical it is, regardless of what benefits we may derive out of the complexity.

We can now turn from our analogy to the direct object, viz., character in man. The question before us is : How do we know that or when integration is complete ? The well-adjusted hypocrite may be perfectly integrated or at least more so than the sensitive soul torn hither and thither by moral scruples of little account. As in the case of adjustment, integration may bespeak character, but it is no criterion of character.

Harbinger of Integration Doctrine. The integration view of character is not by any means novel. It has been foreshadowed, if not actually taught, by Spencer in his *Data of Ethics*, where we read " a greater coherence among its component motions broadly distinguishes the conduct we call moral from the conduct we call immoral . . . Conduct of the lower kind, constituted of disorderly acts, has its parts relatively loose in their relations with one another ; while conduct of the higher kind, habitually following a fixed order, so gains a characteristic unity and coherence ".[1] The phrases " equilibrium ", " coherent heterogeneity ", " establishment of balance " are all forerunners of the theory of integration. But Spencer, at least, does not set up these relations as standards. He merely uses them as auxiliary material to illustrate the uniformity of the principle of evolution throughout the sciences, culminating in the discipline of ethics. To make out of the analogy of equilibrium in physics a moral standard would scarcely have occurred to him. Yet the advocates of integration as a sort of *summum bonum* would erect this *physiological* relation into a standard of character.

Analogy of Lever and Fulcrum. Character, it is true, is mediated by a physiological process, viz. inhibition, but unlike the case of mere integration, the process receives validation only through the regulative principles which, in themselves, bear the symbol of humanity. It is only fitting that *that which is most characteristic of man* (character) *should be grounded in those principles which constitute the essence of humanity.* Inhibition may be likened to the working of a lever, which must have a fulcrum in the shape of the regulative principles upon which the rigid bar (corresponding to the instincts in our analogy) is to rest, or else the mechanism cannot operate. The inhibition itself is merely the force applied to the lever, while the character index is represented by the " mechanical advantage " resulting from this operation.

[1] H. Spencer, *Data of Ethics*, sec. xxvi.

The principle of integration is not satisfactory as a criterion of character for the reason that it purports to serve both as force and fulcrum.

But why then has inhibition been made the basis of character in this book ? Why has character not been directly linked with something positive such as the regulative principles ? My answer is this :

In the first place let us recall that inhibition is not such a negative concept as was supposed at one time. Every act of volition necessitates an inhibition of some sort, and Sherrington's account of the reciprocal innervation of the flexor and extensor muscles should tend to convince us further of the fact that inhibition is an activity, not only useful, but indispensable in bringing about a desired result.

What Differentiates Mankind ? But secondly—and this is the more important reason—the exposition of character, as presented here, is frankly analytic in approach, that is to say, though psychological in method and material, it proceeds from an examination of the concept. I have tried to set forth a theory of character on the basis of what has been generally held to be the essence of character. Character stands for individuality in conduct. It connotes that which distinguishes one person from another in action. Now we notice of course that different people act differently, though they nearly all approve of the same principles ; and even the most hardened criminal who may argue stubbornly that this world is constituted according to the dictum " Every one for himself and the devil take the hindmost " will still shrink at the thought that his son—or, better still, his daughter—may take the same path. What then differentiates individuals so sharply in practice when in theory they form such a close bond—the bond of mankind ? Is it not because of the great divergence of their inhibitions ? **A** cannot check his acquisitive instinct, and so continues to advertise worthless wares. **B** knows he should decry a flagrant malversation, but he is afraid of losing his " bread and butter "—an unctuous attenuative for a comfortable home, fine victuals and entertainments of various sorts. C would like to attend to the task which he undertook on behalf of a worthy cause, but his gregarious instinct cannot be repressed even temporarily ; and so it goes. Primarily then the difference between one degree of character and another is a difference of inhibitability. In order to attain, you must first inhibit. If then inhibition is at least in action (though not in thought; since we must know what to reach out for before inhibition can be put to effective use) prior to the result obtained, are we not justified in regarding it as the *sine qua non* of character, qualified withal by the *direction* of the inhibition ?

An Ingrained Erroneous Belief. The inhibition of an instinct need not necessarily be taken as an indication of the evil inherent in the instinct any more than the inhibition of the extensor muscle when flexing our finger signifies the objectionability of that muscle. Inhibition serves a given purpose, and as such it is entitled to a place among the positive concepts in science.

Inhibition and Deprivation. Inhibition must naturally be looked upon as a deprivation—and that is why character is so admired ; that is to say, because of the restraint, because of the self-denial which only the few care to practise—but the deprivation has been endured in the past. At the moment of acting, there is no great effort exercised, as James and Stout and many others assert. The action is carried out in the line of least resistance just as if there had been no deprivation at all.[1] After the act indicative of character

---

[1] A. A. Roback, " The Interference of Will Impulses," etc., *Psychol. Rev. Monog. Suppl.*, 1918, vol. xxv, pp. 136–137 :

" To the popular mind, virtue is associated with the difficult course of action. Of course, the belief is universal that it is easier to yield to a temptation than to resist it, but this belief cannot be accepted as it stands. It requires further analysis. If it means that the average man or woman more frequently goes astray than not, then the view is

has been carried out, the feeling of deprivation usually is replaced by a feeling of gratification, so that Wotton's felicitous description of the *Happy Life* may be taken to be the picture of the man of character after he had overcome all his inner conflicts, his scruples, and broodings.

How happy is he born and taught
That serveth not another's will ;
Whose armor is his honest thought
And simple truth his utmost skill !

Whose passions not his masters are,
Whose soul is still prepared for death,
Untied unto the world by care
Of public fame, or private breath ;

Who envies none that chance doth raise
Nor vice ; who never understood
How deepest wounds are given by praise ;
Nor rules of state, but rules of good :

*   *   *   *

—This man is freed from servile bonds
Of hope to rise, or fear to fall ;
Lord of himself, though not of lands ;
And having nothing, yet hath all.

certainly not a correct one. What is at the root of this belief is the fact that all people find it easier to yield to a temptation at times than *never* to give way to one. That is an entirely different story. The important point, however, is that whether we yield or not we are *following the lines of least resistance.* Such a conclusion does not seem compatible with the conventional view of morality. One might object that it is putting the hero and the coward, the saint and moral reprobate on a par. We ask : How else can it be psychologically ? The hero is actuated by *his* idea just as the coward is determined by his. What really distinguishes their mode of behaviour is the judgment of value that attaches to their respective ideas. That difference in significance, however, takes us into another sphere entirely. It is no longer a psychological fact but an axiological datum.'' I may add now that there is a difference also in the *genesis* of the act. The praiseworthy act has been released by an idea which it has taken effort, perhaps struggle, to build up.

EPITOME

Although this book has grown far lengthier than originally intended, I cannot represent it as anything but an attempt to indicate the direction in which the study of character is to be undertaken if we wish to retain its original core and at the same time set it down on the solid ground of psychology. It is easy to dispose of character entirely, as some behaviourists are inclined to do, and it is almost as easy to treat it from an exhortative point of view, as religious teachers and moralists are wont to do. But, in making character the function of (*a*) instinctive tendencies, (*b*) certain properties of the nervous organization which facilitate inhibition, and (*c*) principles which claim as their psychological basis a mechanism yet to be investigated, I realize that there will be no end of protests on the ground that antiquated doctrines are being appealed to.

Quantitative Treatment. I am aware, too, that the description of the rating method on the scheme here outlined has been left in its initial stages. It is to be hoped that someone, with a leaning toward quantitative treatment and a knack for the manipulation of charts, will work out on a far more elaborate scale the evaluation of some well-known historical characters in accordance with the definition of character as the psychophysical disposition to inhibit instinctive tendencies in keeping with fundamental principles of action. The stratification of the various characters in an hierarchical system, so as to make allowance for the different levels of principles (legal, social, religious, aesthetic, ethico-logical) would further have to be undertaken at the behest of the conservative critic. Once, however, the method is clear, we should find little difficulty in removing obstacles.

Inhibition—the Technique of Character. Lest some readers still misunderstand my position in the belief that I regard instincts as something to be repressed, as containing the germ of sin and wickedness, I must remind them of what

has already been stated before, namely, that we have nothing
to do with the ascetic doctrine.   This is a point which,
experience has taught me, cannot be reiterated too often.
The machinery of character involves the inhibition of original
or inborn tendencies just as musical composition necessitates
the mastery of a certain technique ; but the inhibition in
itself, just as the technique as such, possesses very little value.
It is the direction which the inhibition or the technique
takes that is all-important.   Both man and beast work along
the lines of least resistance,[1] but it is for *man to change high
resistance into low resistance* by adhering to a rational guiding
principle—a purpose.   The courageous man's very difficult
course is to him a course of least resistance, once he has
firmly espoused his cause.   If time-binding may be considered,
according to Korzybski, the chief characteristic. of man,
we must not neglect the characteristic of resistance-reducing.
In fact, it might be claimed that man is a time-binder only
by virtue of his capacity to reduce resistance.   Consider how
much inhibition was necessary in order to assume permanently an erect posture on the part of our primitive ancestors.
Now, the original tendency to walk on all fours is neither
base nor immoral, but the subsequent change through a
process of inhibition, until the new habit became fixed, may
well be considered a mark of character.

Advocacy of Genetic Studies.   As for the rest, the position
taken in this treatise is based on a view of instincts like the one
described by McDougall, but calling for a more detailed
differentiation and specification in relation to the stimuli
evoking them.   The perceptual determination of the instinct
I should emphasize even to a greater extent than does
McDougall.   And if the numerous " anti-instinctivists "
in the United States were to direct their energies toward
the goal of discovering what tendencies develop in early

[1] Cf. A. A. Roback, " Interference of Will Impulses " : *Psycholog.
Review Monograph Supplements*, 1918, vol. xxv.

childhood, without the aid of education, instead of spending all their efforts in explaining away theoretically and by means of *non sequitur* arguments manifestly instinctive behaviour, we should now be in a more enlightened state regarding one of the most important subjects in a whole group of sciences.

Ordinarily we do not credit young children with the slightest germs of character, but no one who has watched them at play can deny that they exhibit signs not only of the knowledge of right and wrong but even of the observance of certain rules.. The prophets of Israel, and probably those to whom they preached, seem to have evinced a greater interest in that subject than we in the twentieth century, for many are the passages in which an event is prophesied to take place before a symbolic child grows up to know the difference between right and wrong.

Character and behaviour pertaining to the moral sphere can and should be studied genetically and comparatively as in the case of other capacities and behaviour. The sociological researches of men like Westermarck, Lévy-Bruhl, Boas, McDougall and Hose in this regard are valuable indeed, but they cannot take the place of ontogenetic investigations, for the chief reason perhaps that the primitive impulses of the savage tribes are coloured by tradition and custom.

It is only by pursuing an analytic method that we can avoid the nihilistic tendency so current to-day and drawing illegitimate support from modern logistic development—of employing a term in a sense for which it was never intended, and thereby breaking entirely away from the past. The most clear-headed thinker of antiquity, if not of all times, admonishes us in his *Nicomachean Ethics* to consider first the popular notion of a concept before we attempt to define it ; and his suggestion should serve as a methodological beacon-light for all times.

Value of Analytic Approach. By preserving the unitary and essentially unique mark of character instead of breaking it up into a number of unrelated qualities we enjoy the advantage of attaching it to some body of scientific facts and subsuming it under rules and principles, without which even the technical arts are under a serious handicap. The unitary basis of our conception does not prevent us from seeking after elements, factors and determinants, but saves us rather from the fruitless effort of beginning our search blindly or, as in the exuberant mood of some psychologists, contenting ourselves with the feeling that we are looking for what we are looking for—an attitude which may be recommended only for Alice in Wonderland.

There is probably not a single one of the various approaches to the study of character which is without at least a grain of value for the clarification of so complex a subject. The recent experimental methods are particularly hopeful signs. Each point of view may be regarded not only as a contribution *per se*, but should serve as a touchstone for the others. In this way the particles of gold in each finding may be sifted out, but it is necessary to be provided with a field of operation in the form of a general method before the particles can be assembled and properly arranged so as to cohere into a tangible substance.

CHAPTER XL

CHARACTER IN AN ATOMIC AGE

Although the revision, or rather the supplementation, has exceeded the space allotment originally agreed upon, many students would doubtless spot a lacuna were we to omit all reference to the awesome period we are living in. " Awesome " is an unusual word to employ in connection with time, and yet one can confidently declare that there has never been a generation like ours. Apart from the most terrible war in history, and the still more horrible events which were not the direct results of the war, such as the deliberate snuffing out of millions of innocent lives, we have now come to the critical stage as to our very existence. Can we afford to treat our own decade, with its atomic revelations and practices, as any other decade, to which the conception of character might apply ?

Character and Life. During those centuries when science was divorced from life, the great mystic and poet, Luis de León, could resume his lecturing at the University of Salamanca, after years of incarceration by the Holy Inquisition, with the customary opening words " *heri dixi* ". The universities today have possibly gone to the other extreme, making altogether too much of the *idola fori* ; and no sooner does some idea or individual get into the limelight than courses are offered on the subject, in which these figure prominently. The question may now be asked whether there is anything about character that is affected by events of the day ? The answer is : perhaps not, so long as we remain in the abstract realm, but the concept *per se* is of little value until it is attached to human beings who manifest the article which embodies it ; and these individuals do not live in a vacuum, but are influenced by historical occurrences, as well as by their original make-up and environmental experiences.

To Aristotle, the *summum bonum* was contemplation, since that brought happiness to people of the higher class. Happiness was the goal of ethics, and moderation was the hallmark of character. The magnanimous man was the bearer of character in its crystallized shape. The regulative principles had their place in the form of virtues ; but where moderation is the criterion, the weighting of some of the virtues as against others is scarcely applicable ; and temperance retains an almost favored position as compared with truthfulness, sincerity, or liberty-seeking. Aristotle, himself, is alleged to have suffered at the hands of tyranny, yet the tyrant in ancient Greece was looked upon with scarcely more than mild resentment.

Technology without Character Most Dangerous. Standing, as we are now, at the brink of a third global war which, should it take place, is almost bound to destroy civilization, thanks to the acquisition of the mysteries of nature which should have brought us the maximum of happiness instead of destruction on a colossal scale, we are besieged by problems, doubts, regrets, and perplexities of all sorts. The very scientists who have been responsible for the atomic bomb and the development of biological death-cultures and other infernal methods cannot help but wonder many times, and not without mortification, whether they had been true to their calling, whether they did not have a hand in the killing of innocent people in Japan, and might not be the cause of a devastated world.

Not only the physical scientists—each of us who is intelligent enough must assume a definite attitude. It was unfortunately because of the failure to take a stand in the right direction that dictators kept arrogating to themselves more and more power all the while causing the most frightful anguish to millions. The most conservative estimate of the number of people killed, mutilated, or confined in slave labor camps and prisons, as a result of tyranny during the last two decades alone, would aggregate the total of one hundred million souls. The fact that one hundred million human beings have been tortured, maimed, or put out of existence to me is not more tragic, from a personal angle, than, let us say, the rape, torture, and subsequent killing of a single girl by a fiend, for the reason that only one individual feels his or her own pain at such time. When we speak in terms of numbers, it is only because of the social or cultural consequences that such a loss implies. As for the harrowing experience, no summation will make it more terrible. Each pain is an individual pain, unless the bond is so great between close relatives as to cause greater anguish in the surviving individual than in the one who perished, but even in that case, the number must necessarily be very limited.

Disaster Sifts Character.   There are many who, after what has happened, have expressed the opinion that civilization is not worth saving, that the ghoulish acts in the gas chambers and concentration camps have made it clear that under stress, human beings are wolves and tigers and sharks and jackals, and that character then is conspicuous in its absence. The truth is that major catastrophes tend to separate humans into fiends, weaklings, and saints. The third category is, of course, the smallest, but it is by no means negligible. If I have read thousands of accounts of unspeakable brutality, it was, as I thought, because I felt it a bounden duty to know at least how these martyrs fared, how they died, so that somewhere and at some time someone's consciousness registered the fact of their ordeal, their suffering, or their heroism,[1] but I found that in addition to the obligation

[1] Psychoanalysts will, of course, attribute that type of extensive reading to a sadistic streak. Apparently there are few sadists in the world, then. The general tendency has been to brush these horrors aside, to studiously ignore them, on the ground that " we can't do anything about it ".

performed, I was gaining wisdom, obtaining an insight into human or inhuman (as the case may be) differences ; and I discovered the catalyzing properties of calamities such as one cannot detect in everyday life.

On the one hand we have human degradation and depravity such as is not to be found among beasts, but on the other hand, there is such exaltation and sublimity as to make us feel proud of the human race. To familiarize ourselves with the eyewitness descriptions of the concentration camps in Germany and Poland, during the Nazi War, is to become aware that character after all is the touchstone of humanity, and that contrary to pessimistic pronouncements, virtue has not departed from our midst ; and for that very reason we should not abandon all hope in face of future cataclysms.

Poignant Illustrations. Of the hundreds of instances, let me cite only two.

During the Nazi atrocities, one Russian woman of an aristocratic family, who became a nun in Paris, had been helping Jews in their distress, and soon enough was discovered and shipped off to a concentration camp, where again, she was of service to the wretched people who were marked for the gas chambers. When it became known that the so-called labor-camp transports were, in reality, destined for the crematories, many of the women became hysterical in their panic.

Sister Maria, *née* Baroness Durnovo, would do her utmost to console the group individually, allaying their fears and diverting their suspicions. Since one of the transport was beside herself with grief, she assured her that they were all going to be sent to a labor camp, and in order to convince her, she rashly offered to take her place, if she were so skeptical. The wailing woman accepted her offer at once, and the astounded Sister Maria (Lady Durnovo), not to go back on her promise, substituted for her and was soon reduced to a small heap of ashes.[1]

[1] Esther Jesselson : *Oifn Shvel*, March, 1950.

The other story is even more moving. It would be more appropriate to tell part of it in the simple words of the Polish woman, Maria Gorczak (now of London) who was fortunate enough to know such a character in one of the labor camps in far-off Russian Turkestan. The man, who happened to be in Eastern Poland when the war broke out, was arrested by the Russians as a member of the Jewish Socialist Party (Bund) and sentenced to long-term imprisonment, in a camp where, because of conditions, he was wasting away, and yet spent what spare time he had, as a result of the Stalin-Sikorski treaty with regard to prisoners, in assisting his fellow-prisoners and instilling courage into them. He had been a tailor who educated himself and was elected to office in his community.

" Who is this man "—I asked Mr. B., a higher civil servant of my native town.

" You ask about Batist," he answered. " We were together in prison and in labor camps. He suffered more than the others, because he spent a lot of that time in solitary confinement and was treated much worse than any of us. Not only because he is a socialist. His greatest sin was that he always intervened and protected and defended other prisoners. You can imagine it didn't help him too much. You will find me a bit exaggerated," he added, " but he is like a saint. So we called him there. We loved him all and I had not the slightest hope he would survive his trials."

.   .   .   .

Soon the epidemic of typhus spread in the whole county and, as every day new men were coming dirty and with fresh supply of lice, soon we had the epidemic in our asylum.

.   .   .   .

Then came the unhappy case of Mr. K.

Mr. K. was a member of the Bund, too. As there was no place in the ward, so he told us, and all the beds were occupied, he was left for two weeks in the waiting room on the floor. As he was not in bed, nobody cared for his cleanliness and so he was left ill, as he was, lying in his winter coat, without even a wash.

There was a terrible panic when he came back. People knew enough about the implications arising from such a state of dirt, after a typhus disease. So he was shut up in one of the empty spaces around the yard and nobody wanted to get in and to care for him, in fear of infected lice.

Nobody—but David Batist.

He washed him, bedded him up on his own only blanket, cared for his daily food, not an easy task—encouraged him in moments of despair and weakness, until he brought him back to life.

Then he fell ill himself.

At the same time I got typhus too. We were both taken to the hospital by the same dirty droshka (cab). Nobody believed, at least neither of us, that we had much chance to survive. For the first time I saw Batist sad, and for the first time he spoke of himself. He told me that his wife and his little beloved daughter were both in Tarnow. He hoped they could perhaps manage to be saved from the Germans, who then occupied the town.

" Just now I know," he said, " I shall never see them again. But should you survive, as I feel you will, please tell my daughter all about me. Promise me, will you ? "

" Of course," I answered, " but we have equal chances to survive."

" No. I am a dying man, I feel it too well."

I don't remember much more. I had lost consciousness for some time. I awoke being terribly cold and lying on the stony floor in the ante-room of the wards. And Batist in his hospital coat was standing near me shouting :

" I protest, there must be places found when there are

sick people here. I protest against such treatment of the suffering. Go and find a place. I protest ! "

As there was no place in the women's ward, thanks to his intervention I was put in a bed in the men's ward for two days, as I was later told. Only once during this time did I recover my senses for a moment and I caught a glimpse of Batist, sitting on the bed of an Uzbek man and feeding him like a nurse. He was getting food from many people, especially from members of his Party, and he distributed it among other patients without any discrimination, humane in the deepest sense of the word as he was, until his end.

He died on the first of March, 1942, after nine days of illness. As I was later told, the doctors had advised him to lie down quietly and not to be concerned about the other people's fate. But he could not resist being helpful. Until the moment when he himself lost his senses, he was fighting for the welfare of his fellow-men.

He left nothing, when he died, except his plain crooked walking stick, that was taken by Mr. B., his prison friend, as a souvenir.

After the end of the war I tried to find his wife and his child, but I got news they were both destroyed in a German crematorium.

Nothing remains after him, no written words, no clever speeches, no home, no child, not even a grave.[1]

Whenever we are ready to give up in despair and consign this civilization to the doom which has been predicted for it, we need only think of such characters to redeem the name of man. Some are to be found in every country, although it must be said in different proportions, varying perhaps with the traditions of the people inhabiting it, which leads us to the consideration of another matter, viz., the fluctuating value of

[1] M. Gorczak : *Jewish Labor Bund Bulletin*, 1950 (May-June), vol. iii, pp. 4–6.

the regulative principles and its significance in the assessment of character.

Liberty Through the Ages. Only one of these principles will be dealt with at present, since it has come to a focus within the past generation and has been undergoing a serious crisis, the outcome of which is still in the balance. I am referring to liberty. The concept was of course an important one in ancient Greek philosophy, and wars have been fought presumably on behalf of liberty for many centuries, but it was not until recent times that the concept has broadened and deepened so that it embraces equality and democracy.

The first real step toward liberty was the Magna Carta, but that instrument affected only the upper portion of the human pyramid. The French Revolution brought liberty alloyed with terrorism, its very nemesis. In the Russian Revolution, liberty had been achieved only to turn a *salto mortale*. From that period dates the totalitarian state which reached its most terrible form in Nazi Germany. The worst part of this type of rule is that it is not content to remain localized in its own territory, but seeks world expansion under the pretext of some ideology ; and that is the cause of our sorry plight *anno* 1951. In days of yore, tyranny was personal, hence overthrowing it was essentially a step against aggression, but when dictatorship parades under the cloak of a principle or ideology, it is, alas, protected by an impenetrable armor.

There are two other observations one can make in this connection. First, although liberty means so much more to us now than it did, let us say, during the feudal period, it has never been in greater jeopardy than within the last decade or so. It is like meeting with greater and more hazardous obstacles, the higher we climb the snow-capped mountain. Perhaps there is even some cosmic barrier as in the myth of the Towel of Babel to keep man from enjoying in peace his hard-won prize. The shocking farce about it all is that the danger could have been averted easily enough if the regulative principle had been alive in the rest of the world. Not only Hitler, but all dictators could have been stopped by concerted action in a day, a week, or a month.

The second pernicious effect is that totalitarianism is sadly enough integrative. It assimilates and ingests while destroying everything which is inconsistent with its rapid progress, and what is more, by exploiting the most efficient technological devices. Worse still, by setting in full force a powerful propaganda system, it can reach its opponents, through its long arm, thousands of miles away from its field of operation. Thus Theodor Lessing was murdered in Czechoslovakia, Giacomo Matteotti was done away with not in Italy but in France, Leon Trotsky was assassinated in Mexico ; Berthold Jacob was kidnapped in Switzerland and brought to Germany.

What would happen if one power were to conquer the world is too terrible to contemplate.[1] During the darkest ages, whether medieval or not, it would be possible for a nonconformist to take refuge in some other country. Even the unholy Inquisition could not extend its tentacles beyond Spain, Portugal, and their possessions ; and in spite of its extraordinary vigilance, at least a number of " heretics " were able to elude its watchful eye, and worship in their own way. The Gestapo of Nazi Germany and the NKVD of USSR have exercised a stranglehold on almost everyone who dared to differ in the slightest detail.

The most frightening and discouraging aspect of the terroristic monster is that (a) the process of unnatural selection operates in killing off the nobler characters, thus substantiating the proverb " Those whom the gods love die young ", which should really read : " Those whom the Devil hates die young," and (b) in fighting the Monster, we must adopt its

[1] George Orwell, in his *1984*, has presented us with a prevue of what really can happen when the machinery of power dominates the whole world.

methods, and before long, our " realistic " policy, under the pretext of national emergency, makes common cause with the " monsterlings ", and regiments all liberal thought and action.

In a brilliant account of the nihilistic monster, typified by Nechayev and Hitler, Robert Payne offers a most horrendous prospect of a, to all appearances, " perfectly normal " man, who is preoccupied with the problem of destroying the world, and finds the solution—*absit omen*. When, however, in his ambitious, not to say, pretentious programme of averting the catastrophe, Payne proposes vast changes in the present administration of education, which are to be based on the principle of humanness, including among other things, a voice in the government by children, and almost enforced mixing of social groups so that " a student of music should be encouraged to live among lumberjacks; a student of theology should stalk game with hunters," [1] etc., we begin to wonder whether this is not " human—all too human " in the Nietzscheian sense. I wonder how the stalked game would feel about this sort of humanness on the part of hunter and embryo clergyman.

The Shrivelling of Courage. It is because detection of the non-conformist has now become, in totalitarian countries, a certainty that there are very few who would risk their neck, knowing, as they do, that not only would their efforts be futile, but most likely their very disappearance would make less noise than a ripple in a small pond, and their close kin might suffer imprisonment. Many intelligent people must have been puzzled by the fact that while tens of thousands have been willing to forfeit their lives, aside from the even greater numbers who invited terms of long imprisonment or exile to Siberia, opposing the Czarist regime, we hear of no such heroes in USSR. Does it follow that the land of the unfree has also turned into a land of the unbrave ? And yet the

[1] R. Payne : *Zero—The Story of Terrorism*, 1950, p. 256 (Day).

courage displayed during the second World War on the part of the defendants of Stalingrad was second to none. It would take us too far afield to attempt a solution of this problem, but it seems reasonable to suppose that where there is no organization for the purpose, and where an individual and sporadic principle, so insistent under more or less normal conditions, is either repressed or suppressed—and rationalization is employed to keep it submerged, some rebels, who would definitely have committed acts of violence against a reactionary, are somewhat awed by the phrase " dictatorship of the proletariat ", or are reconciled to some extent by the many social reforms which communism has brought to the common people.

Weighting the Regulative Principles. Nevertheless, the thesis set forth in this chapter is that in a totalitarian state or world, just because liberty is crushed, the regulative principle which corresponds to it will have greater weight than some other regulative principle, and thus character is somewhat differently constituted or rated in periods of upheaval. As has been argued elsewhere, prior to the Nazi War :

" Although, truth, for instance, will always serve as an ideal of humanity and will be the goal of science, nevertheless as a regulative principle validating an act as indicative of character, it could not possess the same force in a world where truth is the rule and falsehood the exception. Similarly, justice would take a secondary place as a regulative principle, if it were the most natural thing for people to be just. The just man in such a world would not receive ethical recognition any more than the person who wears his clothes well or takes good care of himself. . . .

" Aside from that, the same question may be raised about genius. Surely, if writing good poetry, or composing fine music were within the power of the average individual, genius would come down a peg. Literature or music would still retain its intrinsic value, but the masters would not be so admired as at present.

" What saves the situation, is of course, the impossibility of such a hypothetical condition ever being realized. Just so is it fatuous to fear that character will lose its great significance when most of the world becomes altruistic." [1]

The dynamic relationships between the concept and the actual conditions which, if disparate, as in a totalitarian state, heighten the value of liberty as a regulative principle may be called *vectors of character*, representing the force from within, in its struggle against the force from without, the resultant contributing toward the estimation of the characterial index. Individual freedom and liberty, or collective freedom, may bear a closer relation to one another than is supposed by philosophers like John Stuart Mill, who somewhat apologetically introduces his classical essay on Liberty with the proviso that his subject is not " the so-called Liberty of the Will—but Civil or Social Liberty ". The question, however, before us is whether there is ever individual freedom in a state that does not allow collective freedom ; in other words, the two are so interdependent that individual freedom and civil liberty, as philosophical problems, cannot be treated the one without the other.

An individual may lead, of course, a spotless life in a totalitarian state. His character is reputed as of the highest, yet unless he contributes to the liberty of the group, not merely by his many beneficent acts or consideration of the rights of others, but by resisting despotism in whatever shape it crops up, his character is not of the first order. It lacks the dynamic coloring which character, viewed in a progressive perspective, must reflect.

On the other hand, the little man, like David Batist, in the squelching atmosphere of the Turkestan labor camp,

[1] A. A. Roback : *Psychology of Common Sense*, 1939, pp. 324–5.

evinced such character as many of the reputedly great were not capable of mustering, when he protested against injustice *to others*, aware of the fact that such intercession meant his own undoing.

The individual who sees injustice about him and either connives at it or feels helpless to do anything, I maintain, is either not free or else he is callous. If he has any human sentiments, he will be undergoing mental conflicts, inner struggles, which in themselves are symptoms of bondage, in Spinoza's sense. Thus do we see that, with due deference to John Stuart Mill, there is a decided kinship between what he calls ' individual liberty ' and ' civil ' or ' social liberty '. You cannot have individual freedom in the sense of self-determinism (what freedom of the will really amounts to) unless you share actively in the attainment of collective liberty. In our dictator-ridden world, the struggle for liberty on the part of the individual becomes the highest virtue, and its goal is the *summum bonum* of society.[1]

[1] A. A. Roback : Loc. cit., p. 334.

POSTSCRIPT TO THE THIRD EDITION

CROWDED as the historical survey is, there is a temptation to include the contributions on character of the past year in the total account, but since this is for technical reasons not feasible, the next best service is, I believe, to take into consideration the points raised by reviewers. Fortunately the critical notices have practically all been very favourable, and it is gratifying to think that *no specific errors of fact* have been thus far pointed out by reviewers. While it is true that the work was prepared under the impression that a second edition would not be forthcoming perhaps for years, there surely must be room for improvement even where considerable care had been bestowed on the work.

Most of the cavils directed at the *Psychology of Character* are of a minor, if not trivial, significance and concern the question of emphasis. Thus one reviewer finds that the volume contains too much historical material ; another that the work is too intellectualistic ; while a third, who is apparently a worshipper of Hegel and his British disciples, would have a work on character dwell almost exclusively on the merits of objective idealism and its relation to ethics. A fourth who seems to have come under the tutelage of Spearman wonders why more has not been made of the statistical views and theories of the London psychologist. A fifth is discontent with the single reference to Rivers. It is obvious that everyone of these would like those features stressed with which he happens to be best acquainted. All the more reason then for the extensive historical treatment of the subject, and the comprehensive review of contemporary theories in relation to character and personality. It would be futile to controvert each of these claims, but there is one review—that of Dr. G. W. Allport in the *Psychological Bulletin* (Dec., 1927, vol. xxiv)—which deserves close attention because of its analysis of the issues involved.

From this review, and others in a less degree, I gather that my theory of character smacks of Puritanism in spite of the emphatic disavowal contained in the book. It is true, as the reviewer suggests, that I see " no good in the expression of the instincts for their own sake ", but neither do I see any *harm* in their expression. The ethical colouring with which character has been saturated seems to be responsible for the misapprehension which is read into my work. The reason for making the inhibition of instincts fundamental to the concept of character, I must repeat, is not because the instincts are bad, but because character connotes, we might say almost *ex vi termini*, the distinguishing mark by virtue of which one individual differs from another in respect of personality minus the intelligence, temperament and physical factors, in other words, in respect of volitional behaviour.

What is at the basis of this view is the fact that although born with propensities in given directions, the man of character has been able to overcome these propensities. If a feeble-minded person could by his own effort make out of himself a genius, he too would be credited with a high degree of character. But while we are on hypothetical cases—in order to drive home the principle of rational inhibitionism—it may be said that if a man were born with tendencies which could never have anything but a good outcome, and this selfsame individual, after a strict discipline, succeeded in modifying some of these inborn dispositions so as to cause mischief, without, however, deriving any pleasure from his acts, he would on the theory outlined be a man of character, although, in practice, we should say his actions were insane. The evaluating criterion would in his case be negative, for the rational guiding principle would be lacking. Nor could he very well be consistent and escape the consequences of his acts.

Those who will sense in this exposition a redolence of Kant's categorical imperative and his rigorous conception of duty must be reminded of the separability of behaviour bespeaking character and conduct of an ethical nature. There is not necessarily a one-to-one correspondence between morality and character ; and I can well conceive of a man with a higher character coefficient being less moral than one with a lower index of character. Fortunately it is in the nature of things that both qualities more or less coincide, but if the discrepancy is wide, the blame must rest with the ethical concepts " good ", " moral ", and the like, which cannot be definitely fixed, and which are apt to depend on previous assumptions and tradition. The relativity of moral or even ethical evaluation in particular cases is too well known to need any further comment. *Per contra*, the criterion of character may be, as I have sought to show, standardized so as to offer few difficulties.

There are three distinctive features about character not to be found in any other phases of personality.

First there is the *universality* of *its possibility*. Thus, although only relatively few are born with a talent for one thing or another, so that, try as they might, the majority of men could not become composers or poets of merit, it is nevertheless theoretically possible for almost anyone to engage in a system of behaviour which would come under the head of character.

By " theoretically possible " is meant that anyone may, in spite of his leanings, say to himself " I am going to check that impulse in me at all costs ", and carry out his plan in a determined manner. There is at least nothing physically which prevents him from so doing. It is true that he is in a sense " charged " or " loaded " to react more in one way than in another, but this predetermination, unless it is so pronounced as to constitute a pathological trait, may be overcome by exhortation and other environmental influences. The extremes, i.e., those who are endowed with a decidedly strong consistency-urge and those tainted with a streak of " moral insanity " are much less susceptible to the influence of public opinion. The social standard in action, however, exercises a wholesome effect on the average person whose consistency-urge is more elastic and pliable.

Secondly we must consider the *range of its locus*. Stature, physique, appearance, and other characteristics are restricted and isolated units, even if they do go to make up the physical side of personality, but character is a dynamic element encompassing so many interrelated acts and motives that it forms a comprehensive system. The third mark which distinguishes our concept of character is the *significance* attached to its concrete manifestations. Surely individuals differ in numerous respects, and there are specialized interests which would single out this or that quality for a certain purpose, perhaps speed of reaction, energy, etc., but these are not significant characterizations of an individual as a member of society.

The next charge involves my taking inhibition to be the basis of character, without explaining its *modus operandi*, " for if inhibition is ' the core of character ' it is a pity to leave the reader inadequately informed as to the nature of its operation."

To this I reply that the inclusion of a chapter on inhibition would scarcely help the theory, for a psychologist should not be required to explore regions which are only timidly approached by physiologists. In 1906, Sherrington wrote : " We do not yet understand the intimate nature of inhibition. In the cases before us now, its seat is certainly central, and in all probability is, as argued above, situated at points of synapsis. I have urged that a prominent physiological feature of the synapse is a synaptic membrane. It seems therefore to me that inhibition in such cases as those before us is probably referable to a change in the condition of the synaptic membrane causing a block in conduction.   But what the intimate nature of the inhibitory change may be we do not know." [1]

Since this declaration was made, our knowledge about nerve conduction has been furthered, but it is doubtful whether the minutiae of the inhibitory process, especially of the more complicated variety which involves ideation, have been satisfactorily explained to this day.

To be sure, theories of inhibition may be advanced aplenty, but it is not my object to commit myself to any one hypothesis at this stage.   Whether the inhibition takes place in the frontal part of the brain, as Loeb·thinks, or is largely a function of the synapses in the cortex as a whole does not affect the inhibition view of character one way or the other.   In the absence of a better hypothesis I am quite willing to subscribe to the drainage theory of McDougall in explanation of what roughly takes place in inhibition.   But must one undertake to explain the mechanism of a motor in order to perceive that an apparatus is driven by a motor ?   Freud and his associates have never found themselves in the least compelled to explain the machinery of their sublimations, fixations, transferences, etc.   No dynamic psychology feels itself under obligation to work out the physiological data of its conclusions.   The conclusion is usually arrived at after surveying the facts. Our analysis of character has shown that in differentiating human beings with regard to their system of volitional qualities, inhibition becomes our psychological guide, wherefore it is for us to accept this result and connect it with other similarly gained results, instead of delving into its physiological mechanism first.   Moreover, even if we were agreed upon what takes place cortically, subcortically or anywhere else in the nervous system, at the time the man of

[1] C. S. Sherrington : *The Integration of the Nervous System*, p. 192.

character performs a meritorious act, or refrains from a reprehensible one, there would be a further demand made to bring to light the nature of the molecular changes in the nerve and other attendant phenomena at the time the inhibition took place. Our theory of character could be invalidated only if the doctrine set forth here were not in accord with the current knowledge of inhibition. Otherwise the *functional* view of inhibition is adequate for our purpose.

It is interesting to note that since the appearance of *The Psychology of Character*, two of the leading American experimental investigators of character, Dr. Hartshorne and Dr. May, of Teachers College, Columbia University, have been working on a method to test the strength of a single type of inhibition, along the lines suggested in chapter xxvi, " The Index of Character."

The reference to inhibition as an " abstract principle " may have been somewhat misleading. Perhaps the word " generic " would have been a more appropriate expression. My meaning is naturally that there are many kinds and degrees of inhibition, so that to label a process as inhibitory does not sufficiently concretize or particularize it in a psychological system.

We are now in a position to understand why " the inhibition of the extensor and flexor muscles is something entirely different from the inhibition of an instinctive urge "—a statement which appears to Dr. Allport somewhat dogmatic in the absence of further expatiation. That both acts come under the head of inhibition is of course incontestable, but I think it is equally undeniable that while the inhibition of a simple muscle like the flexor is a function which requires no resistance and is present soon after birth, the inhibition of an instinctive urge, e.g., running away in the face of danger, does not come about except through the medium of an elaborate system of ideas and sentiments playing against emotions and instincts both individually and severally.

The difference then lies in the complexity of the operation and the ramifications of the process, i.e., the extent of the field or the manifold of the levels involved in the brain, and probably also in the autonomic nervous system. To place the unmotivated opening or closing of the hand, as in the case of the playing infant or the absorbed reader, on the same plane of inhibition as the clenching of the fist, preparatory to striking an opponent on the platform, would hardly occur even to a behaviourist, who will probably see the difference as one between unconditioned and conditioned reflex action, ultimately reducing to the factors of time and the number of repetitions imposed upon the subject.

The difference between the simple motor inhibition and that of an instinctive tendency would, on the other hand, according to my theory, depend in part on the co-operation, and sometimes even the initiative, of the person acting. One impressive incident, one illumination, one hallucination was sufficient in the case of a number of historical celebrities to change their course. In other cases, the conditioning never takes place, even with such powerful stimuli as prison sentences.

Dr. Allport perceives " a strong note of aristocracy in the theory ; it is almost snobbish. It is likewise heavy with fatalism, for the burden is placed almost exclusively upon nativistic determinants. . . . Clearly there is small field here for moral exhortations. It would seem incongruous to blame, to reward, or punish ; and yet the author himself does not refuse to praise and to censor ".

There is a slight misconception in the reviewer's inference, which ought to be corrected. I am prepared to admit a certain snobbishness in the doctrine, but the charge of fatalism is not warranted. Character in its crystallized form is not to be sought in the average man. It is *possible* for most people to develop character, but it is not *likely* that they will do so. There are far more so-called good men and women in the world than those possessing character in the proper sense of the

word, hence the latter class does form a species of aristocracy.
If I were to write a book on the psychology of talent, not to
say genius, certainly the man in the street would not be
prominently featured in its pages. Does it follow, however,
from this premise that a small field is left for moral exhortation ? As well might one say that those who believe in the
native origin of intelligence would dispense with all education.
As a matter of fact, in the chart of points of view (p. 560)
the ethico-religious approach has been set down as one of
the fundamental points of view, and on the previous page
may be found the following statement : " We must remember
that the *normative* method with its *idealization* premises,
serves to stabilize in some degree the constituents of
character. The ethico-religious precepts or maxims form
a centre of reference, never quite attained in actual
life."

Far from decrying the value of traditional impositions in
the development of character, I should rather be inclined to
hold that the most consistent character would, in the absence
of public opinion and social fiats, gradually lapse into inconsistencies owing to the power of the original drives and
the actual circumstances favouring their untrammelled
expression : *a fortiori* would this be true of less consistent
natures. The consistency-urge, in other words, is nourished
by moral exhortation, although at times, when highly
developed, it transcends it and revaluates the commonly
accepted values.

Finally there is to mention the normative colouring of the
theory, which seems to puzzle some reviewers, because, earlier
in the book, a demarcation line was drawn between ethics
and the psychology of character ; and the readers were
promised that the exhortative aspect would not be displayed
in this connexion. It would appear then that the introduction
of absolute principles is somewhat of an inconsistency, or at
least a deviation from the original plan. " As the theory

develops," writes Dr. Allport, " it becomes less psychological and more normative."

Again we have before us a broad issue. There is a tendency in academic circles to identify the normative and the ethical. It is not realized that every *procedure requiring a standard,* every methodological step advances in the direction of a norm and presupposes established canons. Consistency in reasoning is taken for granted ; but it is possible for some modern Gorgias to question the logical necessity of drawing a pertinent or valid conclusion from premises which avowedly imply it. Tertullian's motto *credo quia absurdum* would, if applied to discursive thinking, bespeak such an attitude.

As we approach human problems, the normative method seems to be under obligation to show its credentials, although it is in this sphere that it should be allowed to take a conspicuous place. Yet when we talk of a high intelligence quotient, we are evaluating in terms of a standard, and in spite of the fact that there are divergent definitions of intelligence and many different tests for measuring it, we yet have a relatively absolute conception of intelligence. Even in taste, notwithstanding the dictum *de gustibus non disputandum,* there are absolute principles regardless of the notable disagreement. Shakespeare's genius will be appreciated by the *cognoscenti* of all ages and cultures, even it was berated by Tolstoï ; and Raphael's art is firmly intrenched in the good graces of a dynasty of critics, belittled though it may be by representatives of modernistic coteries.

If the psychology of character cannot be envisaged without invoking the aid of a norm, it is because the psychology of no human function can afford to be without it. In all our contacts with people, we are constantly making appraisals. I find, for instance, that before recalling the person who made a certain statement, I must first reproduce my attitude toward him. In other words, at the time of the utterance, the weight attached to it would automatically depend on what I *marginally* thought about the individual making the assertion : " Is he reliable ? " " Does he usually mean what he says ? " " Are his opinions merely emotional reactions ? " " Do I look up to him, or is he an inferior ? " Never, of course, do these questions occur consciously at the time, but evidently there is a scale of attitudes for the many varieties of people, and later, when recall is necessary, it is through one of these attitudes that the individual's name or face is brought to mind.

To return, however, to the main theme, it would appear that the mention of principles or such terms as " ethico-logical " or " justice " would immediately suggest an ethical atmosphere. That the psychology of character and ethics have certain contacts in common almost goes without saying ; but the confusion of the exhortative and the expository in my book is still to be proven. To conclude that a highly developed character will inhibit all instinctive tendencies in accordance with regulative principles, is surely not the same as an injunction to be moral or heed the " still small voice " in us. Character presupposes the existence of values, but takes precedence of ethics, so that the ethics of character may be undertaken as a separate study alongside the psychology of character.

A CASE OF POETIC JUSTICE

It may now be added that in his own outstanding treatise, Allport ten years later brought the matter to a head by ruling out character altogether from personality. In contradistinction to the general notion that character is the volitional phase of personality, Allport would put the two terms on a par, and courteously give character the congé as outside the psychological universe of discourse ; for to him " Character is personality evaluated, and personality is character devaluated ". " Since character is an unnecessary concept for psychology, the term will not appear again in this volume, excepting in quotations from other writers, or in a clear historical context." [1]

Here we stand before a fundamental difference. Allport's view may be best refuted by showing that personality and character proceed *pari passu*. Character may be treated descriptively, genetically, integrationally, etc., in a word under the same rubrics as personality is discussed in the selfsame book. On the other hand, there is an evaluation to which the whole subject of personality leads up that is unavoidable. To speak of rich personalities, well-integrated personalities, maladjusted personalities, desirable or undesirable traits—what is it but to impress an evaluative stamp on the concept ? And if there were no evaluation to be attained in the final analysis, there would be no need of studying this subject. Hardly an element of personality may be mentioned but it immediately suggests an evaluation. We need not call it ethical, but the goal undoubtedy lies in the realm of the values. If we bow character out of the psychological court, we shall be forced to do the same with personality.

Nor will the authority of John Adams, who is cited as saying " Character is the moral estimate of the individual, an evaluation ", be of any avail here. John Adams would have been the last psychologist to have sponsored this use made of his dictum. If moral evaluation attaches more to character than to any other ingredient of the personality, it is solely because character was presumably to correspond with the will, *which was regarded as the instrument of conduct ; and therefore, improvement even of the other components was ascribable to it alone*, while the physique, the emotions, and even intelligence could not be modified consciously except through the will, or in its broader aspect, character.

Under the circumstances, it is perhaps little short of an irony that Allport should conclude the volume, which was

[1] G. W. Allport : *Personality: a Psychological Interpretation*, 1937 (Houghton Mifflin), p. 52.

studiously to eliminate every reference to character, as beyond the psychological pale, with the following significant sentence : " The individual striving ever for his own integrity ... struggles on ever under oppression, always hoping and planning for a more perfect democracy, where the dignity and growth of each personality will be prized above all else." It is a remarkable demonstration of the fact that although you may have driven character out of your convenient purview, it will catch up with you in the end, forcing you to salute it, in some other guise.

INDEXES

REGISTER OF PERSONAL NAMES [1]

A

Abelard, P., 406, 522
Abraham, K., 290, 295, 297, 298, 301, 302, 306, 359, 527
Ach, N., 105, 106, 147
Adams, John, 713.
Adams, John Quincey, 515
Addison, J., 123
Adickes, E., 218, 219
Adler, A., 119, 264, 327, 332, 338–352, 353, 354, 360, 363, 365, 368, 372, 373, 375, 439, 556
Alceste, 32
Alcmæon of Crotona, 42
Aldington, R., 12 n.
Alexander, Franz, 287, 309, 354, 359
Alexander (the Great), 213, 308, 517, 598
Allport, F. H., 229, 419, 554
Allport, G. W., 465, 529, 532, 535, 537 n., 544, 554, 712, 713
Amiel, H. F., 515, 553, 618
Amsden, G. S., 528, 559
Anaxagoras, 41
Andreas-Salomé, L., 290
Andreyev, L., 613
Anton, G., 283, 341, 375, 376–378
Apfelbach, H., 84, 85, 217, 228–233
Apicius, 171
Apuleius, 653
Areco, H. P., 258, 259
Aristotle, 46, 123, 188, 392, 590, 598, 642, 651 (implied), 688, 691 ; on character types, 8 ; on the humours, 42 ; modifies Hippocrates' doctrine, 43 ; cited by Bacon, 139, 140
Arius, 672
Aschaffenburg, G., 656
Ashmun, Jehudi, 317
Assisi, St. Francis of, 317

Augustine, *see* St. Augustine
Awdeley, John, 13
Azaïs, H., 180, 181, 371, 372, 382
Azam, E., 158, 197, 198, 263, 650, 659, 660, 666

B

Bach, J. S., 341
Bacon, Francis, 133, 134, 135, 139, 141, 142, 303, 372, 373, 512, 599, 649
Bahnsen, J., 66, 67, 216, 273
Bailey, T. J., 146
Bain, A., 146, 182, 183, 185, 186, 200, 205, 512
Baldwin, J. M., 150, 384 n.
Barbellion, W. N. P., *see* Cummings, B. F.
Basedow, K. A., v. 99.
Bashkirtseff, Marie, 518
Batist, David, 694, 701
Bauer, J., 93, 94
Baumgarten, F., 447, 448, 554, 655, 656
Bayes, 245
Beach, F. A., 409
" Beauchamp," Miss, 157
Béclard, P. A., 104, 105
Beethoven, L., 341, 507, 553, 570
Begbie, H., 602
Bekhterev (Bechterew), Vl. v., 248, 250
Benedek, Therese, 287
Beneke, F. F., 94
Ben-Sirach, 8
Bentham, J., 24
Bergler, E., 295
Berlioz, H., 527
Berman, L., 103, 401–405, 486, 651, 652, 666
Bernard, Claude, 480
Bernheim, H., 558
Bertillon, A., 90

[1] Names of characters in *belles lettres* or of persons appearing as titles of books are italicized. Unidentified pseudonyms, as well as sobriquets, are flanked by quotation marks.

24

INDEX OF SUBJECTS